FUNDAMENTALS OF
CLINICAL
MEDICINE

An Introductory Manual

4TH
EDITION

FUNDAMENTALS OF
CLINICAL
MEDICINE:
An Introductory Manual

Humayun J. Chaudhry, D.O., M.S., S.M., FACP, FACOI
Chairman and Clinical Associate Professor of Medicine, and Assistant Dean for Pre-Clinical Education, New York College of Osteopathic Medicine of New York Institute of Technology; Attending Physician, Winthrop-University Hospital, Mineola, New York; Flight Surgeon, United States Air Force Reserve

Anthony J. Grieco, M.D., FACP
Associate Chair and Professor of Medicine, and Associate Dean for Alumni Affairs, New York University School of Medicine, New York; Governor, New York State Chapter of the American College of Physicians

Senior Editors
Roger M. Macklis, M.D.
Chairman and Professor of Radiation Oncology, and Senior Staff Physician, Department of Radiation Oncology, Cleveland Clinic Foundation, Cleveland

Michael E. Mendelsohn, M.D., FACC
Elisa Kent Mendelsohn Professor of Molecular Cardiology and Medicine, Tufts University School of Medicine, Boston
Executive Director, Molecular Cardiology
Research Institute, Tufts-New England Medical Center, Boston

Gilbert H. Mudge, Jr., M.D., FACC
Professor of Medicine, Harvard Medical School; Director of Cardiac Transplant Service, Brigham and Women's Hospital, Boston

Student Editors
Jessica Leung, Harvard Medical School
Liana Spano, New York College of Osteopathic Medicine

 LIPPINCOTT WILLIAMS & WILKINS
A Wolters Kluwer Company
Philadelphia • Baltimore • New York • London
Buenos Aires • Hong Kong • Sydney • Tokyo

Editor: Neil Marquardt
Managing Editor: Amy Oravec
Marketing Manager: Scott Lavine
Production Editor: Christina Remsburg
Compositor: LWW
Printer: RR Donnelly-Crawfordsville

351 West Camden Street
Baltimore, Maryland 21201-2436 USA

530 Walnut Street
Philadelphia, PA 19106

The publisher is not responsible (as a matter of product liability, negligence, or otherwise) for any injury resulting from any material contained herein. This publication contains information relating to general principles of medical care that should not be construed as specific instructions for individual patients. Manufacturer's product information and package inserts should be reviewed for current information, including contraindications, dosages, and precautions.

Printed in the United States of America

Library of Congress Cataloging-in-Publication Data

Fundamentals of clinical medicine / [edited by] Humayun J. Chaudhry, Anthony J. Grieco ; senior editors, Roger M. Macklis, Michael E. Mendelsohn, Gilbert H. Mudge, Jr. ; student editors, Jessica Leung, Liana Spano.-- 4th ed.
    p. ; cm.
Rev. ed. of: Intoduction to clinical medicine, 3rd ed. 1994.
Includes bibliographical references and index.
ISBN 13: 978-0-7817-5192-6
ISBN 10: 0-7817-5192-6 (alk. paper)
 1. Clinical medicine--Handbooks, manuals, etc. 2. Diagnosis--Handbooks, manuals, etc. I. Chaudhry, Humayan J. II. Grieco, Anthony J. III. Macklis, Roger M. Introduction to clinical medicine.
 [DNLM: 1. Clinical Medicine--Handbooks. 2. Internal Medicine--Handbooks. WB 39 F981 2004]
RC55.M24 2004
616--dc22

200365656

The publishers have made every effort to trace the copyright holders for borrowed material. If they have inadvertently overlooked any, they will be pleased to make the necessary arrangements at the first opportunity.

To purchase additional copies of this book, call our customer service department at **(800) 638-3030** or fax orders to (301)824-7390. International customers should call **(301) 714-2324.**

Visit Lippincott Williams & Wilkins on the Internet: http://www.LWW.com. Lippincott Williams & Wilkins customer service representatives are available from 8:30 am to 6:00 pm, EST.

06 07
2 3 4 5 6 7 8 9 10

Contents

PART III: DISEASE PATHOPHYSIOLOGY REVIEW

Contributions from Clinical Faculty

William Berenberg, M.D., FAAP
Professor of Pediatrics, Harvard Medical School; former Director, Division of Cerebral Palsy, The Children's Hospital Medical Center, Boston

Ronald R. Blanck, D.O., MACP
President, University of North Texas Health Science System, Fort Worth, Texas, and Professor of Medicine, Texas College of Osteopathic Medicine; retired Lieutenant General and former Surgeon General, United States Army

Eugene Braunwald, M.D., MACP, FRCP
Distinguished Hersey Professor of Medicine, Harvard Medical School; Chief Academic Officer, Partners HealthCare Systems, Boston; Faculty Dean for Academic Programs, Brigham and Women's Hospital and Massachusetts General Hospital, Boston

John D. Capobianco, D.O., FAAO
Acting Chair and Associate Professor, Stanley Schiowitz Department of Osteopathic Manipulative Medicine, New York College of Osteopathic Medicine of New York Institute of Technology

Robert Coles, M.D.
James Agee Professor of Social Ethics, Harvard University; Research Psychiatrist, Harvard University Health Services, Cambridge, Massachusetts

Brenda J. Connolly, D.O., R.N.
Assistant Professor of Family Practice, New York College of Osteopathic Medicine of New York Institute of Technology; Administrative Director of Medical Education, Long Beach Medical Center, Long Beach, New York

Kenneth H. Falchuk, M.D.
Associate Professor of Medicine, Harvard Medical School; Director, Education Council, Brigham and Women's Hospital, Boston

Rebecca Fishman, D.O.
Chief, Division of Physical Medicine and Rehabilitation, Department of Medicine, and Instructor in Medicine, New York College of Osteopathic Medicine of New York Institute of Technology

Samuel Hellman, M.D.
A.N. Pritzker Distinguished Service Professor of Radiation and Clinical Oncology, Pritzker Medical School of the University of Chicago

Katherine Hochman, M.D.
Teaching Assistant, New York University School of Medicine; Chief Medical Resident, New York University Medical Center and Bellevue Hospital Center

Sandra Kammerman, M.D., FACP
Associate Professor of Medicine, New York University School of Medicine; Attending Physician, New York University Medical Center and Bellevue Hospital Center

Homayoun Kazemi, M.D., FACP
Professor of Medicine, Harvard Medical School; Chief Emeritus, Pulmonary and Critical Care Division, Department of Medicine, Massachusetts General Hospital, Boston

Philip Marcus, M.D., MPH, FACP
Associate Dean for Curriculum Development and Clinical Professor of Medicine, New York College of Osteopathic Medicine of New York Institute of Technology; Chief, Division of Pulmonary Medicine, St. Francis Hospital, Roslyn, New York

David G. Nathan, M.D., FAAP
Robert A. Stranahan Professor of Pediatrics, Harvard Medical School; President Emeritus, Dana-Farber Cancer Institute, Boston

Arnold S. Relman, M.D., MACP
Professor of Medicine, Harvard Medical School; Editor-in-Chief, *New England Journal of Medicine*, 1977–1991.

Cheryl Rosenfeld, D.O., FACP, FACE
Chief, Division of Endocrinology and Metabolism, and Clinical Assistant Professor, Department of Medicine, New York College of Osteopathic Medicine of New York Institute of Technology

Barbara Ross-Lee, D.O., FACOFP
Dean and Provost, New York College of Osteopathic Medicine of New York Institute of Technology; Chair, Board of Directors, Association of Academic Health Centers

Edwin W. Salzman, M.D.
Associate Professor of Surgery, Harvard Medical School; Visiting Surgeon, Beth Israel Deaconess Medical Center, Boston

John Shillito, Jr., M.D., FACS
Former Professor of Surgery, Harvard Medical School; Former Attending Physician, Neurosurgery Unit, Children's Hospital Boston

William Silen, M.D.
Johnson and Johnson Distinguished Professor of Surgery, Harvard Medical School; Surgeon-in-Chief Emeritus, Beth Israel Deaconess Medical Center, Boston

Sidney Simon, D.O., FACOI, FAAAI
Chief, Division of Allergy and Immunology and Clinical Professor of Medicine, New York College of Osteopathic Medicine of New York Institute of Technology

Marshall A. Wolf, M.D., FACP
Professor of Medicine, Harvard Medical School; Program Director, Internal Medicine Residency Program and Vice Chairman of Medical Education, Brigham and Women's Hospital, Boston

From the New York University School of Medicine, Class of 2004:
Vinay Sundaram, Samir Thadani, Marissa H. Kaminsky, Ryan J. Broderick, Michael S. Cohen, Jennifer A. Stein, Ora B. Gewurz Singer, and **Richard Gillespie**

From the New York College of Osteopathic Medicine, Class of 2003:
Tina Khair, Elizabeth Gannon, Katrina DeLeon, and **Enza Mentesana**

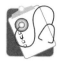# Foreword

In medical school, nothing is quite so bewildering as the first days on the hospital floors as a clinical clerk. Reading through *Fundamentals of Clinical Medicine* brought me back to the excitement and anticipation of those harrowing days almost 50 years ago. Even before you find the lavatories and the cafeteria, you're expected to jump in and work-up patients, write them up, and present them on rounds. The courses in school try to prepare you for this plunge, but they never sufficiently prepare you for these first encounters.

Fundamentals of Clinical Medicine is a handy little book that fills much of the gaps, and it does it well — for students of the health professions who see patients for the first time as part of an Introduction to Clinical Medicine course and, later in training, on medicine clerkships. Years of experience by students and an iterative process of adding, subtracting, and modifying the material by a group of skilled authors will help you make the transition between the classroom and the profession.

Here's some of my own advice. I think you'll find it useful:

- Keep *Fundamentals of Clinical Medicine* with you at all times. Start by reading the terrific introductory sections about the organization of medicine, the clinical environment, and the interactions with patients.
- Work up as many patients as you can. There's no better way to learn clinical medicine.
- Don't be afraid to ask questions. There is no question that's too stupid.
- Don't rely only on textbooks; go back to the original sources of information. You'll be surprised at how much more you'll understand.
- Read at least one weekly journal, cover to cover. It will help you to identify the leading edge of medical practice and medical science.
- Ask for help. Don't be reluctant to ask your intern or resident to show you a physical finding that you missed.
- If you missed pertinent information in a patient's history, try to find out why. Don't make the same mistake twice.
- Dig through old hospital charts on all patients, and call the doctors who have been looking after them. There's gold in them there hills!
- Don't shy away from coming to your own diagnostic conclusions and documenting them in the record. You'll never learn how to diagnose if you don't stick your neck out.
- If you have failed to order a requested test or procedure, or made some other mistake, admit it. No one is perfect.

Clinical medicine is an adventure and a joy. You're lucky to have been chosen to participate in it. Savor the experience.

Jerome P. Kassirer, M.D., MACP

Dr. Kassirer served as Editor-in-Chief of the New England Journal of Medicine *from 1991–1999. After receiving undergraduate and medical degrees from the University of Buffalo in New York, he trained in internal medicine at Buffalo General Hospital. He completed a nephrology fellowship at New England Medical Center, Boston, where he served as Associate Physician-in-Chief and Vice Chairman of the Department of Medicine from 1971 to 1991. He is Distinguished Professor of Medicine at Tufts University School of Medicine in Boston and Adjunct Professor of Medicine at Yale University School of Medicine in New Haven, Connecticut.*

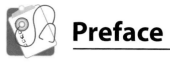

Preface

Much has changed in health care since this manual of clinical medicine was last revised, a decade ago. Managed care in all of its manifestations is now firmly in place across the United States and one consequence, despite the weaknesses and failures of this unique system of health care delivery, has been a greater focus and emphasis on evidence-based medicine and cost savings than ever before. With the emergence of hospitalists, increasing federal and state regulations, rising health care costs, pressure to use disease management algorithms and clinical guidelines, growing public acceptance of complementary and alternative medicine practices, and a greater awareness of the dangers of medical errors, the landscape of the practice of medicine has, in fact, been altered demonstrably and visibly.

We no longer hospitalize every patient with pneumonia nor every interesting patient with a fever of unknown origin if the equivalent work-up, treatment, and follow-up can be done safely on an outpatient basis. We expect the patient with an uncomplicated myocardial infarction to be quickly treated and stabilized, stratified for subsequent risk, prepared for follow-up, and discharged home within days of admission.

This push to have fewer admissions and decrease every admitted patient's length of hospital stay, driven in part by hospitals' desires to minimize health care expenditures but often supported by research showing little adverse risk to patients of such practices, has resulted in one more change. Medical students, residents, and attending physicians are now more frequently challenged by seriously ill patients of all ages with multiple co-morbidities than ever before.

So, too, are changing some of the time-tested methodologies used to evaluate medical students. Medical licensing examinations already include more simulated patient care scenarios, fewer requirements for rote memorization, more emphasis on primary care and the avoidance of medical errors, and the promotion of better communication skills. The Federation of State Medical Boards, the National Board of Medical Examiners and the National Board of Osteopathic Medical Examiners have moved to require that medical students pass a clinical skills examination (CSE) involving one-on-one personal encounters with "standardized patients" for eligibility for medical licensure.

Within this context, the primary duties of the medical student beginning to see patients in the first two years of training or on a medicine clerkship in the final two years have not been made easier, though personal digital assistants (PDA), computerized laboratory data entry and retrieval systems, better diagnostic and therapeutic modalities overall, and ready access to the internet have greatly facilitated and streamlined much of the work. Increased bureaucracy and paperwork requirements (the "hassle factor") resulting from managed care plans' often narrow—and sometimes arbitrary—rules and regulations for specialty referral and prior authorization of patient care, however, have worked against the speed and efficiency that newer technologies offer. The information explosion in medicine, exciting diagnostic advances stemming from the elaboration of the human genome, and overall research in the basic and clinical sciences continues to move forward, meanwhile, to the benefit of the medical profession and a more informed and savvy general public at-large.

Against this backdrop, what the authors of this manual iterated in the preface to the third edition still holds true today, that the fundamental principles of the doctor-patient relationship remain unchanged. The expression of these principles will undoubtedly remain constant even with substantial undergraduate medical curricular reform or additional changes in health care delivery systems.

This edition of *Fundamentals of Clinical Medicine* retains the framework and structure of previous editions, updating clinical and background material where appropriate. The intentional lack of a formal therapeutic emphasis, along with the essentially unchanged approach to the medical work-up, leaves many sections updated but largely the same as before.

The section on the hospital environment and chapters on HIV disease and AIDS, endocrinology, the medical write-up and progress notes, biostatistics and lab results, and the essential clinical library have all been extensively revised. New content areas include an expanded introduction and orientation, an introduction to managed care, professionalism and medical errors, basic head and abdominal radiography, preventive medicine screening recommendations, a listing of common herbal remedies, summaries of common evidence-based complementary medicine modalities, a listing of common drug-drug and drug-herb interactions and, for osteopathic medical students, a useful review of the basic musculoskeletal structural examination.

A handy medical compendium—in a format that summarizes quickly and easily the vast practical and clinical knowledge students are expected to utilize in an Introduction to Clinical Medicine course or master on a busy clinical medicine clerkship—remains an important commodity and a crucial supplement to formal, didactic undergraduate medical education. Though written with the medical student in mind, students of the allied health professions (e.g., nurses, physician assistants, medical technicians) will also find the manual useful as an introduction to the medical profession and as preparation for their own training and employment in hospital settings. The need for all these individuals to have such a basic manual should be paramount, and we hope readers will find this work a useful adjunct to their learning.

This manual began in 1984 as a wonderful effort by two students at Harvard Medical School (R.M.M. and M.E.M.), under the guidance of one of their teachers (G.H.M.), to provide a helpful introductory guide for medical students taking their Introduction to Clinical Medicine course. The breadth and depth of the material originally presented has been greatly expanded as we have sought to preserve the best attributes of the manual: its readability, accessibility, and utility. We are indebted to Drs. Macklis, Mendelsohn, and Mudge—the authors of the first three editions—for their useful and supportive commentary and review. Their contributions to this manual cannot be overstated, and we are grateful for their continuing involvement and counsel. We are also grateful to our families (Nazli, Shaun, Haris, Audrey, Regina, and Matthew) and friends for their continuous support and encouragement.

We thank Dr. Sandra Kammerman for allowing us to use her write-up protocol for medical students at New York University. We thank Stacey Brand for her assistance in researching the medical literature whenever called upon. We are indebted to Neil Marquardt, Amy Oravec, Christina Remsberg, and their able colleagues at Lippincott, Williams and Wilkins for helping us masterfully move this project to completion. Finally, we are indebted to the multitude of medical students, colleagues, and patients—at Harvard Medical School, New York College of Osteopathic Medicine, and New York University School of Medicine—who have directly and indirectly provided the authors the inspiration and energy for this manual and for our life's efforts.

H.J.C.
A.J.G.

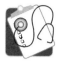

Acknowledgements

We would like to thank Drs. Chaudhry, Grieco, Macklis, Mendelsohn, and Mudge for giving us the opportunity to review and comment on this edition of their excellent manual. With so many changes underway in undergraduate medical education and in health care, a manual like this should be extremely useful for medical students—and students of nursing and other health fields—who are just beginning to see and examine patients.

J.L.
L.S.

Notice. The indications and dosages of all drugs in this book have been recommended in the medical literature and conform to the practices of the general medical community. The medications described do not necessarily have specific approval by the Food and Drug Administration (FDA) for use in the diseases and dosages for which they are recommended. The package insert for each drug should be consulted for use and dosage as approved by the FDA. Because standards for usage change, it is advisable to keep abreast of revised recommendations, particularly those concerning new drugs.

The practices, suggestions, and advice in this manual do not represent the policies and views of the United States Department of Defense or the United States Air Force.

PART I

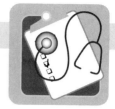

The Hospital Environment

CHAPTER 1

Introduction and Orientation

A n air of excitement and some measure of anxiety mark the transition from the pre-clinical to clinical years. The anxiety may be openly expressed or hidden by a white coat of cultivated sophistication. It may range from passive bewilderment to uncomfortable levels of assertiveness. You are leaving the tidy world of the library, the seminar, and the laboratory to face the infinite variations of illness and the human condition. You are a student and something more; you are a doctor and something less. You are no longer merely a spectator; as an observer you become part of another person's life, for good or ill.

You will make mistakes that others will forgive but you will remember. You have weathered many years of academic competition; now for these all too brief years of medical school, enjoy what you have earned.

J. Gordon Scannell, M.D. (1914–2002)

A graduate of Harvard Medical School and cardiac surgeon, Dr. Scannell was chosen in 1949 to develop the Cardiac Surgery program at Massachusetts General Hospital. He was a leader in the development of open-heart surgery and active in undergraduate medical education.

I. Introduction. Most medical students will get their first taste of clinical medicine as part of an **Introduction to Clinical Medicine** course, when they are gradually introduced to the art and practice of the clinical encounter, in the first and second years of medical school. In addition to learning how to perform a physical examination and the ways in which to start generating a differential diagnosis for a spectrum of presenting signs and symptoms, they will learn how to introduce themselves and how to earn their patients' trust while dutifully recording their findings.

Beginning courses of this type, regardless of how they are named or managed at different schools, generate much interest and excitement among students because they give a more **practical, hands-on approach** to what it's actually like to be a physician than, say, a course in biochemistry or genetics. The material learned, particularly the art of the **physical examination**, is readily and willingly practiced on fellow students and courageous family members. As the course progresses, lecture time will give way to more practical time just as students are getting a handle on how to apply what they've been taught on real patients.

The formal transition from the classroom to the clinical setting, between the second and third years of undergraduate medical education, is one of the most important and dramatic steps in the long road to becoming a physician. Though in many ways an incredibly exciting period, it can be a very challenging transition as well, with unclear expectations at times, long hours and little sleep, and sometimes unpleasant encounters with patients, other health care providers, and ancillary personnel.

As the medical historian and internist Kenneth M. Ludmerer has observed, any physician will recognize that **learning to heal the sick and infirm is in actuality a lifelong process** that only begins with what one learns in medical school, in the classroom, on the inpatient wards, and in outpatient settings. While you "learn the ropes" and expand your fund of medical knowledge at every turn, you will be amazed at how much more there is still to learn. The feeling is at once inspiring and daunting, yet one that you will ultimately overcome in time with an appropriate mixture of confidence and humility.

While one of your goals is to have a medical diploma conferred upon you that gives you the right to call yourself a doctor, it is prudent to remember that the best physician is one who is actually a **medical student for life**, one who constantly strives to learn, to earn the respect of patients and peers, and to advance the profession.

In every clinical setting in your first years of medical school and on every student clerkship, as you make your way through your assigned hospital's wards and corridors, you will quickly establish working relationships with interns and residents only a few years more senior than yourself as you work hard to establish your credentials. Every time you complete a clinical assignment or finish a clerkship, you will have developed a higher level of confidence and comfort in your abilities, made friends with graduates from other schools, felt a respect for your supervising residents, and, hopefully, departed with a lifelong admiration of the attending physicians who will serve as your educators and role models. Those who may not be able to achieve, or display, their full professional or academic potential need not worry too much since the process starts anew, offering more opportunities and perhaps a different set of challenges, with the next clinical encounter, the next clerkship, and the next hospital.

II. Orientation

    A. About this manual. This manual has remained popular over the last two decades among medical students, residents and others because of the simplicity of its format and the practical usefulness of its content, clinical and informational. Many a medical student has carried the manual in his or her white lab coat, or kept it as a reference nearby or at home, throughout the four years of medical school and often into residency.

    To ensure that it is as current as possible, this edition includes content areas that are new and which, many academic and clinical faculty now agree, should be *de rigueur* in undergraduate medical education—the principles of managed care, a recognition of the dangers of medical errors, preventive medicine screening recommendations, commonly used herbal remedies, and a familiarity with evidence-based complementary medicine modalities. While these essential areas are covered succinctly in the same outline format as the other chapters and sections, they are intentionally addressed cursorily and generally. Readers are welcome to review outside sources—authoritative textbooks, medical journals, and websites—for more exhaustive, and critical, analyses of these areas.

As a preparatory approach to clinical medicine, medical students may find it beneficial to approach this manual methodically. Carefully read **Part I (The Hospital Environment)**, browse the items in **Part II (The Medical Work-Up)** to ensure recall of material usually already taught in the classroom, and review the content in **Part III (Disease Pathophysiology Review)** as necessary. Areas under **Part II** that should be particularly helpful to review before setting foot on the hospital wards are Chapters 13 (Electrocardiography) and 15 (Arterial Blood Gases and Acid-Base Disorders). **Part III** is also handy as a quick review just prior to formal attending, or resident, rounds on the wards to refresh one's memory of a particular differential diagnosis or disease pathophysiology.

Part IV (Complementary and Alternative Medicine) and the **Appendices** are available as quick and handy reference resources when managing patients who utilize such practices and to recall commonly used drugs and drug-drug interactions, respectively. The essential clinical library (in Appendix F) lists some important sources of educational material readers may wish to review. All students are strongly advised to familiarize themselves with the medical abbreviations and acronyms found on the inside front and back covers because they are a part of the written, and spoken, language of modern medicine and ready recall of them will greatly facilitate and maximize your communication with others and, ultimately, the care your patients receive.

B. **Primary care medicine** is perhaps best described as comprehensive and preventative longitudinal medical care of the general population that involves a continuum of care, from a patient's first visit for a check-up or presentation of a medical symptom to subsequent management in sickness and in health. Such care is usually supplemented by the assistance and counsel of a variety of medical and surgical specialists (secondary care providers) or subspecialists as needed. The primary care physician typically sees patients initially for every illness and formally consults with specialists for those cases that cannot be fully or successfully managed alone. According to Peter Sam of the University of California at San Francisco, a primary care physician should be able to treat most of the top diagnoses that make up a majority of office visits for such care **(Table 1-1)**.

Internists (physicians trained in internal medicine) and **family practitioners** have traditionally been recognized and designated as primary care physicians and continue to serve in this capacity. Recognizing that many patients today use specialists and other health care providers for their primary health needs, the definition of primary care has expanded in recent years to include **pediatricians** (who primarily see children and adolescents), **geriatricians** (who primarily see the elderly), **obstetrician-gynecologists** (whose practice is limited to women's health but who may not always provide a full complement of comprehensive primary care), and **emergency medicine** physicians (who have become primary care physicians by default in areas of the country where access to a primary care doctor is not readily available or where there are a large number of uninsured individuals).

In recent years independent **nurse practitioners** have also been recognized as providers of some, though certainly not all, components of primary care.

TABLE 1-1. Top 20 diagnostic categories for primary care. (National Ambulatory Medical Care Survey)

Rank	Diagnosis
1	Hypertension
2	Acute upper respiratory illness
3	General medical exam
4	Sinusitis
5	Acute lower respiratory illness
6	Otitis media
7	Depression, Anxiety
8	Diabetes mellitus
9	Acute sprains, Strains
10	Arthritis
11	Ischemic heart disease
12	Asthma
13	Low back pain
14	Lacerations, Contusions
15	Fibrositis, Myalgia, Arthralgia
16	Nonfungal skin infection
17	Headache
18	Abdominal pain
19	Bursitis, Tenosynovitis
20	Chronic rhinitis

Rosenblatt RA, Hart GL, Gamliel S, et al. Identifying primary care disciplines by analyzing the diagnostic content of ambulatory care. *J Am Board Fam Pract*. 1995; 203: 1-20. (Reproduced with permission).

All medical specialists (**cardiologists, geriatricians, gastroenterologists**, etc.) have completed training in internal medicine and a significant number of them practice primary care medicine in addition to their specialty. The vast majority of family practitioners are primary care providers, though some have received additional fellowship training in sports medicine, geriatrics, or women's health.

C. **Internal medicine.** An **internist** is a specialist in adult medicine who has completed three years of residency training in internal medicine approved by the Accreditation Council on Graduate Medical Education or the American Osteopathic Association, or both. Many of the faculty involved in Introduction to Clinical Medicine courses and most of the faculty on medicine clerkships you will interact with are internists or medical specialists so it is useful to have an understanding of their background and training.

Sometimes confused with interns (a first-year resident), internists have actively worked with their specialty colleges on publicity campaigns to better educate the public of their role and function. Unlike family practitioners, who are trained to also treat children and perform obstetrical deliveries, internists are considered experts in the acute and chronic health care of adults only and do not treat children or deliver babies.

An internist's residency training includes in-depth exposure to all the specialties of internal medicine (e.g., cardiology, gastroenterology, pulmonary and critical care medicine, infectious diseases, nephrology, hematology and oncology, rheumatology, allergy and immunology, geriatrics, etc.) and experience managing patients in a hospital's emergency department and intensive care units. In parts of the country that lack medical specialists, the general internist may also fulfill those patient care needs usually reserved for medical specialists.

A recent survey of internists indicated that the following personality traits tend to characterize them: thoroughness, constancy, and deliberateness. More thoughtful and cautious than active and aggressive, the internist is also characterized as a problem solver who likes challenges and is a good listener. Those who enjoy direct patient care tend to choose general internal medicine while those who prefer the more complex and difficult cases, or are procedure-oriented, tend to gravitate to the specialties of internal medicine.

At least 24 concepts have been identified that every internist must know well including those that serve as the foundation for much of the practice of internal medicine (**Table 1-2**). Students will find that one or more of these areas come up for discussion on teaching rounds or at the bedside on practically a daily basis in every clinical encounter. A full and comprehensive understanding of each of these areas by the student would be prudent.

TABLE 1-2. Twenty-four areas every internist must know well

Heart murmurs	HIV disease
Electrocardiography	Glaucoma and cataracts
Hemodynamic monitoring	Basic biostatistics
Peripheral smears	Urinalysis
Arterial blood gas analysis	Sexually-transmitted diseases
Role of ACE inhibitors	Fluids and electrolytes
Paraneoplastic syndromes	The arthritides
Renal cell carcinoma ("The internist's tumor")	Pulmonary flow-volume loops
Inflammatory bowel disease and manifestations	Ethnic and geographic associations of disease
Skin cancers	Collagen vascular diseases
Criteria for PPD positivity	Thyroid function tests
Viral, fungal, and parasitic infections	Diagnosing Cushing's and Addison's diseases

(Modified from Chaudhry HJ: How to Prepare for the Boards. In: New York Internal Medicine Board Review Course Syllabus. Philadelphia: American College of Physicians, 2000: 178.)

Medical specialists (cardiologists, gastroenterologists, etc.) first complete residency training in internal medicine and then pursue fellowship training in their chosen specialty that may last from one year (as in geriatrics) to four years (as in interventional cardiology). A **hospitalist** is a relatively new breed of inpatient medical specialist in the United States, usually trained in internal medicine, who spends at least 25% of his or her professional time serving as the physician-of-record for hospitalized patients of primary care physicians and who returns such patients back to the care of these physicians at the time of hospital discharge. Benefits to patients and hospitals of having such a specialist include more careful supervision and oversight of a hospital stay and cost savings; drawbacks include a lack of continuity of care and some patient dissatisfaction at being handed over for admission to a physician who does not have the same bond and trust that may have been carefully nurtured by a comprehensive physician provider of primary care.

D. **Medical specialty societies.** The **American College of Physicians (ACP)** is the largest medical specialty society in the United States. Founded in 1915, the organization today has more than 115,000 members, including 15,000 medical students. Its mission is to enhance the quality and effectiveness of health care by fostering excellence and professionalism in the practice of medicine. The ACP (www.acponline.org) sponsors continuing medical education (CME) programs for physicians, the Medical Knowledge Self-Assessment Program (MKSAP)—a popular program utilized by many internal medicine residents to help prepare for internal medicine and specialty board examinations—and more than 50 postgraduate courses annually. A new medical knowledge self-assessment program for medical students includes a printed collection of 400 patient-centered, self-assessment questions specially selected for medical students on their medicine clerkship. The College's flagship journal is *Annals of Internal Medicine*.

The ACP also publishes *Impact*, a quarterly newsletter about internal medicine for medical students, for whom membership in the College is free if they are enrolled in U.S. or Canadian medical schools or in medical schools outside the United States where an ACP Chapter exists.

Fellowship in the College (designated by the letters "FACP" after a physician's name) is an honor achieved by those recognized by their peers for personal integrity, superior competence in internal medicine, professional accomplishment, and demonstrated scholarship. Mastership in the College ("MACP") is an even higher honor bestowed upon only a few internists every year.

The **American College of Osteopathic Internists** (www.acoi.org) is osteopathic medicine's counterpart to the ACP. Founded in 1940, the College seeks to advance the practice of internal medicine within the osteopathic profession through excellence in medical education, patient advocacy, clinical research, and opportunity for community service. Membership in the College for osteopathic medical students is free. Fellowship in the College (designated by the letters "FACOI" after a physician's name) is bestowed upon an active member who has successfully passed the examination of the American Osteopathic Board of Internal Medicine or the American Board of Internal Medicine at least four years prior to application and who has made significant contributions to the College, the osteopathic profession, and the community. Mastership ("MACOI") is the highest honor bestowed by the College.

E. **National licensing and specialty board examinations.** The National Board of Medical Examiners and the Federation of State Medical Boards sponsor the **United States Medical Licensing Examination (USMLE)**, and successfully passing all three Steps of this examination is required of allopathic medical students for state medical licensure. The National Board of Osteopathic Medical Examiners administers the **Comprehensive Osteopathic Medical Licensing Examination (COMLEX)**, and successfully passing all three Levels of this examination is required of osteopathic medical students for state medical licensure. The first of these Steps/Levels is usually taken at the end of the second year of medical school and emphasizes the basic medical sciences. The second and third Steps/Levels, which have greater emphasis on the clinical sciences and will soon include a clinical skills examination, are usually taken before graduation from medical school and at the completion of one full year of postgraduate training, respectively. The designation of **diplomate** is conferred after successful passage of either, or both, of these examinations.

Internal medicine specialty and subspecialty **board examinations** are administered near the completion of residency training by the American Board of Internal Medicine and the American Osteopathic Board of Internal Medicine. Once physicians have successfully passed either of these examinations, they are known as "board certified" in internal medicine. Long considered a mark of academic excellence rather than a mark of clinical competence, board certification is now required by employers and managed care plans and has become a surrogate marker of qualification and basic competence. Re-certification every 10 years is now also required of all new internists and internal medicine specialists.

REFERENCES

Chaudhry HJ. *How to Prepare for the Boards.* In: *New York Internal Medicine Board Review Course Syllabus.* Philadelphia: American College of Physicians, 2000, pp. 170–182.

Taylor AD. *How to Choose a Medical Specialty.* 3rd ed. Philadelphia: W.B. Saunders Company, 2000, pp. 80–84.

Wachter, RM. The emerging role of "hospitalists" in the American health care system. *N Engl J Med* 1996;335:514–7.

http://medicine.ucsf.edu (official website of the Department of Medicine at the University of California, San Francisco).

www.acponline.org (official website of the American College of Physicians).

www.acoi.org (official website of the American College of Osteopathic Internists).

CHAPTER **2**

The Inpatient Ward and Outpatient Clinic

For many **first** and **second year medical students**, patient encounters on the inpatient wards or outpatient clinic are carefully arranged beforehand and enough time is allotted to perform a comprehensive history and physical examination. The chief advantage of interviewing and examining patients in the inpatient setting is the availability of relatively more time than in a busy, outpatient clinic or practice where patients are eager to be cared for quickly so they can return home or to their place of employment.

At many teaching hospitals, a semi-formal orientation process greets medical students on a **third** or **fourth year student clerkship**. The process may be led by a welcome from the hospital's Director of Medical Education, Vice President for Academic Affairs, Residency Program Director, Chief Resident, or other designated faculty member or resident assigned to supervise medical students. As you will be given a significant amount of specific information, including contact information and instructions in case of unexpected or planned absences (which you will need to arrange residency interviews), it will be to your advantage to note such information (either in a small notebook or, electronically, in a Personal Digital Assistant) and as much background material as possible about the hospital, faculty and staff, resources, and training programs. Such information may come in handy when you subsequently sit down to contemplate where you want to apply for residency training and how you wish to rank various hospitals where you completed clerkships.

As you proceed through these clinical settings in the third and fourth years, the prospect of **clerkship subject exams** and **national licensing board examinations** may loom at the back of your mind. While medical educators and students ahead of you will recommend formal studying for these standardized examinations, keep in mind that what you take away from managing patients under supervision at the bedside, careful attention and participation at lectures and discussions (e.g., Morning Report, Resident Rounds, Attending Rounds, Grand Rounds, Daily Conferences), and reading about your patients' conditions and the medications they have been prescribed will likely stay with you longer than what you read on your own without any connection to a patient or patient management experience.

Experience shows that the most successful medical students, and physicians, are not necessarily those who are able to retain all knowledge first imparted to them. Being a physician is more than being able to quickly memorize the differential diagnosis of hypokalemia or knowing how to determine the existence of acute hepatitis by deciphering liver function test results precisely. It includes developing a genuine empathy for your fellow human, learning to work harmoniously with others on a team, and learning to teach other students as well as your patients as you learn yourself.

John M. Maxwell has identified 17 essential qualities of a **team player** that can be tailored to reflect the traits that every member of a health care team should constantly espouse **(Table 2-1)**. Consciously emulate as many of these traits as you possibly can on your busy, sometimes chaotic, inpatient ward or outpatient setting and you will cement your value to the other members of the team and thrive. While adoption of work-hour limitations across all residencies has eased workloads to some extent (interns and residents are now required to work no more than 80 hours a week, on average), any assistance you can provide a busy intern or resident will be greatly appreciated.

Take careful notes for yourself on the patients you see, on the clinical pearls passed on to you in discussions and at lectures, and on the peculiarities of how your hospital functions. Remember to maintain patients' privacy, as mandated by the 2003 implementation of the **Health Insurance Portability and Accountability Act** of 1996, and avoid any detailed patient identifying information in your personal notes. Many students will see patients in an outpatient clinic or faculty practice in addition to the inpatient wards; take notes on what you learn regardless of setting. Review these notes regularly and often to maximize your learning, facilitate board exam review, and master the science and art of medicine.

This chapter discusses your roles and responsibilities, and those of the other members of your team on the wards and in the outpatient clinic, as well as a crucial topic for your own safety—universal precautions.

TABLE 2–1. The 17 essential qualities of a health care team player

Adaptable	Adapt, innovate, and overcome
Collaborative	Help others and they'll help you
Committed	Go beyond the 9-5 mentality
Communicative	Ask questions!
Competent	Study every day; stay sharp
Dependable	Be trustworthy and responsible
Disciplined	Be punctual; get the job done
Enlarging	Add value to your teammates
Enthusiastic	Be excited and show it
Intentional	Make every action count
Mission conscious	Treat the patient, not the lab result
Prepared	Back-up everything
Relational	Get along with others
Self-improving	Read, Read, Read
Selfless	There is no "I" in team
Solution oriented	Don't complain; offer solutions
Tenacious	Keep looking for solutions

Modified from Maxwell JM: *The 17 Essential Qualities of a Team Player.* Nashville, Thomas Nelson Publishers, 2002. (Used with permission.)

I. Roles and responsibilities

A. Your role. One of the biggest changes in going from learning in the classroom to learning on the wards (and clinics) is that on the wards you have a much larger responsibility to others—to your patients and to members of your team. In the words of George Washington, "Sleep not when others speak, sit not when others stand, speak not when you should hold your peace, and walk not on when others stop." Your particular responsibilities will change from service to service and year to year, as you gain experience. Always ask, early on, what is expected of you. Your role as a student on the wards, for instance, may be demonstrably different from your role in the outpatient clinic.

1. As a **first** or **second-year student** in medical schools that provide early exposure to patients, your role will be to master the art of interviewing and examining patients. These exercises may be a part of your Introduction to Clinical Medicine or Introduction to Physical Diagnosis course. Frequently you will be given the name of a patient and asked to write a comprehensive **H&P** (history and physical) or perhaps to give an oral presentation of your findings. Such an exercise may be asked of you in a variety of clinical settings, including a physician's quiet private office, a hospital's busy medical clinic, or a bustling emergency department.

2. As a **third-year student** on a formal hospital clerkship (also known as a rotation), you are more integrated into the team that is taking care of patients. You will do admission histories and physicals, follow your patients' progress and perhaps write orders (which will be countersigned by an intern or resident) for tests and interventions, present your patients on teaching rounds, and be expected to read about their problems. You will also be asked to accompany members of the inpatient team to see patients in the emergency department or in the hospital's outpatient clinic.

3. As a **fourth-year student**, more will be expected of you in terms of your fund of medical knowledge, confidence, and overall comfort as you complete either an elective within a specialty of internal medicine or surgery or a sub-internship or acting internship (abbreviated "Sub-I" or "A-I") where you get more hands-on experience in the management of medical patients under supervision.

B. The **other members of the team** on the inpatient wards will most certainly include:

1. The **Intern**, who is in his or her first year of post-medical school training (sometimes called PGY-1, or postgraduate year 1), is responsible for most of the day-to-day work of taking care of patients on the service. Though often feeling overworked, interns are great sources from whom to learn the details of patient management. Remember, they were in your shoes not very long ago.

2 The **Resident**, who is in the second year or higher of post-medical school training, is responsible for supervising the interns. It is usually the resident's responsibility to teach the medical students as well, and he or she will be able to answer broader questions about your patients.

3. **Fellows** have completed their residency and are undergoing further specialty training. With their advancing knowledge, most are happy to answer any questions, especially in their field, about your patients.

4. The **Attending Physician** is an experienced doctor who is responsible for all the patients on the service, and most major decisions on management are discussed with him or her before they are made. The attending is also the person generally responsible for teaching and evaluating the medical students, interns, and residents.

5. **Nurses** can be your best allies on the wards. Though you will no doubt hear stories of nurses occasionally taking out their frustrations concerning doctors on medical students, if you treat them like colleagues they will no doubt treat you similarly. As a second-year student, always check with a patient's nurse before examining or interviewing the patient — this can alleviate many interruptions later. As a third-year student, learn the names of the nurses caring for your patients and remember that they have a lot to teach you as well. Time permitting, learn also to share with nurses any major new findings or diagnostic test results about patients both of you are following. This will help them maximize understanding of their patients and also leave them appreciative of your thoughtfulness. It helps to know the different types of nurses involved in the care of patients:

   a. A **Registered Nurse (RN)** is defined as a professional who can diagnose and treat human responses to actual or potential health problems through such services as case finding, health teaching, health counseling, and the provision of care supportive to, or restorative of, life and well-being, and executing medical regimes *prescribed by a licensed physician.*

   b. A **Licensed Practical Nurse (LPN)** is a nurse who can perform tasks and responsibilities within the framework of case finding, health teaching, health counseling, and the provision of supportive and restorative care *under the supervision of a registered nurse or licensed physician.*

   c. A **Nurse Practitioner** is a professional certified to provide the diagnosis of illness and physical conditions and the performance of therapeutic and corrective measures within a specialty area of practice, in *collaboration with a licensed physician qualified in the specialty.*

   d. A **Certified Nurse Midwife (CNM)** is a certified registered nurse who is trained to provide care for *essentially normal* expectant mothers and to handle abnormal cases by referring the patient to physicians or by consulting physicians or working jointly with them.

   e. **Nursing Assistants (NA), Medical Technicians,** and **Medical Assistants** are individuals who receive basic training in a hospital or other center of learning in order to be able to complete certain specific tasks. While they are not required to apply for licensure or certification, these assistants are invaluable ancillary health care personnel whose services are needed.

6. **Other health care professionals**. Physician assistants, respiratory therapists, physical therapists, clinical nutritionists, discharge planners, pharmacists, infection control personnel, and others are also part of the patient care team. They, too, can be a huge resource for you on particular aspects of patient care. As a second year student, your patient examinations will frequently be interrupted by therapists and others. Ask them politely if they can return later, but remember that, like you, they are very busy and that they play an important role in the health of your patient.

II. Universal precautions

A. Your own safety is one of the most important things to keep in mind when you are on the wards or in the clinic. While a medical student, you will almost inevitably come into contact with many patients who have transmissible diseases, including HIV and hepatitis. You are at risk for contracting these diseases through contact with bodily fluids. You should make sure that you have been immunized against hepatitis B before you enter the wards, but remember that even the full series of immunizations is not always 100 percent effective. Because of this, and because of the presence of HIV, for which there is still no vaccine, you need to observe certain precautions while on the wards.

B. Since it is impossible to tell at all times who is infected and who is not, you should practice **universal precautions**—that is, you should act as if every patient you encounter is potentially infectious. Specifically, you should wear protective clothing and use devices to prevent contamination of your skin and mucous membranes whenever you handle certain bodily fluids. It is crucial for you to understand how the HIV virus can be transmitted and how it cannot. Blood, semen, vaginal secretions, and lab preparations of cerebrospinal, amniotic, synovial, pleural, peritoneal, and pericardial fluids have all been implicated in the transmission of HIV. It is thought that feces, nasal secretions, breast milk, sweat, tears, urine, and vomitus carry a very low risk of transmitting the HIV virus. Hepatitis B, while formerly thought to be transmitted only parenterally and through sexual contact, is thought to be infectious through the oral route as well, though much more rarely.

C. **Specific measures you should take** while on the wards include:

1. **Gloves** should be worn whenever handling any blood or body fluid. After each use, gloves should be discarded carefully, without touching the outside of the gloves with your bare hands. Most hospitals have gloves available in each patient room; if not, carry some with you.

2. **Wash your hands**, with soap, before and after each patient contact. Patients especially like to see their doctor washing his or her hands before examining them. Get into the habit of doing this early; it's good for both you and your patients.

3. Be extremely careful with **sharp instruments** like needles and scalpels. They should be disposed of immediately after use, in a puncture-resistant container. **Do not recap needles under any circumstances.** Be especially careful during codes, when chaos reigns and inadvertent nee-

dle sticks are more likely. Always check for sharp objects before handling used materials after a procedure. If you use any sharp object, it is your responsibility to dispose of it.

4. **Wear protective eyewear and a mask** if there is potential for blood or body fluids to splash into your eyes, nose, or mouth. In some cases, you may be fitted with a portable high-efficiency particulate air (HEPA) filter respiratory mask, which is not only useful protection against suspected cases of tuberculosis but also is recommended by the Centers for Disease Control and Prevention as useful in protecting against a number of airborne biological pathogens, including spores produced by *Bacillus anthracis* (anthrax).

5. To avoid contamination during **mouth-to-mouth resuscitation**, use a barrier device or a resuscitation bag; these should be available on every ward.

D. All of this is meant not to scare you but to stress the importance of **protecting yourself**. Some providers trained in the pre-AIDS era may not follow these safety guidelines, and you may feel pressure to follow their example. Do not. These recommendations could save your life, so get into good habits early and practice universal precautions.

E. **If you do get splashed**, wash the area immediately. If you think you have been exposed, for example through a needle stick, you should **act on it immediately**. Data indicate that the chance of getting HIV from a single contaminated needle stick is about 1 in 250. Make sure you know the procedures at your institution for reporting exposures. If you do not, begin by contacting your supervising resident and the hospital's infection control coordinator. Appropriate medications given within a few hours after an exposure to the HIV virus might reduce the risk of infection. Treat this incident as a **crisis** and seek assistance immediately.

III. Some words of advice

A. **Your role as a medical student** on the wards performing histories and physicals is a particularly difficult one, as you may frequently feel your presence is simply a burden, and at times patients may even refuse to talk to you. Remember that they are not feeling well; think back to the last time you were sick and remember how miserable you felt. Though at times you may not think so, **your presence is really valuable**. Learning to do interviews and perform physicals on actual patients is an important part of your training. Patients will also benefit from your work; it is rare that anyone in a busy hospital takes the time to talk with them at length and hear their story.

B. You need to **take control of your own education**. Never be afraid to ask questions, whether about your patients, your responsibilities, or medicine in general. There is a lot you need to learn and experience before you graduate, so take advantage of every opportunity. To do well on the wards, try to be enthusiastic and dependable, an advocate for your patients, well prepared and, especially, a team player. Being regularly punctual and always completing tasks, however mundane, asked of you will win you more praise than any correct answer you give to a complicated academic question on teaching rounds.

C. Finally, in the midst of taking care of all the patients, remember to **take care of yourself.** Work on the wards can expand to take up your whole life if you allow it to. Try to eat and sleep well, exercise, and keep up with at least one aspect of your life outside the hospital. The road ahead is a long one, and this is a good time to learn to balance your life inside and outside of medicine.

REFERENCES

Chaudhry HJ. Working Less, Training Harder. Letter. *J Am Ost Assoc* October 2002;102(10): 522–523.

Maxwell JM. *The 17 Essential Qualities of a Team Player*. Nashville: Thomas Nelson Publishers, 2002.

Washington G. *Rules of Civility and Decent Behavior in Company and Conversation*. Boston: Applewood Books, 1988.

CHAPTER 3

Managed Care, Medicare, and Medicaid

> Had the medical profession not been a "profession," that is, if its members had been free to set up combinations of skills and types of personnel without the formal restraints of licensing laws and medical ethics and the informal restraints of guild fraternalism, the most congenial American pattern for organizing health services would almost certainly have been independent, voluntary associations of specialists and other health personnel, organized on efficient business lines and offering a clearly specified range of services.
>
> As it was, the diffuse system of practice organization stimulated demands for a centralized governmental role in paying for medical care.
>
> *Rosemary Stevens, Ph.D.*
>
> *Dr. Stevens is the Stanley I. Scheerr Professor of History and Sociology of Science at the University of Pennsylvania. She is the author of* In Sickness and in Wealth: American Hospitals in the Twentieth Century *and* American Medicine and the Public Interest.

A decade ago, most people in the United States received health care from a personal physician who practiced privately or in a small group, with health insurance provided by their employers. That hasn't changed much, though patient charges for health insurance associated with such visits (in the form of co-payments, premiums, and deductibles) continue to rise as managed care organizations find themselves unable to stem increases in health care costs in the face of a backlash from patients, physicians, hospitals, and employers.

Whereas the proportion of the population enrolled in managed care plans has increased from 13.5% in 1990 to 30% in 2000, most of this growth has actually been through what are known as preferred-provider organizations (PPOs), or loosely structured health maintenance organizations (HMOs), as opposed to staff-model HMOs. But what is a PPO? What is a staff-model HMO? To any casual observer of the changes occurring in health care delivery, and certainly to most patients, there is an abundance of confusion about the terms and acronyms used to describe managed care. To compound matters, most students are not introduced to managed care concepts, let alone what Medicare and Medicaid are, until they have graduated, are nearing completion of residency training, and are about to enter practice.

This chapter will provide a brief summary of managed care, Medicare and Medicaid, and a handy listing of commonly used health care terms. All patients you encounter in your Introduction to Clinical Medicine course or on your medicine clerkship should get equal treatment and care from your attending physicians and yourself, regardless of which managed care plan they belong to or which health insurance policy they possess (if any, for that matter). A cursory understanding of managed care principles and the realities of today, to be sure, will go a long way to explain why certain medications may not be available to some of your patients upon discharge or why there is a need to convince a managed care plan's representative to allow your patient to stay in the hospital longer than originally intended.

I. Managed care

A. **Definition.** Managed care has been defined as a system of health care delivery that attempts to influence or control the utilization of health care services and the costs associated with such services. The degree of influence depends on the model. For example, a PPO requires its members (patients) to share less of the cost of their care if they use the providers (physicians) enrolled in the PPO. Health maintenance organizations, on the other hand, may choose not to reimburse health services received from providers with whom the HMO does not have a contract.

B. **Introduction.** Managed care essentially expresses a new relationship between the purchasers, insurers, and providers of health care. Traditionally, a patient's physician alone decided how much care a patient would receive, of what kind, and by which providers; these providers often unilaterally decided how much to charge. The insurers simply paid the bills, and if the bills were too high, the insurers would charge higher premiums to the purchasers the following year. Under managed care, **organizations that foot the bill for a patient's care take on the role of managing that patient's care, deciding how much care a patient receives, of what kind, and by which providers**. Moreover, these managed care companies decide how much money providers will receive and how that money is paid.

Early models of managed care existed as organized practices of groups of physicians established during and immediately after World War II—the Kaiser Permanente Plan on the West Coast and the Health Insurance Plan in New York are two of the earliest examples. Although opposition by organized medicine, mainly the American Medical Association, to prepaid group practices of this type eased in the late 1950s, there was no large, continuing movement for such practices until the early 1970s.

The Nixon administration embarked on a landmark health care strategy of restructuring the "medical marketplace" around decentralized, private, competitive institutions in place of governmental institutions that were felt to be bogged down, uncreative, and inefficient. Under the administrations of Presidents Ford, Carter, and Reagan, managed care was allowed to flourish and command ever more control of health care, generally, and its delivery, specifically.

Health care costs in the United States, after a brief period of cuts in growth in the mid-1990s attributed in part to the success of managed care, have since resumed their upturn. National health care spending in 2001 was $1.4 trillion, or 14.1 percent of the gross domestic product (total economy). While the bureaucracy of managed care is certainly here to stay, resentment against the system's restrictive policies (limiting, for example, which physician a patient can see) and narrow interpretations of which therapeutic modalities should be "covered" or not, has so far helped maintain traditional, fee-for-service financing and wide-open networks that promise a choice of providers for patients.

A 1999 survey revealed that negative views of managed care are widespread among medical students, residents, faculty members, and medical school deans. Realizing that managed care is here to stay, several medical schools have instituted elective clerkships at managed care settings for their students to better understand how care can be delivered efficiently and comprehensively within such systems.

II. Medicare and Medicaid

A. **Introduction.** In 1965, Congress created Medicare for the elderly and Medicaid for the poor as amendments to the Social Security Act of 1930. This resulted in a **compulsory health insurance program for the elderly**, financed through payroll taxes (Medicare Part A), a voluntary insurance program for physicians' services subsidized through general revenues (Medicare Part B), and an **expanded means-tested program** administered by the states (Medicaid).

Responsibility for managing Medicare was initially vested in the Social Security Administration with Medicaid subject to both federal oversight and state control. Congress grew dissatisfied with the performance of the Social Security Administration when it failed to constrain Medicare expenditures and, in 1977, the Health Care Financing Administration (HCFA) was created to manage both Medicare and Medicaid. Since 1996, HCFA has also been responsible for implementing some 700 provisions of five major laws related to health care costs, insurance, benefits, and overall accountability.

The Balanced Budget Act of 1997, the most controversial of these laws, reduced Medicare payments to virtually every clinical laboratory, hospital, skilled nursing facility, and home health care agency in the United States, with an estimated reduction of $112 billion for the period from 1998 to 2002. Subsequent legislation reversed a small proportion of those cuts but not before some hospitals closed, merged, or downsized.

The **Centers for Medicare and Medicaid Services (CMS)** is the new name for HCFA and remains the **single largest purchaser of health care in the world**, with an estimated $476 billion paid for health care services in 2001 on behalf of 70 million disabled, elderly, and poor beneficiaries. The agency also has a fiduciary role as guardian of tax revenues that represent 15 percent of the federal budget.

B. **Medicare** is a federal entitlement program created in 1965 that provides medical benefits, at a cost of $257 billion in 2002, to 40 million people **over the age of 65**, or those who have received Social Security **disability** payments for more than two years, or those who have **end-stage renal disease**. In 2003, President Bush signed into law a major Medicare reform package, estimated to cost $400 billion over 10 years, providing prescription drug benefits for beneficiaries.

C. **Medicaid** is a means-tested federal program created in 1965 that is administered and operated by all 50 states and the District of Columbia and which provides medical benefits to 51 million **eligible low-income persons**: 24 million children, 14 million adults, and 13 million disabled and elderly persons. It is the **nation's largest health insurance program**. Disabled and elderly persons who are eligible for both Medicare and Medicaid receive the full Medicaid benefit package as a supplement to Medicare. The costs of the Medicaid program are shared by the federal government, states, and, in New York, counties. The federal government and the states spent more than $259 billion on Medicaid in 2002, with the federal share accounting for 57 percent. Medicaid favored institutional care for its recipients until 1981, when Congress authorized home and community care as an alternative.

III. **Commonly used health care terms.** A comprehensive understanding of common health care terms is essential in today's world to understand how the business side of medicine impacts patient care, individually and globally. Through medical specialty societies and national organizations of physicians and students, greater opportunities to advocate on behalf of patients exist than ever before. Plenty of examples exist of how an individual medical student's, or physician's, advocacy of an important health care issue can impact health policy changes locally and nationally. Before you can advocate for your patients, however, you have to know the alphabet soup of health care:

A. **Accreditation** is the process for determining whether an organization or program is in substantial compliance with established standards as promulgated by the accrediting body. Accreditation is often a necessary condition for participation in other programs, such as eligibility for Medicare reimbursement. For hospitals and long-term care facilities, the largest accrediting body is the Joint Commission on the Accreditation of Healthcare Organizations (JCAHO). Individual programs or units within a hospital may also be separately accredited by other nationally recognized accrediting bodies.

B. A **benchmark** is an outcome with which a subject compares its own performance. It is merely a reference point. It can also be, but is not necessarily, a goal, ideal, or best practice.

C. **Capitation** is a payment method in which a pre-set amount is paid to a provider to deliver care to an individual. The payment is generally made monthly and the provider is responsible for delivering or arranging for the delivery of a specific range of health services for this set payment, regardless of the actual cost of services.

D. **Current Procedural Terminology (CPT)** refers to a classification system developed by the American Medical Association in which unique codes are assigned to procedures and services (but not diagnoses) performed by providers.

E. A **diagnosis-related group (DRG)** is a diagnosis-based classification system used by Medicare and Medicaid to reimburse hospitals for inpatient costs on a per-discharge basis, regardless of length of stay or actual cost.

F. The **Employee Retirement Income Security Act (ERISA)** was enacted by Congress in 1974 to set national standards for employers who voluntarily offered pension plans to their employees. An ERISA plan is any plan created by a private employer, group of employers, or union, with a few exceptions, to offer pensions, health coverage, or other benefits to employees.

G. Evidence-based medicine (EBM) describes the process of researching and applying information presented in the medical literature to improve patient care. The process involves trained clinicians who transform knowledge deficits into specific clinical questions, research and evaluate the medical literature related to the clinical question, apply the literature to improve patient care, and share new information with their colleagues.

H. Fee-for-service (FFS) represents a method of payment that provides reimbursement, usually in pre-determined amounts, to physicians for a specific service. Fee-for-service payments occur each time a service is rendered, as opposed to capitated payments, which are paid on a regular schedule regardless of whether or when services were rendered.

I. The **Health Insurance Portability and Accountability Act (HIPAA)** of 1996 seeks to improve the portability and continuity of health insurance for groups and individuals, extend fraud and abuse measures to all types of insurers, and achieve administrative simplification by creating a framework for the standardization of electronic data interchange in health care, including protections for the privacy and security of individually identifiable health information.

J. Hospice is a program of care that treats terminally ill patients and their families. The program, which is designed for patients with a prognosis of six months or less to live, provides coordinated, interdisciplinary inpatient and home care services, and emphasizes pain control and psychological well-being.

K. Depending on a state's regulation, an **independent practice association (IPA)** is typically a certified organization of providers that contracts with HMOs to arrange health care services for its enrollees. Although an IPA is generally thought of as a group of physicians, it may comprise other providers or combinations of various types of providers.

L. The **International Classification of Diseases (ICD)** is a classification system developed by the World Health Organization listing diagnoses using six-digit numerical codes. The codes are used by health care providers to specify primary, secondary, or other diagnoses on insurance claim forms. The National Center for Health Statistics and CMS released changes to these codes, effective October 1, 2002, that have been described as the most numerous affecting primary care providers in eight years.

M. A **peer review organization (PRO)** is any organization that undertakes reviews of provider quality, utilization, or management of care. However, under Federal law, PROs are a specific type of organization with which CMS or its fiscal intermediaries or carriers contract to undertake reviews of the Medicare program. A newer term for a PRO is a Quality Improvemnt Organization (QIO).

N. A **physician-hospital organization (PHO)** is an organization formed by physicians (either individually or as represented by a group) and a hospital for the purpose of joint ventures, such as managed care contracting.

O. A **point-of-service (POS) plan** is a managed care product offered by an HMO that provides enrollees the option of receiving services from participating or non-participating providers. The benefits package is typically designed to encourage the use of participating providers by imposing deductibles and/or co-insurance fees for services provided by non-participating providers.

P. A **preferred provider organization (PPO)** is a managed care product that is offered by indemnity insurers or self-insured plans that provides enrollees the option of receiving services from participating or non-participating providers.

Q. Congress in 1997 enacted the **State Children's Health Insurance Program (SCHIP)**, which provides coverage to 4.6 million children whose families earn incomes that are too high to allow them to qualify for Medicaid but too low to permit them to afford private health insurance.

R. A **Staff-model HMO**, also known as a Group-model HMO, is a type of managed care entity in which providers (physicians and others) are employees salaried by the health maintenance organization to provide and deliver care to enrollees, utilizing guidelines and policies set by the HMO.

S. **Supplemental Security Income (SSI)** is a means-tested Federal program, created in 1974 and administered and operated by individual states, that provides a monthly cash benefit to low income elderly, the blind, or the disabled who cannot afford to meet their basic needs of food, clothing, and shelter. The amount of income received depends on the individual's living arrangements and any other income.

REFERENCES

New York Healthcare Terms: A Compendium. New York: Greater New York Hospital Association, 2001, pp. 2–34.

Stevens R. *In Sickness and in Wealth: American Hospitals in the Twentieth Century.* Baltimore: Johns Hopkins University Press, 1999, pp. 244, 301.

Stevens R. *American Medicine and the Public Interest.* 2nd ed. Berkeley: University of California Press, 1998, p. 422.

CHAPTER **4**

Professionalism and Medical Errors

> **B**illions of dollars are spent on heroic efforts to "save" lives, but very little money is allocated for the kind of compassionate patient care that was the hallmark of the profession.
>
> This is the crisis of contemporary medicine: billions for cures, peanuts for care. No wonder people are frustrated. No wonder we see daily news stories about some new disaster connected with medical care—too many errors, too many denials of care, and too little concern for patients, who are mere numbers to be counted, checked off, and disposed of. But guess what: cures are still elusive, and the need for care is still pervasive.
>
> *George D. Lundberg, M.D.*
>
> *Editor-in-Chief Emeritus of Medscape—a provider of medical information on the internet—and Special Healthcare Advisor to the Chairman and CEO of WebMD, Dr. Lundberg was editor of the* Journal of the American Medical Association *(JAMA) for 17 years.*

Many medical students of today get a formal introduction to the concepts related to medical jurisprudence and bioethics while still at school. Such didactic learning is sometimes delivered as a separate course or included in a seminar or symposium. The subject matter is dutifully memorized, regurgitated for examinations, and quickly forgotten so as to better focus on "real" medicine. Most textbooks of medicine compound matters by barely mentioning ethics.

This chapter reminds students of their important role as junior members and future leaders of a learned profession and reports on the real dangers of medical errors.

I. Professionalism

A. **Definition.** The word "professional" implies a degree of **commitment, training, and competence**, but it does not by itself encompass the special responsibilities and obligations of the medical professional. Law, religion, and medicine have been described as the three traditional learned professions because attorneys, clergymen, and physicians need to be trusted with the most private and intimate secrets of a person's mind, soul, and body.

B. The 1957 **Principles of Medical Ethics** of the American Medical Association neatly address the need to serve humanity justly, improve medical knowledge, assure physician competence, maintain confidence, and protect patient vulnerability. Physicians could make these commitments then, it has been said, because they were the center of medical practice. With the advent of managed care, physicians now feel the need to reassert their authority and capture once again the medical high ground.

The **Medical Professionalism Project (MPP)**, formed by the American Board of Internal Medicine, the American College of Physicians, and the European Federation of Internal Medicine in 2000, has developed a physician charter on professionalism that seeks to help guarantee a more committed relationship between patients and their doctors.

The MPP is a collaborative effort that cites **10 qualities of medical professionalism** in its charter, qualities students should also be mindful of as they focus on the mechanics of clinical reasoning and manage the health care needs of patients assigned to them:

1. **Professional competence.** Doctors must understand their business and improve upon their competencies by partaking in continuing educational and evaluative opportunities. Students must strive to learn as much as possible to provide quality care for their patients.

2. **Honesty with patients.** Physicians and students must obtain complete informed consent (explaining the indications, attendant risks, and probable outcomes and side effects of any planned intervention) prior to, during, and after patient treatment. Doctors and students should also acknowledge medical errors to patients and peers. Admitting mistakes is never easy, especially during training, and the best place to start is with your supervising resident or attending physician.

3. **Patient confidentiality.** Preserve confidentiality despite technological and scientific advances as well as public health pressures.

4. **Maintain appropriate relations with patients.** Avoid establishing financial or personal relations with patients.

5. **Improve quality of health care.** Physicians must work to reduce medical errors, increase patient safety, minimize overuse of health care resources and encourage living wills and proxy-decision making—documents that anticipate situations where patients may be unable to make health care decisions for themselves.

6. **Advocate for improved and equitable access to care.** This includes uniform and sufficient care for all patients as well as elimination of discrimination and barriers to access. At the student level, this may take the form of signing a petition or calling your local Congressman to express your concern for, support of, or opposition to pending legislation on a health care matter.

7. **Promote a just distribution of scarce resources.** Here, a balance must be reached between individual patients' needs and those of the wider public.

8. **Scientific knowledge.** Maintain scientific integrity and standards and promote valid research agendas.

9. **Manage conflicts of interest.** Doctors have an obligation to disclose all legitimate conflicts of interest.

10. **Professional responsibilities.** Participate in self-regulation, remediation, standard setting, and assessments.

II. Medical errors. The Institute of Medicine, in its landmark 2000 report, *To Err Is Human*, reported that more than 1 million preventable adverse events occur each year in the United States, of which 44,000 to 98,000 are fatal—more than are killed annually by automobile accidents. The report also notes that our health care system fails with embarrassing frequency to provide medical interventions known to benefit patients. The **three main types of medical errors are underuse, overuse, and misuse.** Although the accuracy of the magnitude of errors has been challenged, there is general agreement among physicians and regulators that the problem is serious. An important issue is whether these errors represent failures of humans or systems. The continuous quality improvement (CQI) model of William Deming that is utilized at most hospitals assumes that most adverse events are system failures and that the design of work processes should aim to detect and eliminate the human error that inevitably occurs.

The Quality Improvement Group at the Centers for Medicare and Medicaid Services leads the quality improvement organizations (QIO)—formerly known as peer review organizations (PROs) but also including other related review organizations—and uses 24 quality clinical indicators that have relatively strong evidence to support them.

Interest in developing new voluntary and mandatory systems that would allow physicians and other health care personnel to report adverse events, or even "close calls," without fear of punishment is high. The primary purpose of reporting adverse events ideally should be to learn from these experiences and many hospitals and medical institutions have moved ahead to create a **Chief Safety Officer**, or other equivalent, to address the issue.

As Thomas H. Lee, M.D., a Chief Medical Officer of Partners Healthcare System in Boston has observed, "The credibility of the systems of accountability that physicians support will help determine the level of trust the public has for our profession in the years to come."

Every hospital you work in will likely have its own process of reporting adverse events, accidents, and serious errors that do or do not cause harm. Such reporting information will usually be provided to you during your orientation; if it is not, and a medical error is recognized during the course of your medicine clerkship, begin the process by contacting your supervising resident or attending physician. Sharing openly with your patient care team your experience with a medical error, however difficult, is an important part of your learning and it is likely your candor and maturity in speaking up will be appreciated and everyone will gain from the educational value of your experience.

REFERENCES

Bodenheimer TS, Grumbach K. *Understanding Health Policy: A Clinical Approach.* 3rd ed. New York: McGraw-Hill, 2002, pp. 2–3.

Chaudhry HJ. The Shifting Faces of Power: A Book Review of Howard Brody's *The Healer's Power. The New Physician* 1995;44(5):36.

Crippen DL. *Impact of the Balanced Budget Act on the Medicare fee-for-service program.* Testimony before the House Energy and Commerce Committee, Washington, D.C., September 15, 1999.

Employee Retirement Income Security Act of 1974, 88 Stat. 829 (as amended and codified at 29 U.S.C.).

Health, United States, 2001: urban and rural health chartbook. Hyattsville, Maryland, National Center for Health Statistics, 2001.

Hsia DC. Medicare Quality Improvement: Bad Apples or Bad Systems? Editorial. *JAMA* 2003;289(3):354–356.

Iglehart JK. The American health care system—Medicare. *N Engl J Med* 1999;340:327–332.

Iglehart JK. The American health care system—Medicaid. *N Engl J Med* 1999;340:403–408.

Iglehart JK. The Centers for Medicare and Medicaid Services. *N Engl J Med* 2001;345:1920–1924.

Iglehart JK. The Dilemma of Medicaid. *N Engl J Med* 2003;348:2140–2148.

Kohn LT, Corrigan JM, Donaldson MS, eds. *To err is human: building a safer health system.* Washington, D.C.: National Academy Press, 2000.

Leape LL. Reporting of Adverse Events. *N Engl J Med* 2002;347:1633–1638.

Lee TH. A Broader Concept of Medical Errors. *N Engl J Med* 2002;347:1965–1967.

Levit K, Smith C, Cowan C, et al. Inflation spurs health spending in 2000. *Health Aff* (Millwood) 2002; 21(1):172–181.

Ludmerer KM. *Learning to Heal: The Development of American Medical Education.* Baltimore: Johns Hopkins University Press, 1985, p. xi.

Lundberg GD. *Severed Trust: Why American Medicine Hasn't Been Fixed.* New York: Basic Books, 2000, pp. 2, 162–163.

McDonald CJ, Weiner M, Hui SL. Deaths due to medical errors are exaggerated in the Institute of Medicine report. *JAMA* 2000;284:93–95.

Patel K, Rushefsky ME. *Health Care Politics and Policy in America.* 2nd ed. Armonk, New York: M.E. Sharpe, 1999, pp. 36–41.

Pear R. Report Criticizes Federal Oversight of State Medicaid. *NY Times*, July 7, 2003, p. A1.

Pear R. Spending on Health Care Increased Sharply in 2001. *NY Times*, January 8, 2003, p. A12.

Reiser SJ, Banner RS. The Charter on Medical Professionalism and the Limits of Medical Power. Editorial. *Ann Intern Med* 2003;138:839–841.

Sandy, LG. Homeostasis without reserve—the risk of health system collapse. *N Engl J Med* 2002;347(24):1971–1975.

Simon SR, Pan RJD, Sullivan AM, et al. Views of Managed Care: A Survey of Students, Residents, Faculty and Deans at Medical Schools in the United States. *N Engl J Med* 1999;340(12):928-936.

www.professionalism.org (official website of the Medical Professionalism Project).

PART II

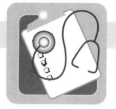

The Medical Work-Up

It is a truism of philosophy that a complete knowledge of a thing can only be obtained by elucidating its causes and antecedents, provided, of course, such causes exist. In medicine it is, therefore, necessary that causes of both health and disease should be determined.

Avicenna (980–1037)

Born Abu Ali ibn Sina, Avicenna (as he became known in the West) began writing his monumental Canon of Medicine *in 1012. Translated into Latin and many other languages from its original Arabic, this treatise remained the world's premier textbook of medicine for more than 500 years.*

The *medical work-up* is a term used to refer to the sequence of diagnostic inquiries and laboratory tests that are implemented during the evaluation of any specific medical problems. The primary job of the student starting clinical work is to become familiar with the work-up process and to learn to conduct a patient work-up thoroughly and efficiently.

Although the specific details of the work-ups for various problems may be quite different, the **sequence of data acquisition and analysis** is always the same: first a **history** is taken, then a **physical examination** is performed, then **diagnostic tests** are conducted and analyzed, and finally an **assessment and a therapeutic plan** are formulated. This sequence of history, physical examination, diagnostic tests, assessment, and plan is at the heart of every work-up.

Part II of this manual is organized in a sequence roughly parallel to that of the work-up. Chap. 5 outlines the content and technique of the medical interview, while Chap. 6 presents a brief outline of the general physical examination. Chap. 7 contains a detailed description of the physical exam, arranged by organ system. Finally, Chap. 8 describes how you alter your basic exam when seeing children of different ages.

Turning from the bedside work-up to the clinical laboratory, the next seven chapters present, first, a general discussion of biostatistics and when to order lab tests, and then brief overviews of the principles and interpretation of the six most common diagnostic tests: the hematologic screen, the serum chemistry battery, the urinalysis, the electrocardiograph, diagnostic imaging of the head, chest, and abdomen, and the arterial blood gas determination. In each of these chapters, an attempt has been made to simplify the interpretation of the lab results and to concentrate only on the more common and significant findings. These chapters do not, of course, take the place of the more rigorous treatments found elsewhere.

Chap. 16 is a discussion of the medical case write-up and includes sample student write-ups as well as specific advice on how to construct a good write-up. The medical case presentation is described in Chap. 17, which contains specific advice on how to present medical cases on hospital resident and attending rounds and in formal didactic sessions.

Because the information in many of these chapters is of two types, objective and subjective, some chapters are divided into two sections: Sec. I, which contains generally objective information and will be useful as a memory aid and pocket reference; and Sec. II, which contains subjective advice and the kind of pragmatic information that traditionally has been passed informally from student to student. The purpose of Sec. II in these chapters is to help students "learn the ropes" of clinical work early in their careers, to give them more time to concentrate on the factual information that must be mastered. As much as possible, Sections I and II of each chapter parallel each other and should be read together.

This book contains no specific therapeutic information; for this the student is referred to the *Washington Manual of Medical Therapeutics* (also published by Lippincott Williams & Wilkins). For the novice clinician this latter book is indispensable.

CHAPTER 5

Taking a History

> M̲ost people have a furious itch to talk about themselves and are
> restrained only by the disinclination of others to listen. Reserve is an
> artificial quality that is developed in most of us but as the result of innu-
> merable rebuffs. The doctor is discreet. It is his business to listen and no
> details are too intimate for his ears.
>
> *W. Somerset Maugham (1874–1965)*
>
> *English novelist, short story writer, and playwright, Maugham was trained as a*
> *physician at St. Thomas' Hospital in London. He wrote more than 60 books,*
> *including the autobiographical novel* Of Human Bondage *(1915). This excerpt*
> *appears in* The Summing Up *(1938).*

The patient interview, usually referred to as the history, is the **first step** in the
diagnostic work-up. Taking a good history is probably the **single most important
task** in the work-up. Both because of its importance in diagnosis and because the
history is the portion of the work-up in which the **physician-patient relationship**
is first established. The job of the medical student is not only to learn how to conduct a thorough interview but also to develop a professional manner that will put
the patient at ease. Whether the patient will regard the student as an unnecessary
third party or as a vital member of the medical team often depends on the tenor
and style of the initial interview.

Section I of this chapter is a point-by-point review of the subjects and style
of each part of the formal medical interview. Section II contains a collection of
practical advice intended to help the student conduct and interpret the interview.

The parts of the medical interview that should be memorized early in a clinical career are outlined in **Table 5-1**. Chap. 16 presents information and formats
useful in subsequently writing up the case for the medical record.

I. The history and review of systems

A. **Introductory information.** Begin by collecting the identifying data about
a patient from both the existing medical record and the patient, especially
the patient's name, age, sex, race, occupation, and, if the patient has been
referred from elsewhere, the source of and reason for the referral.

B. **Chief complaint and its duration.** The chief complaint is traditionally
defined as that problem or set of problems that makes the patient decide to
seek medical attention. Questions concerning the chief complaint follow
the physician's greeting of the patient (see p. 43) and the brief questions
about introductory information. The chief complaint is elicited by asking

TABLE 5.1.   Outline of the patient interview

    I. Introductory information

   II. Chief complaint (CC)

  III. History of present illness (HPI)

  IV. Past medical history (PMHx)

       A. Other medical problems

       B. Injuries, hospitalizations, operations

       C. Medications

       D. Habits

       E. Allergies

       F. Major childhood illnesses

       G. Immunizations

    V. Family history (FHx)

   VI. Social history (SHx)

       A. Lifestyle

       B. Home life

       C. Occupational life

       D. Sexual history

  VII. Review of systems (ROS)

 VIII. Conclusion

an open-ended question, such as "What brings you here today?" "What made you decide to come to the hospital (or clinic)?" "What seems to be the trouble?" or simply "How can I help you?" Letting the patient answer such an opening question without jumping to interrupt with closed-ended questions is an art form you will master in time. The **duration** of the chief complaint provides an important temporal framework for the physician and should be inquired about at this time.

C. **History of the present illness.** The logical continuation and expansion of the chief complaint is the history of the present illness (HPI). The HPI is recounted by the patient to the interviewer, who is predominantly a listener at this point in the interview, and, when appropriate, interjecting questions or phrases that may facilitate the flow of information.

   1. **Symptoms.** The crux of the HPI is a detailed exploration of the symptoms that constitute the chief complaint. Each symptom is subjective by definition and should be investigated thoroughly, first by listening to the patient's unfolding story and then by asking specific questions to discover any dimensions of the symptoms that may have been omitted. The dimensions to be explored are detailed in **Table 5-2.**

   2. **Review of pertinent organ systems.** The chief complaint and HPI usually suggest the involvement of one or more organ systems in the

TABLE 5-2. Symptom analysis

Dimension	Typical question	Synonyms and related ideas
1. Location	Where is the pain located?	Main site, region, radiation
2. Quality	What is it like?	Character
3. Quantity	How intense is it?	Severity, frequency, periodicity, degree of functional impairment
4. Chronology	When did it begin and what course has it followed?	Onset, duration, frequency, periodicity, temporal characteristics
5. Setting	Under what circumstances does the pain take place?	Relation to physiologic functions
6. Aggravating-alleviating factors	What, if anything, makes the pain worse or better?	Provocative-palliative factors
7. Associated manifestations	What other symptoms or phenomena are associated with this pain?	Effects of disease, related concerns

patient's illness. It is useful to inquire about other symptoms that relate to the organ systems involved while discussing the present illness. This implies that inferences about the disease process must be made during the history-taking procedure (probable organ systems involved must be identified). It is also therefore necessary to be familiar with the topics and symptoms related to the various organ systems, in order to review the pertinent systems during the HPI (**Table 5.3**). The purpose of reviewing the pertinent organ systems at this point is to accumulate further support for, or evidence against, diagnoses being considered by the interviewer. For example, if a patient enters with a chief complaint of "spitting blood," the interviewer will inquire about each topic in the respiratory systems review. It then becomes diagnostically useful to note a recent history of tuberculosis (TB) exposure (a pertinent positive) or to discover that the patient does not smoke cigarettes (a pertinent negative).

3. **Concluding the HPI.** To close this part of the interview, you should summarize your understanding of the patient's story and ask him or her if this is accurate. You should end with a question that gives the patient a further chance to air concerns, such as, "Is there anything else about these recent pains that you would like to bring up?"

D. **Past medical history.** The past medical history (PMHx) is devoted to defining and describing medical problems that may be related to the pre-

TABLE 5.3. Review of systems (ROS)

System	Master list	Clinical points
Constitutional	Weight change	Recent change important.
	Anorexia	Acute or chronic?
	Fatigue	
	Weakness	
	Fever	Pattern (intermittent, remittent, sustained, or relapsing)? How documented?
	Sweats	Night? Drenching or mild? Frequency?
	Chills	Goose bumps vs. shaking (rigors)?
	Insomnia	Acute or chronic? When during night?
	Irritability	
Skin	Rashes	Local or generalized? Characterize.
	Itching	Diffuse?
	H/O skin trouble	Occupational? Allergic?
	Sores that do not heal	Squamous cell carcinoma? Poor diet? Drugs (e.g., steroids)?
	Bruising	Recent change?
	Bleeding disorders?	FHx?
Head	Headaches	
	Loss of consciousness	Cardiovascular vs. neurologic? Hx crucial.
	Seizures	Focal vs. general? Motor vs. absence?
	H/O trauma	When? Sequelae?
Eyes	Vision	Recent change? Glasses?
	Date last eye exam	
	FHx of glaucoma	Glaucoma often asymptomatic; hereditary with high penetration.
	Photophobia	Meningeal irritation?
	Pain	
	Redness	
	Irritation	
	Excessive tearing	
	Diplopia	
	Scotomata	
Ears	Hearing	Recent change?
	Discharge or pain	H/O otitis? Trauma?
	Vertigo	Sensation of movement (vertigo) vs. dizziness.
	Tinnitus	Drug-related (aspirin)?

(Continued)

TABLE 5.3. Review of systems (ROS) (Continued)

System	Master list	Clinical points
Respiratory Upper	Frequent colds	
	Sinus trouble	
	Postnasal drip	
	Nosebleeds (epistaxis)	Trauma? Other bleeding problems?
	Obstruction	Snoring history?
Lower	Cough	Chronic? A.M.? Productive? Recent change? Smoking history?
	Sore throat	
	Sputum	Amount? Color? Character? Recent change?
	Shortness of breath	Dyspnea? Rest or exertional? Accompanying chest discomfort?
	Wheezing	Seasonal? Episodic? Known allergens?
	Hemoptysis	Oral (e.g., dental) vs. pulmonary (e.g., bronchitis) vs. cardiac (e.g., mitral stenosis). Frank blood vs. tinged sputum vs. pink sputum?
	H/O chest illness	TB exposure? Bronchitis? Emphysema? Asthma? Pneumonia(s)?
	H/O smoking	Quantitate no. of pack-years. If "no," quit recently?
Lymphatic	Increased node size	Tender vs. painless? Location? Reactive (infections? systemic disease? drug?) vs. infiltrative? How first noticed? Any AIDS risk factors?
Breasts	Swelling	Unilateral or bilateral? Associated changes? Tender?
	Lumps	Recent change? Transient or persistent? Menstrually related?
	Pain	Unilateral or bilateral? Trauma?
	Discharge	Milk (galactorrhea) vs. serous vs. blood? Unilateral or bilateral?
	Do you do self-exam?	Be able to teach during PE.
Cardiovascular	Chest pain or discomfort	Major DDx: cardiovascular vs. gastrointestinal vs. musculoskeletal.
	Palpitations	If ⊕, ask patient to tap out rate and rhythm. Syncope history? Any particular time when increased?
	Blood pressure	Usual range? H/O ↑ or ↓? FHx? Medications?

(Continued)

TABLE 5.3.   Review of systems (ROS) (Continued)

System	Master list	Clinical points
	Shortness of breath	Paroxysmal nocturnal dyspnea? Exercise tolerance? Exertion induced?
	Orthopnea	No. of pillows? If ⊕, what happens when patient reclines without pillows?
	Edema	Generalized (e.g., CHF, liver disease, nephrotic syndrome) or localized?
	Leg pain, cramps	Relieved by rest (intermittent claudication) vs. unremitting or night time (muscular)?
	Other cardiac Hx	H/O murmur(s), thrombophlebitis, "blood clots," varicose veins, "large" heart. Other cardiac medications? Rheumatic fever?
	Risk factors	Smoking, hypertension, hypercholesterolemia, DM, gout, obesity, FHx?
	Nocturia	Quantitate.
Gastrointestinal	Dentures, problems with teeth, oral lesions	Bleeding gums, ulcers, sores.
	Dysphagia	Where? (Have patient point and describe.) Invariably heralds organic disease.
	Heartburn (pyrosis)	How does patient find relief?
	Other symptoms of indigestion	Bloating, belching, flatulence; food-related Hx critical.
	Nausea	Relation to food. H/O GI disease and surgery, associated symptoms and signs.
	Vomiting	All medication, H/O weight loss, psychosocial factors.
	Hematemesis	Color? H/O ulcer disease? H/O gastritis? (Lesion usually proximal to ligament of Treitz.)
	Abdominal pain, discomfort	Hx critical. Acute vs. chronic? GI vs. reproductive?
	Food intolerance	Milk products? Gluten-containing fried or fatty foods? H/O gallbladder disease?
	H/O GI disease	Hepatitis, ulcer disease, gallbladder disease, pancreatitis, diverticulitis, hemorrhoids?

(Continued)

TABLE 5.3. Review of systems (ROS) (Continued)

System	Master list	Clinical points
	Hematochezia	Often suggests distal lesion; hemorrhoids most common, but R/O neoplastic.
	Jaundice	FHx? Viral-drug exposure? Associated Sx and/or signs?
	Change in stool	Color, consistency, unusual odor, oiliness, mucus? Caliber?
	Diarrhea	Acute vs. chronic? Infectious, drug or laxative? Dietary, inflammatory?
	Constipation	Mechanical vs. systemic illness vs. drug-induced vs. neurologic?
Genitourinary		
Urinary	Polyuria	Recent change? (Common causes: DM, renal disease, iatrogenic.)
	Dysuria	UTI "triad" (dysuria, frequency, urgency), but R/O genital disease.
	Hematuria	Painless (primary renal disease) vs. painful (e.g., UTI, stones, renal infarct)?
	Nocturia	How often? Recent change?
	Hesitancy	In older men, along with ↓ stream, dripping, incontinence, consistent with prostatic hypertrophy. Medications?
	Other renal Hx	UTIs? Stones or gravel in urine? Flank pain?
	Testicular swelling	Painful vs. painless?
Menstrual	Menarche	Cycle length, regularity, duration and amount of bleeding.
	Amenorrhea	Primary vs. secondary?
	Menorrhagia (profuse)	
	Metrorrhagia (intermenstrual)	
	Date last period	
	Date last Pap smear	
	Pregnancies	Gravida ___ Para ___ Abortions ___ Miscarriages ___
	Vaginal discharge	H/O vaginal infections? Itching?
Venereal disease	H/O VD	If ⊕, what Rx did patient receive?
	H/O penile discharge	
	H/O chancre	
Sexual history		Must be tailored to patient (see p. 48). AIDS risk?

(Continued)

TABLE 5.3. Review of systems (ROS) (Continued)

System	Master list	Clinical points
Musculoskeletal Joints	Pain	Location? Acute vs. chronic? H/O trauma? H/O previous infection? Present medication? FHx? H/O gout? Morning vs. evening stiffness?
General	Weakness	
	Cramping	
	H/O back difficulties	Low back strain, osteoarthritis, and disc disease are common causes.
	H/O trauma, fracture	
	H/O endocrine disease	
	Diabetic symptoms	Weight change, polyuria, polyphagia, polydipsia.
	Thyroid symptoms	Goiter, heat-cold intolerance, change in metabolic rate.
	Change in head, glove, shoe size	Acromegaly; change in head size only may be consistent with Paget's disease.
Nervous system	Neuro. difficulties in past	H/O stroke, seizures, childhood illness.
Motor	Atrophy	Location, time course, change in normal function.
	Weakness	Location, asymmetries? (Quantitate.)
	Involuntary movements	Tremor, fasciculations, seizure Hx.
Sensory	Anesthesia	Recent burns?
	Paresthesia	
	Hyperesthesia	
Mental status	Cortical function change	Memory change?
	Reading, writing change?	

Note: *At the end of the ROS, it is useful to ask two questions:* (1) "Is there anything else bothering you?" (2) "Is there anything you would like to bring up or ask about before I do a physical exam?"

sent illness, problems that are active but unrelated to it, and problems that existed at one time but are inactive at present. Although some patients may remember and provide much of the information during this part of the interview, portions of the past medical history are often discovered in, and elaborated by, the existing medical record.

1. **Other medical problems** are sought by the interviewer, with a particular effort toward discovering any existing medical problems that may relate to the present illness. For instance, a 10-year history of hyperten-

sion may be of particular interest in a patient who enters complaining of chest pain. This is the point to get the patient to elaborate on any other medical problems that may have been identified during the review of pertinent organ systems.

The interview for other problems should include questions concerning date of onset and any diagnostic procedures and/or major therapies for the problem in question. For each medical problem discovered, it is also important to gain an understanding of the current status of the problem. For the patient with hypertension, for example, it would be important to inquire about how well the hypertension has been controlled since its diagnosis and treatment 10 years before and to ask for the most recent blood pressure measurement.

2. **Injuries, hospitalizations, and surgical operations** are also sought in this portion of the interview. Included is any history of auto or other accidents, broken bones, trauma, or surgery. Information about previous hospital admissions should be sought, and the reason for the admission, the date and year, and the hospital involved should be systematically explored.

3. **Medications.** The name, dosage, and regimen of each drug the patient is using should be discussed. Any drugs that have been recently discontinued or used intermittently should be inquired about as well. Patients frequently need to be reminded about their use of birth control pills, over-the-counter analgesics (aspirin, acetaminophen), laxatives, sleeping medications, diet pills, and herbal products.

4. **Habits.** Tobacco smoking should be quantified (and significant or prolonged exposure to second-hand smoke noted), as should ethanol intake. Also ask about the use of recreational drugs as well as habits that may be relevant physiologically, such as coffee, tea, and other products containing caffeine. See p. 46 for some hints on how best to approach this subject.

5. **Allergies** should be documented carefully, and the patient should be specifically questioned about drug reactions and reactions to prior blood transfusions or hospital procedures. When a patient notes an allergy, it is extremely important to obtain a description of the specific allergic reaction. Is a penicillin allergy manifested with a rash on the upper trunk or with spasm of the larynx and difficulty breathing? Sometimes patients will mistake a minor side effect, such as gastrointestinal irritation, for an allergy and this should be explored so that you only list real, or presumed, allergies.

6. **Major childhood illnesses** such as tuberculosis, rheumatic or scarlet fever, polio, chicken pox, mumps, measles, rubella, and whooping cough should be investigated.

7. **Immunizations** for polio, chicken pox, measles, mumps, rubella, diphtheria, pertussis, tetanus, hepatitis B, *Haemophilus influenzae* type B, smallpox, influenza, pneumococcus and so on are inquired about in the PMHx portion of the patient interview.

E. Family history. The history turns to questions about the family after the patient's medical problems have been explored. This part of the interview has two goals: to find out about the health of immediate family members, and to discover certain common diseases with a familial pattern.

1. The age and health of the patient's parents, siblings, spouse, and children are first discussed. If a family member is deceased, the cause of death is noted.

2. The occurrence of any disease like that described in the patient's HPI is sought in other family members. Important diseases with a strong hereditary component or a tendency for familial clustering are also sought, including atherosclerotic heart disease, diabetes mellitus, high blood pressure, stroke, asthma, allergies, arthritis, anemia, cancer, kidney disease, and mental illness.

F. Social history. Although some of the information sought in this portion of the interview emerges from simply speaking with the patient while taking the history, several goals exist for the social history. Specifically, insights into the patient's lifestyle, home life, occupational life, and attitude toward the disease and the hospitalization or office visit are sought. This is also the portion of the interview in which many physicians choose to take the sexual history.

1. **Lifestyle.** An attempt should be made to understand what constitutes a typical day for the patient, what recreation the patient engages in, and what religious beliefs he or she holds, if any. The patient's school and military experience may be discussed at this point.

2. **Home life.** Housing, the emotional atmosphere at home, marriage and family, and significant others should be briefly explored. An attempt should be made to identify factors that have influenced the relationship between the patient's disease and home life. Such questions may range from concerns about the physical layout of the home to the impact of the disease on the family.

3. **Occupational life.** Two goals exist here. First the nature of the patient's occupation is explored, and second, when relevant, the likelihood of a toxic exposure related to the patient's job is investigated.

   a. **Nature of the occupation** is evaluated through questions about what the patient does for work and by attempting to gain insight into the relative satisfactions and dissatisfactions associated with the work and the workplace.

   b. **Toxic exposures** may be especially relevant in patients with respiratory or dermatologic disease without obvious etiology (e.g., silicosis in a cement plant worker or contact dermatitis on a surgeon's face or hands). Occupational exposures may occasionally be associated with disease of the liver (e.g., hepatitis in a hospital worker), central nervous system (e.g., polyneuropathy in an insecticide worker), and other organ systems. Exposures may also play a role in oncologic illness (mesothelioma in a shipyard worker with brief asbestos exposure, or hematologic malignancy in a worker exposed to radiation).

4. **Sexual history.** The sexual history is one of the hardest parts of the patient interview for most students, but is also one of the most important. It may be taken during the psychosocial history, the genitourinary part of the review of systems, or the past medical history. The goal is to find out about the patient's sexual preferences and habits, sexual history, and any physiologic or psychological concerns he or she might have. The sexual history is particularly important in cases with possible venereal, gynecologic, or psychological problems, but it should be addressed with all your patients.

    a. **Questions to ask** in a matter-of-fact, non-judgmental fashion include: Are you sexually active? Have you engaged in sexual relations with men, women, or both? Is there any history of sexual difficulties or sexually transmitted diseases? Do you engage in any high-risk sexual behavior? What type of birth control, if any, do you use? Do you have any concerns about your sexual functioning? Ask especially about the effect of any chronic diseases (like diabetes) or medications (e.g., antihypertensives) on the patient's sex life.

    b. Section II of this chapter contains further discussion of how to conduct this important and difficult part of the patient interview.

G. **Review of systems.** In this portion of the history interview, all organ systems not already discussed during the HPI are systematically reviewed. The review of systems (ROS) is the **last portion** of the interview, and it serves three purposes: (1) to provide a thorough search for further, as yet undiscovered disease processes, (2) to remind the patient of possible, as yet unmentioned symptoms or difficulties he or she may be experiencing, and (3) to remind the physician in a logical manner of points of inquiry that may have been inadvertently omitted. The ROS purposely contains some redundancy in the interest of thoroughness, and it is a final methodic inquiry prior to the physical examination. **Table 5-3** contains a master list of the topics in the ROS, as well as selected clinical points of emphasis. Performance of the ROS and usage of the ROS table are discussed further in Section II of this chapter.

H. **Conclusion of the history.** After the ROS, the physician concludes the history by offering the patient an opportunity to question or comment further, by asking a question such as, "Is there anything else you would like to discuss before I examine you?"

" $\mathbf{L}$ isten to the patient. He will tell you the diagnosis." This well-known admonition of Dr. Hermann Blumgart to generations of medical students underscores the importance of an empathetic and sensitive history, but the patient will teach the receptive physician more than the simple identity of his illness. Given a prepared and responsive listener, the patient will also reveal for his examiner the most intimate workings of his disease process.

The patient who manifests an unusual feature of his illness, no matter how humdrum the diagnosis, or the patient who presents with an uncommon diagnosis, or the patient with a mystifying illness and no clear diagnosis—any of these may provide the acute observer with new understanding of a previously stubborn and frustrating question. The patient is prepared to teach the professor and student alike; they must be prepared to be his pupils.

Edwin W. Salzman, M.D.

An Associate Professor of Surgery at Harvard Medical School and Visiting Surgeon at Beth Israel Deaconess Medical Center, Boston, Dr. Salzman has served as a Deputy Editor of the New England Journal of Medicine.

II. Practical points concerning the patient interview

A. Introduction: Before the interview

1. **Patient's chart.** The patient's medical record is still known as the *chart* in many institutions, a holdover from the days when all information was recorded on a chart kept at the foot of the bed. Often you will be assigned a patient who has accumulated a substantial chart from previous admissions that includes recent notes concerning the present admission. Should you read the chart before seeing the patient, and if so, how much of it should you read?

   a. In general, it is not a good idea to read the information concerning the **present admission**, especially when first learning how to interview and take a history.

   b. There is nothing wrong with having knowledge of **previous admissions** or problems, provided that the HPI is respected and faithfully taken. The present admission may be for new disease processes; it may also concern new nuances of previous problems. Being forearmed with some knowledge of the patient's prior problems may be an advantage and can prompt further insightful questions during your interview.

   c. The chart that has accumulated during the present admission may be especially useful after you have finished your HPI and physical exam. Use it to compare your understanding of the patient's story, as well as your physical findings, with those of more experienced physicians.

   d. Despite **(a)** above, as you become more comfortable with interviewing and begin to do admissions, you will realize that the chart can be very useful for gaining a rapid introduction to a patient's case. Do not assume that something has been "unfairly provided" —the work-up is not a test. Similarly, realize that your responsibilities as an interviewer and as a caregiver are not lessened by the chart and by another person's input into the patient's care. Always confirm with the patient any information you read in the chart before assuming it is true.

2. **Approaching the patient.** Although the patient in a teaching hospital generally knows that he or she may be seen by a student, you are still obligated to explain your status. This is usually done by introducing yourself and saying, for instance, "Hello, Mr. Jones. I'm Wendy Morgan, the medical student who will be working with Dr. Thomas on your case." Remember, however, that the hospitalized patient is undergoing a threatening and uncomfortable experience and that your visit may be seen as an irrelevant intrusion. If you sense hostility, it may be prudent to have the patient's main doctor introduce you as a member of the team. Adamant refusal to see a medical student is uncommon, and if you encounter it often, it may be time to reevaluate your approach.

3. When first learning to interview, you will occasionally be sent to interview a patient who is **clearly too ill** to be subjected to yet another history and physical examination. At such time it becomes necessary to take the initiative and, after a brief visit with the patient, return to your preceptor, explain the situation, and find a new patient to interview.

4. **Do not introduce yourself as a doctor.** If the patient wishes, he or she may call you "doctor" after you have explained your medical student status, but it is **misleading and legally unwise** to introduce yourself as a physician. Patients will respect you for being a medical student; the discomfort students feel when explaining this is a part of the natural insecurity involved with learning to be on the wards. It will not be uncommon for other physicians to introduce you as a doctor; in general, that moment is not the time to redefine your position. However, you may explain to the patient at a later time that you are, in fact, a medical student.

5. **Greeting the patient.** When you first enter the room and greet the patient, begin with an introduction of yourself, followed by a brief conversation that is not medical but is rather an exchange of pleasantries, an attempt to find out how the patient is feeling in general without yet pursuing the specific. The point here is to help both you and the patient feel a bit more at ease before you begin with the introductory information and your questions about the chief complaint. If there are family members present, introduce yourself to them and get their contact information (this may not always be recorded elsewhere) in case you need to contact them later for questions or to notify them of the patient's progress. Politely ask family members to wait elsewhere as you proceed with your history and physical exam.

6. Always call a patient by the proper title and his or her last name (e.g., Mr. Jones or Ms. Jones), unless they tell you to do otherwise.

7. It is your responsibility to ensure a good setting for the interview.

Though this is difficult in a crowded, busy hospital, try to find a quiet, private place in which to talk to your patient. (This may require asking visitors to leave, or moving to a location other than the patient's room, if that is possible.) Always sit down when interviewing a patient, and make sure that you are both comfortable.

8. In the course of your clerkships you will inevitably have to interview some patients who do not speak English. The best solution to this problem is to get an official translator, usually available at every hospital for most common foreign languages, who will translate everything that is being said. It is better not to depend on fragmentary conversations and broken English, and one should be careful about having family members translate, as they may change the meaning of what the patient said.

9. It is a good idea to take a clipboard and scratch paper into the interview so that you can jot down brief notes during the HPI, record information that will be difficult to remember, and note points to which you wish to return. You will find such notes especially useful when inquiring about the past medical history, the family history, medications and habits, and the review of systems. In the beginning, you will find yourself writing down much of what is said, but try to devote yourself more to the patient than to the notes. When discussing particularly sensitive or emotional topics, it is best to put your clipboard down and simply listen.

B. Chief complaint and its duration

1. Many clinicians recommend using the **patient's own words** to describe the chief complaint (CC) in the write-up. This is the time to record just what is said in response to your questions about why the patient has come to the hospital.

2. **The chief complaint may not be immediately obvious**, since patients will not uncommonly complain of several things. Listen for a minute and try to pinpoint or determine the main problem that caused the patient to seek medical attention. **Taking a stance** is central to developing clinical skill. Therefore, choose a chief complaint and record other complaints to be placed after the HPI in your own write-up (see Chap. 16). Drawing conclusions that prove to be erroneous and emphasizing inappropriate data are expected consequences of learning to organize a case, and thoughtful mistakes will be respected.

3. Realize that the chief complaint may be very different from what you subsequently consider to be the patient's **most serious problem**. When a patient with a history of leukemia enters with a mouth ulcer, you may be more concerned about a possible relapse, while the chief complaint remains "my mouth is very sore."

C. History of present illness

1. As a student, your primary goal in taking the HPI should be to get the patient to relate for you a clear **sequence of events** that led the patient to seek medical attention. This information should be both **specific** and **quantitative** ("I felt pain all across my chest and down my left arm"; "I can only walk half a block before I get short of breath"). To obtain this sort of HPI, you will have to use a combination of careful listening and skillful, goal-oriented questioning.

2. At first, when the interviewing process seems overwhelming, and later, when time is precious, it is easy to be too tired or harried to **listen well**. We cannot overemphasize that respect for and attention to the patient's story are central to any thoughtful work-up. Failure to listen to the patient's story and then to react with refining questions is perhaps the most common difficulty for the beginning clinician. Do not allow the history to drown in the flood of concerns about further diagnostic steps (physical exam, lab work) that it rightfully sets in motion.

   Let the patient do as much explaining as possible without interrupting. Interject to clarify and prompt, but avoid leading questions. **Give your patient several uninterrupted minutes** before you delve into a dissection of the symptoms or attempt to order the events.

   Also, be wary of patient's use of medical jargon; ask about symptoms, not about diagnostic phrases that may be offered by the patient. A patient complaining of what he thought was a "peptic ulcer" some time ago may, in fact, have had a small heart attack.

3. There are specific **techniques in interviewing** that will help you encourage and maintain the flow of information. Basically, the interviewer can follow the patient's own lead by using these techniques, which include facilitation, echoing, reflection, clarification, validation, reassurance, responding with empathy, summarization, interpretation, and, occasionally, confrontation. We recommend the discussion on "Techniques of Skilled Interviewing" in *Bates' Guide to Physical Examination and History Taking* (also published by Lippincott Williams & Wilkins).

4. In your mind, try to **organize the evolving story around calendar days and clock times**. Realize that your first clue in this regard is the duration of the chief complaint. The history (and its subsequent write-up) is built on a chronological foundation. If you are clear about the course of the patient's problems, two things result. First, the case will be logically organized for yourself and later for your readers or listeners. Second, you will have further insight into the tempo of the disease, one of the cornerstones of diagnosis.

   In the timeline you use to describe the sequence of events surrounding the chief complaint or HPI, it is prudent to avoid descriptions of time that will not be easy to interpret days or weeks later ("The patient states that his pain began last Friday") and instead **use descriptions of time that will always be easy to understand** in relation to the initial presentation ("The patient states that his pain began eight days prior to admission.").

5. **Symptom analysis** is explained in detail in Section I of this chapter. The scheme for symptom analysis in **Table 5-2** is thorough and worth learning, and a helpful mnemonic (created for the attributes of the symptom "pain") is presented in *DeGowin's Diagnostic Examination*. The mnemonic is **PQRST**:

   Provocative-palliative factors
   Quality of the pain
   Region/Radiation of the pain
   Severity of the pain
   Temporal characteristics

6. Do not be afraid to **re-question** the patient about points that are unclear or that seem crucial to your understanding of the case. People forget to mention things and may be reminded of them the second time, or they may have dismissed what seemed unimportant to them. Generally, the first time you ask a question you will take an open-ended stance ("Did you have any blood in your urine?"), the second time you can be more direct ("And you have seen blood in your urine only once?").

7. It is useful to stop and **summarize** your understanding of the details the patient has recounted at select points during the interview and especially as you conclude the HPI and get ready to begin the past medical history. Say something such as, "Let me see if I have this straight," then pause and summarize aloud the patient's HPI, as you understand it. This will encourage you to construct the story in a concise, uncluttered form, and it allows the patient to edit out errors and supplement areas of omission. Once you become good at the summarizing process, the write-up of the HPI will be a lot easier.

8. At some point during the interview you should ask directly **what the patient thinks is wrong** and what features of the symptoms are causing the most worry. If the patient's fears are not addressed, the patient will undoubtedly leave the interview with some measure of anxiety. In addition, you may gain a new insight into the nature of the problem.

D. Past medical history

1. The best way to **begin the past medical history** (PMHx) is to ask a question such as, "Now, have you had any other medical problems or illnesses besides what we just discussed?" Often patients, especially older ones, will have trouble recalling their earlier medical history and will forget to mention illnesses that are chronic and treated, such as diabetes. It may help to prompt them with questions about prior admissions, but it will often be necessary to refer to the old chart. Turn to the PMHx section of the discharge summary from the previous admission, which provides a good place to begin constructing a list of other medical problems.

2. Although other medical problems may have been brought up during the discussion of the present illness, **specific discussion of each problem** identified takes place at this point. Make a quick note of various diagnoses or problems poorly remembered by the patient, and consult the chart later for further details.

3. Patients commonly deny any **allergies**, but there are instances when more specific questions are important. For instance, if you think antibiotics may be important in a patient's management, you might ask, "Have you ever taken penicillin before?" Because penicillin and penicillin derivatives are extremely useful and allergic reactions are their biggest disadvantage, a specific inquiry is merited. Similarly, patients admitted for cardiac catheterization should be asked about past allergic reactions to shellfish. It is also important to distinguish between drug allergies and allergies to environmental factors. You need to make it clear whether you are asking about allergies to drugs or allergic triggers (e.g., ragweed, pollen, dust mite) of asthma.

4. **Childhood illnesses** may be revealed with a general question such as, "Were you ever seriously ill as a child?" If the patient gives a positive response, it is important to determine how the diagnosis was made, how long the problem lasted, and whether there were any sequelae. Patients who claim to have had rheumatic fever, for instance, should be asked whether they have had a rash (erythema marginatum), painful joints, uncontrolled movements especially of their hands (Sydenham's chorea, or St. Vitus' dance), or any evidence of heart difficulties since that time.

5. In gathering information about previous hospitalizations, a question that seeks a specific history of prior surgery often will jog the patient's memory.

6. As the patient lists medication out loud, jot down each entry on a note pad in three columns. For example:

Drug name	Dose	Regimen
Propranolol	40 mg	bid

   a. If a patient cannot remember the name of a medicine, ask for a description of the medicine and the reason for its use; you can later describe it to a more experienced clinician, who may be able to identify the drug. Also, you can ask patients if they have brought along their pill bottles, on which you will find the information you seek.

   b. **Appendix C** contains a list of common drugs and their actions, which may be helpful in this part of the interview, and the **inside covers** of this manual list some common abbreviations found on medication labels.

7. While it is important to quantitate your patient's **alcohol intake**, realize that many patients may underestimate this number. A more sensitive set of screening questions for problems with alcohol is called the *CAGE* questions:

   "Have you ever felt the need to **C**ut down on your drinking?"
   "Have you ever felt **A**nnoyed by criticism of your drinking?"
   "Have you ever had **G**uilty feelings about drinking?"
   "Have you ever taken a morning **E**ye-opener?"

   One positive answer to these questions should lead to further inquiry about problem drinking, and two should be considered good evidence for a diagnosis of alcohol abuse or dependence. CAGE questions are considered more accurate in men than in women, who may express guilt about drinking even if they don't abuse alcohol.

8. Quantitate **cigarette** smoking in pack-years (1 pack-year equals 1 pack per day for 1 year). For example, a patient who smoked 2 packs per day for 3 years but cut back to 1 pack every other day for the past 2 years has a 7 pack-year history.

E. **Family history.** Record the information given about the patient's family by constructing a quick, simple **pedigree diagram.** Males are represented with squares, females with circles. Living relatives' ages are recorded within the circles or squares, and deceased relatives' circles or squares have slashes drawn through them. Specific diseases are noted next to the appropriate symbol for the relative with the history of that disease. The patient is included on the diagram and identified with an arrow. For examples, see the family history (FHx) portion of the sample write-up in Chap. 16.

F. **Social history**

1. The social history is perhaps the most variable portion of the medical history. It is the section of the interview that focuses on the patient's lifestyle, home life, work, and anxieties, in an effort to develop a more complete idea of the patient as a person. Because you may have gained some of the information in a less formal manner during the course of your conversation, the time required for the psychosocial history varies. **The key insights are those that relate to the ways in which the patient's daily life may interact with his or her disease and treatment, both physiologically and psychologically**. A sedentary 70-year-old man with occasional back pain when bending will have very different therapeutic needs from those of an active 40-year-old with similar pain.

2. As in other portions of the history, asking general, open-ended questions is a good way to initiate a discussion. For example, "How do you spend a typical day?" or "Tell me about your life at home" may be a useful starting point. In asking about occupation, both general questions ("What sort of work have you done in your life?") and directed questions ("Have you ever worked in a place where you were exposed to fumes or chemicals?") may be appropriate.

3. In beginning the **sexual history**, the ease with which the patient is able to discuss his or her private life will be related to your own ease in discussing and asking questions about sexual matters. It is important to not make any assumptions in asking questions. Do not assume people are attracted to others of the opposite gender, or that they have a traditional family structure. Questions like "Who are the important people in your life?" are better opening questions than "Tell me about your wife." Also, do not assume that just because someone is elderly he or she is no longer sexually active. Nor should you assume that because a patient has never married that they do not have children.

   In asking about people's sexual lives, it is crucial to pay attention to both verbal and nonverbal responses. Generally you will be able to sense whether or not people have more to say on the subject; if they do, you can facilitate the discussion by being receptive and understanding. On the other hand, a patient who is comfortable with his or her sexual life will usually make that fact clear. It is well worth reading a more thorough discussion concerning the sexual history, such as that found in *Bates'*.

G. **Review of symptoms**

1. Conduct this portion of the history **quickly and efficiently**. Explain to patients that you must ask a long series of questions, but that they may simply answer "no" after each question that does not apply to them. Some people like to conduct this review of systems as they are doing each part of the physical exam.

2. **Avoid unnecessary repetition.** Although some redundancy will occur, as explained earlier, it is not necessary to review the organ system(s)

you covered during the HPI interview unless there is a particular point you want to clarify.

3. **Recent changes** are the most important points to glean from the ROS. Has the patient's exercise tolerance decreased recently, or has climbing stairs fatigued her for several years? Did the patient begin to have night sweats this year, or has he always had them in the summertime? Patients may bring up several issues in one or more organ systems. It takes experience to know which complaints are more significant, but those that have not appeared or changed recently will usually assume a lower place on your list of priorities as you organize the case.

4. If a patient points to a lesion during the ROS, state that you will return to it while doing the physical exam, and continue your questioning.

H. Concluding the history. The patient is offered a chance to ask questions at the end of the history. Realize that you can always return to history questions later, during the physical exam or on a subsequent visit. The sequence explained in this chapter is designed to help retrieve most of the important data necessary for considering the case. The next step in that framework is the physical examination.

REFERENCES

Avicenna. *The Canon of Medicine*. Adapted by L. Bakhtiar. Chicago: Kazi Publications, 1999, p. 11.

Bickley LS, Szilagyi PG. *Bates' Guide to Physical Examination and History Taking*. 8th ed. Philadelphia: Lippincott Williams & Wilkins, 2003.

Braunwald E, Fauci AS, Kasper DL, et al. *Harrison's Principles of Internal Medicine*. 15th ed. New York: McGraw-Hill, 2001.

DeGowin RL, Brown DD. *DeGowin's Diagnostic Examination*. 7th ed. New York: McGraw-Hill, 1999.

Maugham WS. In *On Doctoring: Stories, Poems, Essays*. Reynolds R and Stone J, eds. 3rd ed. New York: Simon and Schuster, 2001, pp. 45–50.

Mayfield D, McLeod G, Hall P. The CAGE Questionnaire: Validation of a new alcoholism screening instrument. *Am J Psychiatry* 1974;131:1121–1123.

CHAPTER **6**

The Physical Exam: An Overview

> The advice I would give to young clinicians is the advice I was lucky enough to receive from a wonderful doctor and poet, William Carlos Williams. I accompanied him on his "house rounds" in the industrial cities of northern New Jersey, and he kept saying this to me: "Watch and listen and let these men and women and children, these patients, teach you, and they will (boy will they!)"
>
> Old Doc Williams he was called, and never did he fail to heed his own advice. He would say, "What's the matter?" Something in his face, his manner, his very soul, indicated that he meant the question. He got his answers—and did his best, thereafter, to earn the trust and confidence given him. "Technique is part of the game," he once told me, "but heart is what really matters." Yes, indeed.
>
> *Robert Coles, M.D.*
>
> *A child psychiatrist and author of more than 50 books, Dr. Coles received the Pulitzer Prize for his* Children of Crisis *series. A graduate of Harvard College and Columbia University College of Physicians and Surgeons, he has been recognized by* Time *magazine as the "most influential living psychiatrist in the United States."*

The best physical exams are quick, thorough, and follow a logical sequence that maximizes both efficiency and the patient's comfort. A **minimum number of position changes** during the physical exam, especially when examining sick individuals, is highly desirable. The purpose of this chapter is to lay out the physical exam in broad strokes so that a formalized structure can be developed and used in the future. The hope is that by internalizing this broad schematic of the physical exam, through repetition your physical exam will begin to flow smoothly.

Before the specific details concerning the examination of a particular organ system are learned, it is an absolute imperative that the examiner know **when each organ system is examined** over the course of the physical exam and **what the appropriate patient position is** for examining that organ system. A useful analogy here would be to think of the physical exam as a tree. The trunk and largest branches are the information in this chapter. In Chapter 7, a detailed account of the physical exam, we will add the leaves that cover the tree. Remember: **Make your tree, then add the leaves.**

I. **Exam sequence: head to toe**

   A. **Patient position 1.** Patient is sitting on the edge of the examining table, stretcher, or bed, and you stand in front of the patient, moving to either side as needed. **Exam segments:**

1. **General inspection**
2. **Vital signs**
3. **Skin**
4. **HEENT** (head, eyes, ears, nose, and throat) and **neck**, including cervical nodes and cranial nerves
5. **Breast exam** (inspection with patient's hands on hips and over head), with examination of axillary and epitrochlear nodes. Because of the need for a female chaperone (typically a busy nurse) to be present during the breast exam, this portion is sometimes fully completed later in, or at the completion of, the full exam depending on the timing of the chaperone's availability.

B. **Patient position 2.** Move behind the sitting patient. **Exam segments:**

1. **Thyroid gland**
2. **Posterior thorax** and **posterior lung fields**
3. **Back**

C. **Patient position 3.** Patient is supine; you should stand on the patient's right side. **Exam segments:**

1. Continue **breast exam** (palpation)
2. **Anterior thorax** and **anterior lung fields**
3. **Cardiovascular system** (jugular venous pressure [JVP], heart, radial, and brachial pulses)
4. **Abdomen**, and palpate inguinal nodes and femoral pulse
5. **Musculoskeletal system**, and palpate dorsalis pedis, posterior tibial, and popliteal pulses

D. **Patient position 4.** Patient is standing; you should sit in a chair or stool. **Exam segments:**

1. Continue **musculoskeletal system** exam; examine alignment of back, legs, knees, and feet
2. **Rectal exam** for men
3. **Genital exam** for men
4. Screening **neurological exam** (gait, Romberg's test)

E. **Patient position 5.** Patient is sitting. **Exam segments:** Continue **neurological exam** (sensory, motor, cerebellar, and deep tendon reflex [DTR] exams).

F. **Patient position 6.** Lithotomy position. **Exam segments: Pelvic** and **rectal exams** for women.

II. **Summary**
   Patient position 1 and 2: **sitting**
   Patient position 3: **supine**
   Patient position 4: **standing**
   Patient position 5: **sitting**
   Patient position 6: **lithotomy**
   (Remember: head to toe)

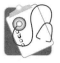

CHAPTER **7**

Annotated Physical Exam

In taking a history from a patient in the hospital, always sit down in a chair at the bedside. Taking the history standing up gives the patient the impression that you are in a hurry. It takes no more time and the patient is more at ease if you sit while taking the history.

Eugene Braunwald, M.D., MACP

Author of more than 1,000 publications, and Editor-in-Chief of Harrison's Principles of Internal Medicine *(15th ed.), Dr. Braunwald graduated from New York University School of Medicine and completed his internal medicine residency at the Johns Hopkins Hospital. From 1972 to 1996 he was the Chairman of the Department of Medicine at the Brigham and Women's Hospital, Boston. He is currently the Distinguished Hersey Professor of Medicine at Harvard Medical School and Vice President for Academic Programs for the Partners Healthcare Systems, Boston.*

The physical examination follows and complements the history in the sequence of the patient work-up. Chap. 6 described the general **head-to-toe** flow of the exam and discussed how to conduct the exam with the minimum of inconvenience. In this chapter we will more fully discuss each part of the exam, what to look for, and how to address some common problems faced by students new to the wards.

Section I of this chapter is an outline of the physical examination arranged by organ system, presented telegraphically for bedside use. It parallels the order in which the exam is usually presented in both written and oral form, and it contains comments on exam procedure and on positive and normal findings. Its goal is not to explain how to do the exam, which is carefully detailed in the recommended physical diagnosis textbooks (see **Appendix F**), but rather to answer some questions and address some concerns that frequently emerge during the specific exam sequence. Section II of this chapter contains some practical advice concerning the physical exam for the student who is inexperienced in physical diagnosis. It gives hints both on the general conducting of the exam, as well as on particularly difficult sections of it.

I. Annotated outline of the physical exam

   A. General exam

      1. Appearance

         a. State of **health and nourishment**

         b. Obvious **distress or affect (mood) problems**

         c. Apparent **age and vigor**

         d. Grooming and expression

         e. Hair distribution

         f. State of consciousness

    g. Note speech patterns, lethargy, stupor, coma, intoxication, or anything else that will affect interpretation of the rest of the physical examination.

  2. Vital signs and measurement

    a. Respiratory rate and character. Note any respiratory patterns while taking the pulse. Do not announce your intention to "count breaths," which may increase the patient's anxiety and alter the normal breathing pattern.

    b. Oral or rectal temperature. Fever means infection until proved otherwise. Normal oral temperature fluctuates diurnally between 35.8°C (96.4°F) and 37.3°C (99.1°F).

    c. Pulse strength, rate, and rhythm. Taking the radial pulse is an unthreatening way to initiate physical contact. Note if irregularities are regularly irregular or irregularly irregular. Do beats drop occasionally? Sporadically? Note if the pulse is strong or weak. Compare to apical pulse during the cardiac exam.

    d. Blood pressure. Hypertension is defined as > 140 mm Hg systolic and/or > 90 mm Hg diastolic. In patients with possible or known asthma, pericardial effusion or tamponade, or emphysema, check for pulsus paradoxus (an inspiratory fall in systolic arterial pressure that exceeds 10 mm Hg). In patients with suspected hypotension, check pressure sitting or lying down as well as standing. If the initial reading is elevated, check pressure in the other arm, and recheck at some later point in the exam.

    e. Height and weight. Weight is useful for following nutritional status and fluid balance. The most widely used method to gauge obesity is the **body mass index** (BMI), measured as the weight/height^2 (in kg/m^2). A BMI of 30 is most commonly used as a threshold for obesity in both men and women.

  3. Hands. Note temperature, color, appearance, nails, clubbing, nodes, contractures, and any degenerative changes.

    a. Compare general **palm color** to your own, especially if considering anemia. Try to describe any **degenerative changes** seen. Note which **interphalangeal joints** are involved and which are spared. Note location of any **nodules, swelling, or contractures**; presence or absence of **tenderness**; and **degree of motion** remaining in the affected digits.

    b. Examine and describe for yourself changes in the nails, especially clubbing, deformities, or discolorations. **Clubbed nails** are consistent with (c/w) numerous pulmonary, cardiovascular, and other diseases. **Spoon nails** (koilonychias) are c/w iron deficiency or hypochromic anemias. **Mees' lines** are c/w renal insufficiency, MI, infectious fevers, and poisonings, among other conditions.

  4. Integument. Note skin color, temperature, turgor, moisture, and any lesions.

    a. Skin color. If suspicious of cyanosis, check for blue especially around the mouth, nails, and lips. Look for the yellow of jaundice especially in the sclera. Decreased **skin turgor**, best examined over the sternum or forehead, is c/w dehydration and old age.

b. Skin lesions. Note type (**Fig. 7-1**), shape (round, irregular), arrangement with respect to each other (discrete, clusters), and distribution on body (legs, trunk, face). Note especially lesions with irregular borders, heterogeneity of colors, and inflammatory regions. The majority of skin malignancies do not cause pruritus or pain. If a suspicious lesion is found, ask the patient: How long has it been present? Has it changed? Does it seem not to heal? (See also color-plates.)

The skin exam may be continued throughout the physical exam. Draw quick diagrams on your clipboard and qauntitate size and distribution when possible.

B. HEENT

1. Head

a. Skull shape, scalp, hair distribution, lesions

b. Characteristic facies, including the edematous, myxedematous, cushingoid, acromegalic, and parkinsonian

2. Ears

a. External ear exam; check for any discharge, or pain on movement.

b. Otoscopic look at the auditory canal, tympanic membranes; check for a light reflex and for fluid behind the eardrum.

c. Hearing (you can use whispered numbers, a tuning fork, or rub fingers); perform ancillary tests, if indicated:

(1) Test for lateralization (**Weber test**) by placing the base of a lightly vibrating tuning fork firmly on the top of the patient's head or on the midforehead. Ask where the patient hears it: on

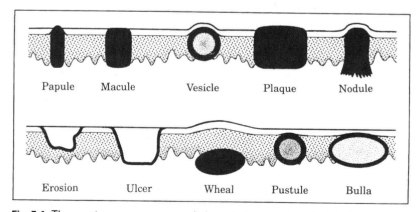

Fig. 7-1. The most common structural changes in the skin. (Modified from Judge RD. Zuidema GD, Fitzgerald FT. *Clinical Diagnosis*, 5th ed. Boston: Little, Brown, 1989.)

one or both sides. Normally the sound is heard in the midline or equally in both ears.

   (a) In **unilateral conductive hearing loss**, sound is heard better in the impaired ear. Causes include otitis media, perforated tympanic membrane, and an ear canal obstructed by cerumen.

   (b) In **unilateral sensorineural hearing loss**, sound is heard in the good ear.

(2) Test air conduction versus bone conduction (**Rinne test**). Place the base of a lightly vibrating tuning fork on the mastoid bone, behind the ear and level with the auditory canal. When the patient no longer hears the sound, quickly place the tuning fork close to the ear canal and determine whether the patient hears the sound again. Normally, sound is heard longer through air than through bone.

   (a) In **conductive hearing loss**, sound is heard through bone as long as or longer than it is through air.

   (b) In **sensorineural hearing loss**, sound is heard longer through air. (See discussion in *Bates'*, pp. 196–197.)

3. **Eyes**

   a. **Eyelids, conjunctivae, and sclera.** Look for xanthelasma (suggests hypercholesterolemia), unequal palpebral fissures (clue to ptosis), scleral yellowing (implies jaundice), redness of eyes, discharge, congestion of lacrimal glands.

   b. **Visual acuity.** Measure with and without glasses. You can use a pocket **Snellen's or Rosenbaum's chart** or, if one is not handy, ask the patient to read an excerpt from any printed matter for gross visual testing.

   c. **Pupils.** Check size, symmetry, direct and consensual papillary reaction to light, and accommodation. **Anticholinergics** cause dilated pupils. Opiate intoxication causes pinpoint pupils. **Argyll-Robertson** pupil (reacts to accommodation but not to light) is c/w syphilis, diabetes, or central nervous system (CNS) disease.

   d. **Extraocular movements.** See **Figure 7-2** for muscles and nerves associated with each direction. Check for **nystagmus**; remember, a few beats of nystagmus on horizontal gaze is within normal limits.

   e. **Visual fields.** Use the confrontation technique with the tip of a pen, looking for gross field deficits.

   f. **Ophthalmoscopic exam of fundi.** Note opacities of the lens and fundoscopic abnormalities (arteriovenous nicking, hemorrhages, exudates, arteriolar narrowing); check for papilledema. The fundoscopic exam is especially important in diseases with microvascular sequelae, such as hypertension and diabetes mellitus (DM). See hints on this exam, p. 72.

4. **Nose**

   a. Note **septal position, nasal discharge, sinus tenderness, turbinate exam**, and **airway patency.**

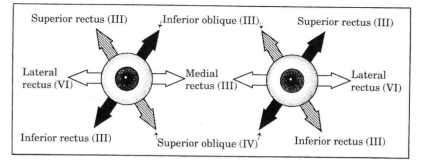

Fig. 7.2. Extraocular movements and their controlling nerves. Cranial nerves noted in parentheses. (Modified from Judge RD. Zuidema GD, Fitzgerald FT. *Clinical Diagnosis*, 5th ed. Boston: Little, Brown, 1989.)

 b. Sinusitis may be brought out by having the patient flex his or her neck and lower the head and tapping over the ethmoid, maxillary, and frontal sinuses. If it is suspected, ask the patient whether sinus difficulties have been a problem. **Transillumination** of sinuses using a pen light, or otoscope without a disposable earpiece attached, should be performed to test for sinus opacification if tapping the sinuses elicits tenderness.

 c. The most common cause of **epistaxis** is nose picking.

5. Mouth and throat

 a. Lip conditions, cheilosis, gum and mucous membrane condition. Check for **mucosal lesions** (petechiae, aphthous ulcers, and areas of induration). **Gingival hypertrophy** is c/w puberty, pregnancy, dilantin therapy, leukemia, and gingivitis. Note any **bleeding of gums**.

 b. Tongue color and condition. An abnormally smooth, red tongue is c/w vitamin B_{12} or iron deficiency (atrophic glossitis).

 c. Dentition. Note the state of the teeth and whether any are missing.

 d. Oropharynx. Note especially any unusual breath odor, hoarseness, lesions, and excessive salivation (ptyalism) or redness (injection).

C. Neck and axilla

 1. Lymphadenopathy. Characterize cervical and axillary adenopathy: note number, location, size, tenderness or lack of tenderness, texture (rubbery versus soft), and mobility. Recall that some "shotty" adenopathy is common, especially in the inguinal area and in children. Remember to check supraclavicular nodes (a Virchow's node can indicate thoracic malignancy).

 2. Trachea position. Tracheal deviation may suggest a mass effect, pneumothorax, loss of lung volume, or fibrotic change.

 3. Thyroid. Note thyroid size, mobility, and symmetry. It is often easier to see and feel the thyroid when the patient swallows (provide a cup of water). The thyroid may be palpated either from in front of or even when standing behind the patient, though most clinicians palpate it from behind.

4. **Carotids**. Listen for bruits and palpate pulses for thrills. Be careful when palpating older patients, and only check one carotid artery at a time.

D. **Back**

1. **Spinal column curvature and tenderness**. Forward flexion of the trunk may make scoliosis and kyphosis more obvious. **Appendix H** contains an abbreviated osteopathic musculoskeletal examination.

2. **Costovertebral angle (CVA) tenderness**. Extreme CVA tenderness is c/w acute kidney disease. Minor CVA tenderness is c/w low back pain of any etiology.

E. **Respiratory exam**

1. **Inspection**

   a. **Symmetry and shape of chest** (note how it moves with inspiration).

   b. **Respiratory pattern**. Note rate, rhythm, regularity, and depth. Normal rate is 12–18 cycles/min for adults; it may be 25–40 cycles/min in infants. Resting shallow tachypnea is c/w restrictive lung disease. Hyperpnea (or tachypnea) is commonly c/w anxiety or exertion. Rapid, deep **Kussmaul** breathing is seen in metabolic acidosis. Decreased respiratory rate is c/w a CNS respiratory depression. **Cheyne-Stokes** breathing (alternating hyperpnea and apnea) is c/w normal sleep, congestive heart failure, uremia, and CNS dysfunction.

2. **Palpation of thoracic wall.** Note by inspection and palpation the presence or absence of symmetry and excursion of the thoracic wall. In trauma patients check for pneumothorax, tension pneumothorax, hemothorax, flail chest (paradoxical inward buckling of chest during inspiration).

3. **Percussion**

   a. **Diaphragmatic descent**. Normal descent is approximately 3–6 cm with full inspiration. Compare both sides and note any gross asymmetries in movement.

   b. **Resonance**. Compare percussion notes of right and left lung fields. Dullness is often caused by pleural thickening or consolidation. Palpate for tactile fremitus if consolidation is suspected.

4. **Auscultation**

   a. **Posterior chest**. Compare the corresponding sites in right and left lung fields. Check for presence of breath sounds at both bases and for adventitious sounds (crackles, wheezes, rhonchi, or rubs). Listen for egophony ("E to A" changes), bronchophony ("99" sounds louder), and whispered pectoriloquy (a whispered "99" sounds louder) if consolidation is suspected.

   Airway deflation and pulmonary consolidation often lead to egophony, crackles, and/or increased fremitus. Bronchitis and asthma often cause crackles, wheezes, and an increased expiratory-inspiratory ratio.

   b. **Anterior chest**. Always check apices of lungs; some diseases have primarily apical findings (e.g., TB). If you are suspicious of an apical abnormality, you will need to consider obtaining a chest x-ray with an **apical lordotic** view.

F. Breast exam

1. **Inspection**. Have the patient perform several maneuvers: arms at the side, over her head, pressed against her hips. Dimpling, contour asymmetry, venous prominence, redness, and nipple retraction or discharge may all be c/w breast cancer.

2. **Palpation**. Use a systematic manner of palpating. Note tenderness, nodularity, or nipple discharge. Nodules may be c/w fibrocystic breast disease, benign fibroadenomas, or carcinoma. Malignant lesions are typically firm, irregular, and neither well encapsulated nor mobile. Superficial signs of breast tissue retraction may be present. Draw diagrams indicating findings and specifying position with respect to the nipple.

G. Cardiovascular exam

1. **Inspection**

    a. **Jugular venous pulsation (JVP) level**. Often best performed when the patient's upper body is elevated with pillows to a 30-degree angle **(Fig. 7-3)**. The normal JVP meniscus, measured at this angle, can be seen one-third to one-half of the way up the neck. Increased JVP is c/w elevated right-side pressures (consider elevated pul-

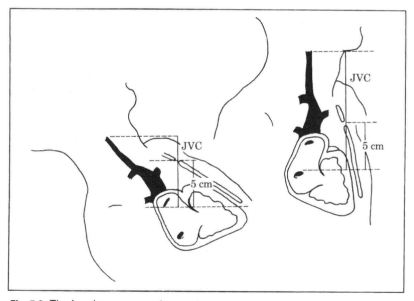

Fig. 7.3. The jugular venous pulse can be used as a manometer to measure right atrial pressure. Since the distance from the right atrium to the sternal angle is 5 cm, regardless of the patient's position (see above), right atrial pressure can be estimated by measuring the distance in centimeters from the sternal angle to the top of the jugular venous column (JVC). Then, right atrial pressure = 5 cm + JVC (cm). (Modified from R. Judge and G. Zuidema, *Methods of Clinical Examination: A Physiologic Approach*, 3rd ed. Boston: Little, Brown, 1974.)

monary pressures, right ventricular failure, pericardial tamponade or constriction, or tricuspid valve disease).

b. **Point of maximal impulse/intensity (PMI), or apex/apical beat.** Search for the apex beat visually before palpating. It is normally located at the 5th intercostal space along the mid-clavicular line.

2. **Palpation**

   a. **Apex/apical beat (PMI).** Note the position and character of the apex beat. An enlarged, prolonged, or displaced apex beat may indicate right or left ventricular hypertrophy or dilatation.

   b. Note any other impulses or palpable thrills, and whether they occur in systole or diastole.

3. **Auscultation**

   a. **Heart sounds**

      (1) The **first sound (S$_1$)** is created by closure of the mitral and tricuspid valves.

      (2) The **second sound (S$_2$)** is created by the closure of the aortic and pulmonic valves. Note splitting of the sound, heard best at the left sternal border (third intercostal space).

      Normally, S$_2$ splits **(physiologic splitting)** during inspiration, as increased venous return slows closing of the pulmonic valve. **Fixed splitting** occurs with any condition that delays closure of the pulmonic valve, like pulmonary stenosis, atrial septal defect (ASD), or right bundle branch block (RBBB). **Paradoxical splitting** (split disappears on inspiration) occurs with delayed closure of the aortic valve, as with aortic stenosis (AS), left ventricular (LV) myopathy, and left bundle branch block (LBBB). **See Fig. 7-4.**

      (3) The **third sound (S$_3$)** is a low-pitched sound in early to mid-diastole, heard best at the apex using the bell of the stethoscope, with the patient in a left lateral decubitus position. The S$_3$ is generated by the sudden termination of excessively rapid filling of the left ventricle, usually in the dilated heart. While an S$_3$ may be heard in children and adolescents with normal hearts, in mature patients it is considered pathologic and can indicate ventricular failure, MI, or valvular heart disease. When S$_1$, S$_2$, and S$_3$ are heard in sequence, the sound has a cadence like the syllables of the word "Ken-tuc-ky," in which the final "ky" represents S$_3$. A pathologic S$_3$ is frequently called a **ventricular gallop.**

      (4) The **fourth sound (S$_4$)** is a low-pitched sound in late diastole, also heard best with the bell at the apex, with the patient in the left lateral decubitus position. S$_4$ is generated by decreased ventricular compliance and the atrial systole, which ejects an atrial jet of blood against the stiff ventricle and thus generates a sound. An S$_4$ implies myocardial disease. When S$_4$, S$_1$, and S$_2$ are heard in sequence, the sound has a cadence like the syllables of "Ten-nes-see," with S$_4$ represented by the initial "Ten." A pathologic S$_4$ heard in the setting of tachycardia is commonly called an **atrial gallop.**

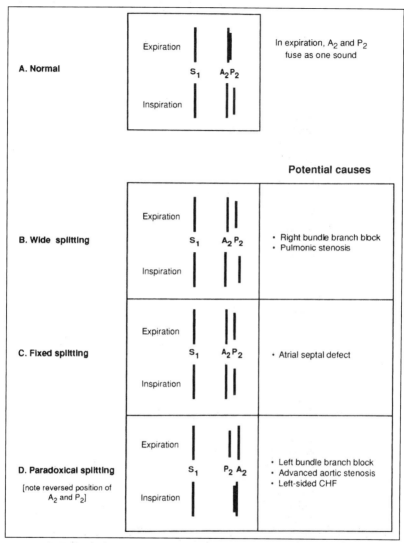

Fig. 7-4. Splitting patterns of the second heart sound (S_2). S_1 = first heart sound; A_2 = aortic component of S_2; P_2 = pulmonic component of S_2. (Reproduced with permission from Lilly LS. *Pathophysiology of Heart Disease.* Philadelphia: Lea and Febiger, 1993.)

(5) **Rubs** usually indicate pericardial inflammation. They sound like squeaky leather, heard both in systole and diastole. Rubs are heard best with the diaphragm over the sternum, with the patient sitting up, leaning forward, and holding his or her breath after exhaling.

(6) Other sounds to listen for include: **opening snap** (rheumatic involvement of mitral or tricuspid valves; heard in diastole), **pericardial knock** (constrictive pericarditis), **tumor "plop"** (especially with left atrial myxoma), and **ejection clicks** (heard in systole; represents most common valvular disease). See **Fig. 7-5** for a diagram of the relationship of some of these sounds to the cardiac cycle.

b. Murmurs. Describe the timing, location and radiation, loudness, pitch, duration, quality (crescendo/decrescendo, musical, etc.). **Table 7-1** shows how to grade murmurs by loudness.

(1) Systolic murmurs (Fig. 7-6)

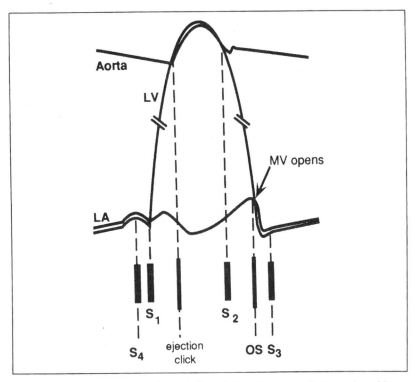

Fig. 7-5. Timing of extrasystolic and diastolic heart sounds. S_4 is produced by atrial contraction in the case of a "stiff" left ventricle (LV). An ejection click follows the opening of the aortic or pulmonic valve in cases of valve stenosis or dilation of the corresponding great artery. An S_3 occurs during the period of rapid ventricular filling; it is normal in young individuals, but its presence in adults implies LV contractile dysfunction. The timing of an opening snap (OS) is shown for comparison, but it is not likely that all of those sounds would appear in the same individual. LA = left atrium; MV = mitral valve. (Reproduced with permission from Lilly LS. *Pathophysiology of Heart Disease.* Philadelphia: Lea and Febiger, 1993.)

TABLE 7–1. Grading of heart murmurs

Grade	Description
I/VI	Heard only after special maneuvers and "tuning in"
II/VI	Faint, but readily heard
III/VI	Loud, but without a thrill
IV/VI	Associated with a thrill, but stethoscope must be fully on chest to be heard
V/VI	Heard with stethoscope partly off the chest; palpable thrill
VI/VI	Heard with stethoscope entirely off the chest; palpable thrill

Reproduced with permission from Judge RD. Zuidema GD, Fitzgerald FT. *Clinical Diagnosis,* 5th ed. Boston: Little, Brown, 1989.)

(a) **Midsystolic.** Usually ejection murmurs, caused by valve stenosis (aortic or pulmonic), increased stroke volume (SV), or dilation of vessel just distal to the valve.

(b) **Holosystolic.** Regurgitant murmurs; commonly mitral regurgitation/tricuspid regurgitation (MR/TR) or ventricular septal defect (VSD).

(c) **Late systolic.** Heard in mitral valve prolapse, usually preceded by a click.

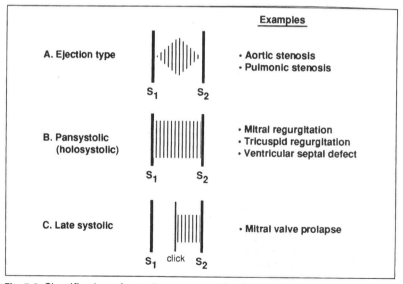

Fig. 7-6. Classification of systolic murmurs. Ejection murmurs are crescendo-decrescendo (or "diamond-shaped") in configuration, whereas pansystolic murmurs are homogenous throughout systole. A late systolic murmur often follows a midsystolic click, and suggests mitral-valve (or tricuspid-valve) prolapse. (Reproduced with permission from Lilly LS. *Pathophysiology of Heart Disease.* Philadelphia: Lea and Febiger, 1993.)

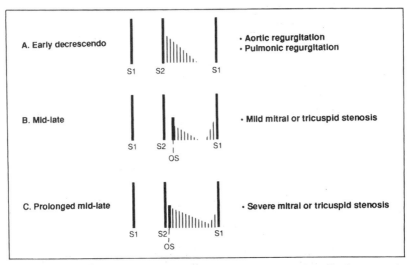

Fig. 7-7. Classification of the diastolic murmurs. A. An early diastolic decrescendo murmur is typical of aortic or pulmonic valve regurgitation. B. Mid or late low-frequency "rumbling" murmurs are usually due to mitral or tricuspid valve stenosis, which follows a sharp opening snap. Presystolic accentuation occurs in patients in normal sinus rhythm, because of forceful propulsion of blood across the stenotic valve by atrial contraction. C. In more severe mitral or tricuspid valve stenosis, the opening snap and diastolic murmur occur earlier, and the murmur is prolonged. (Reproduced with permission from Lilly LS. *Pathophysiology of Heart Disease.* Philadelphia: Lea and Febiger, 1993.)

(2) **Diastolic murmurs (Fig. 7-7)**

   (a) **Early diastolic.** Aortic regurgitation (AR) or pulmonic regurgitation (PR). AR is high-pitched and heard best with the diaphragm at the left sternal border while the patient is sitting up and holding his or her breath after exhalation. PR is of similar quality, heard better at the pulmonic area.

   (b) **Mid to late diastolic.** Mitral stenosis (MS) or tricuspid stenosis (TS). MS gives a low-pitched rumble heard best at the apex with the bell, and the patient lying on the left side; falls then rises in intensity during diastole. TS has similar quality, is louder on inspiration, and is heard best at the tricuspid area (4th intercostal space at left sternal border).

(3) **Continuous and to-and-fro murmurs (Fig. 7-8).** Continuous murmurs begin in systole, and continue without interruption into diastole; seen in patent ductus arteriosus and other arteriovenous (AV) fistulas. To-and-fro murmurs do not extend through S_2 and have discrete systolic and diastolic components.

(4) **Maneuvers.** Various maneuvers that can alter hemodynamics to help differentiate murmurs and heart sounds are described in section II of this chapter. **Fig. 7-9** demonstrates the position of the heart and aorta in relation to the sternum and diaphragm.

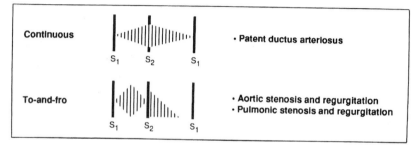

Continuous	S₁ S₂ S₁	• **Patent ductus arteriosus**
To-and-fro	S₁ S₂ S₁	• **Aortic stenosis and regurgitation** • **Pulmonic stenosis and regurgitation**

Fig. 7-8. A continuous murmur peaks at and extends through the second heart sound (S_2). A to-and-fro murmur is not continuous; rather there is a systolic component and a distinct diastolic component, separated by S_2. (Reproduced with permission from Lilly LS. *Pathophysiology of Heart Disease*. Philadelphia: Lea and Febiger, 1993.)

H. Abdominal exam

1. **Inspection.** Draw a brief diagram on your clipboard on which to note data from the abdominal exam (see p. 143). Note any distention, scars, superficial lesions, or venous prominence. Venous prominence is seen with portal hypertension.

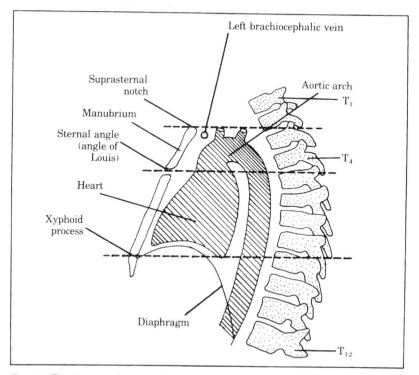

Fig. 7-9. The heart and aorta. (Reprinted with permission from R. S. Snell, *Clinical Anatomy for Medical Students*, 2ⁿᵈ ed. Boston: Little, Brown, 1981.)

2. Auscultation.

   a. Note: Auscultation **precedes** palpation and percussion in the abdominal exam, so that you can listen to the bowels while they are undisturbed.

   b. Listen for **bruits** (especially over the liver, spleen, and abdominal aorta) and **bowel sounds**; absence of bowel sounds for up to 1 minute may be normal. Absence of bowel sounds beyond that time suggests serious pathology and needs to be addressed immediately.

3. Palpation. Palpate first lightly, then more deeply. Start away from any painful areas. Note any rigidity, guarding (if present, whether voluntary or involuntary), tenderness, rebound tenderness, organomegaly, or masses; watch the patient's face for change in expression as you palpate, to help quantify the degree of tenderness. Note any kidney tenderness or enlargement. Palpate the liver edge for texture, contour, and tenderness. Remember that the spleen is usually not palpable in the adult.

4. Percussion

   a. Percussion note. Note the character of the percussion note (gas percusses with a hollow, tympanitic sound; fat, fluid, and underlying tissue percusses with dull sounds).

   b. Liver and spleen. Percuss for size of the liver and spleen. Many clinicians report hepatomegaly as the extent to which the liver is percussed below the right costal margin in centimeters or "finger breadths"; this exam method may falsely estimate liver enlargement, however, in patients with chronic obstructive pulmonary disease (COPD) whose hyperinflated lung fields result in a liver that is situated lower than normal. It is preferable to "percuss out" the liver and record it in centimeters. Liver size can also be determined by the scratch test.

   c. Shifting dullness. In cases with possible ascites, check for dullness that shifts as the patient changes position. Look also for a fluid wave.

I. Peripheral vascular pulses

   1. Note carotid, brachial, radial, femoral, popliteal, dorsalis pedis, and posterior tibial pulses.

   a. Weak pulses (**pulsus parvus**) are c/w shock, congestive heart failure, and aortic stenosis.

   b. Increased pulse pressure is c/w aortic regurgitation and high-output states like thyrotoxicosis, fever, and anemia.

   c. Delayed carotid upstroke is c/w significant aortic stenosis (**pulsus tardus**).

   d. Alternating strong and weak pulses (**pulsus alternans**) are c/w LV failure. Right-left asymmetries in pulses suggest vascular diseases or shunts.

   2. Bruits. Listen for bruits, which may be heard with atherosclerosis or aneurysms. Check the carotid and femoral arteries, and listen in the abdomen for aorta and renal artery bruits.

J. Hematopoietic system. Check for **adenopathy** in cervical, axillary, epitrochlear, and inguinal areas. Note the location, size (use a ruler), degree of tenderness, fixation to underlying tissue, and texture (hard, soft). Usually each set of nodes is examined when examining its region of the body (e.g., cervical nodes are checked during the neck exam).

K. Musculoskeletal exam. This exam is one in which it is particularly important to **focus on the symptomatic or suspicious areas** pinpointed by the general screening questions and exam. For example, complete, quantitative range-of-motion testing is warranted when there is a specific history, or findings, consistent with musculoskeletal disease. (Osteopathic medical students should see **Appendix H** for a review of the osteopathic musculoskeletal examination.)

Ask again about joint or bone pain, and have the patient point to the specific area involved. Listen throughout this exam for crepitations; inspect for joint swelling or deformities; and evaluate strength and range of motion.

1. **Head and neck.** If neck pain is present, especially with headache, suspect meningitis. After making sure there is no injury to the cervical vertebrae or cervical cord (this may require evaluation by radiographs if you suspect trauma to the area), check for the following:

   a. Flex the patient's leg at both the hip and knee, and then straighten the knee. Pain and increased resistance to extending the knee are a positive **Kernig's sign** and, when bilateral, suggests meningeal irritation.

   b. Have the patient lie supine. As you flex the neck, watch the hips and knees in reaction to your maneuver. Flexion of the hips and knees is a positive **Brudzinski's sign** and suggests meningeal irritation.

2. **Shoulders.** Pain may be generated from or referred to local structures (e.g., processes involving the diaphragm may be referred to the shoulder).

3. **Elbows.** Warm, tender joints with subcutaneous nodules around the olecranon process suggest rheumatoid arthritis.

4. **Hands and wrists.** Palpable enlargement of bones in the hands and **Heberden's nodes** on the distal interphalangeal (DIP) joints are seen most commonly in degenerative joint disease (osteoarthritis). Bilateral wrist swelling and proximal interphalangeal (PIP) involvement is seen usually in rheumatoid arthritis.

5. **Spine.** Always inspect contour carefully and test range of motion.

6. **Hips.** Pain and limitation of motion are common arthritic sequelae.

7. **Knees.** Note any presence of **genu varum** (bowlegs) or **genu valgum** (knock knees).

8. **Feet and ankles.** Gout commonly affects the metatarsophalangeal joint of the first (big) toe. Note any fungal-appearing infections of the toenails (onychomycosis).

L. Neurologic exam

1. **Mental status.** Use the mnemonic **"looks-speaks-feels-thinks"** to remember the four main parts of the exam.

   a. **Looks** – general appearance and behavior. Check the level of consciousness, posture, dress and grooming, facial expressions, and manner; orientation to person, place, and time.

b. Speaks – speech and language. Note quantity, rate, volume, fluency, and modulation of speech. Note especially circumlocutions, neologisms, dysarthria, pressured speech, perseveration, clanging, and echolalia.

c. Thinks

  (1) Thought process and content. Check thought content (hallucinations, delusions, and obsessions), thought process (loose associations, tangentiality, flight of ideas, and confabulation).

  (2) Cognitive functions

    (a) Attention. Check with serial sevens or threes, or digit span.

    (b) Memory. Test recall: give the patient three items to remember and explain that you will ask for them again in 5 minutes, and then do so; recent memory: ask about occurrences in the past 24 hours; remote memory: ask about date of marriage, childhood events, or the name of their high school principal.

    (c) Construction ability. Ask the patient to draw a cube or a house. Ask him or her to copy a figure you draw.

    (d) Higher functions. Test **judgment** ("What would you do if you found a stamped, addressed envelope on the sidewalk?"); **proverbs** (ask the patient the meaning of common proverbs, like "A stitch in time saves nine"); **calculations**; **fund of knowledge**.

2. **Cranial nerves.** The cranial nerves that have not yet been tested are examined at this point (all may have been tested earlier in the exam, while examining the head and neck.)

  a. I, Olfactory. Smell; not routinely tested. Use nonirritating scents, not alcohol swabs. Most significant in unilateral loss.

  b. II, Optic. Vision; test acuity, visual fields, and pupils.

  c. III, Oculomotor. Most extraocular muscles; papillary constriction.

  d. IV, Trochlear. Movement of the eye down and in (superior oblique muscle).

  e. V, Trigeminal. Sensory to the face; motor to the temporal and masseter muscles. Palpate the masseters on forced closure of the jaw; touch cornea for corneal reflex; test all three divisions for sensation on the face.

  f. VI, Abducens. Lateral movement of the eye (lateral rectus muscle).

  g. VII, Facial. Motor to most of the facial muscles; anterior tongue taste. Check smile, strength of eye closure, symmetry of forehead wrinkling and nasolabial folds.

  h. VIII, Auditory (Vestibulocochlear). Hearing and balance. Use a 256-cps or 512-cps tuning fork for low frequency, a ticking watch for high frequency, a whispered voice or rubbing of the fingers for medium frequency.

  i. IX, Glossopharyngeal. Pharynx, sensory and motor; posterior tongue taste.

   j. X, Vagus. Motor to the palate, pharynx, and larynx; sensory to the pharynx and larynx. For nerves IX and X, test swallowing, phonation ("me," "la," ga"); check the gag reflex and for a midline uvula.

   k. XI, Spinal Accessory. Motor to the sternocleidomastoid and trapezius muscles. Test shoulder shrug, turning of the head, and head flexion.

   l. XII, Hypoglossal. Motor to the tongue. Check symmetry of tongue protrusion and look for tongue fasciculations, strength in pushing the tongue against the cheeks.

3. Sensory exam. Check symmetric areas in both right and left limbs; symmetric loss is c/w peripheral neuropathy. With pinprick and vibration, if sense is intact in the distal extremity you need not proceed proximally.

   a. Pinprick. Use only a broken tongue depressor, not reusable pins.

   b. Vibration. Use a 128-cps or 256-cps tuning fork on joints. Be sure the patient is really sensing vibration (check this with a "sham" vibration caused by pressing the extremity with a nonvibrating tuning fork).

   c. Position sense. Grasp the sides of a toe or finger and move it up or down, asking the patient which way you moved it.

   d. Light touch. Use a cotton wisp.

   e. Temperature. Differentiate between a tuning fork (cold) and the rubber of a reflex hammer (warm). This usually corresponds to pinprick sensation.

   f. Cortical discrimination. Examples of tests include graphesthesia (blindly identify letter or number "written" on the palm), stereognosis (blindly identify an object, like a coin or key, placed in the hand).

4. Motor Exam

   a. Muscle strength. Strength is usually graded on a scale of 1 to 5 **(Table 7-2)**.

   b. Tone. Test the resistance to passive motion. For Parkinson's disease, look for "cogwheel" rigidity.

   c. Bulk. Compare one side of the body to the other, but remember to allow for handedness and occupation-induced differences. Look for fasciculations, tenderness, and wasting.

5. Reflexes. Note any right-left asymmetries. Record the findings on a clipboard by drawing a stick figure (see the sample write-up in **Chap. 16**).

   a. Biceps (C5, C6), **triceps** (C6, C7, C8), **brachioradialis** (C5, C6), **patella** (L2, L3, L4), and **Achilles' tendon** reflexes (S1, S2). Upper motor neuron lesions cause spasticity; lower motor neuron lesions cause flaccidity. Leg reflexes can be reinforced by isometric, opposed arm pulls. Graded 1+ to 4+ (1+ means present but difficult to elicit; 2+ means average; 3+ means hyperactive but not necessarily pathological; 4+ means very hyperactive, with clonus.)

TABLE 7–2 Testing for muscle strength

100%	5	N (normal)	Complete range of motion against gravity with full resistance
75	4	G (good)	Complete range of motion against gravity with some resistance
50	3	F (fair)	Complete range of motion against gravity
25	2	P (poor)	Complete range of motion with gravity eliminated
10	1	T (trace)	Evidence of slight contractility; no joint motion
0	0	0 (zero)	No evidence of contractility

    b. Babinski reflex. A positive Babinski reflex is c/w upper motor neuron disease.

    c. Other reflexes not routinely tested include: **upper abdominal** (T7, T8, T9), **lower abdominal** (T11, T12), **cremasteric** (T12, L1), **jaw**, and **anal wink**. The presence of grasp, suck, or rooting reflexes usually indicates frontal lobe disease.

  6. Cerebellar. Test finger-nose, heel-shin coordination.

  7. Gait. Include heel-to-toe walking and Romberg's sign (have the patient stand with feet together and eyes closed: if the patient sways enough to require shifting his or her feet to maintain balance, the test is positive).

M. Genital and rectal exam

  1. Male

    a. Penis. Note the presence of any penile lesions or discharge.

    b. Scrotum. Check for scrotal lesions and varicosities; palpate the spermatic cord.

    c. Testes. Check the testes bilaterally, and evaluate the shape and firmness.

    d. Hernia. Inspect for hernia; this is best done with the patient standing. Ask the patient to cough, and feel for weakness of the wall.

    e. Rectum. Anal lesions, sphincter tone, stool color, and prostate size. Prostate exam is especially important in men more than 50 years old. Always check for occult blood with a stool guaiac test.

  2. Female

    a. External exam. Labia, urethral orifice, introitus, and perineum. A careful inspection is conducted here for irritation, discharge, and lesions.

    b. Speculum exam. Cervix and os specimens (endocervical swab, cervical scrape, and vaginal pool) and a vaginal canal exam. The Pap smear and gonococcal cultures are taken here. The vaginal canal may be inspected as the speculum is removed.

    c. Bimanual exam. Cervix, fornix, uterus, and ovaries.

    d. Rectal exam. The rectal exam is often done with simultaneous placement of a finger in the vagina to palpate the interposed tissue. Change gloves before doing this exam, to decrease the likelihood of spreading infection.

II. Practical points for the physical exam

A. General advice

1. Many patients have negative expectations about physical exams, and it is important that you **make patients comfortable** throughout the process. Patients should be completely disrobed, except for underwear, to allow for proper exposure, but parts of the body not being examined should be kept covered for modesty's sake. Get into the habit of washing your hands before and after each exam; patients are reassured if you do this in their presence. Make sure your hands and stethoscope are warm before allowing them to touch the patient. Always let the patient know what you are about to do, and why.

2. The physical examination is an art that is learned only by constant repetition. You will learn a great deal through careful study of one of the many available physical examination manuals, but the only way to get comfortable with the techniques of the exam is to practice. The best way to learn physical diagnosis is through **repeated proctoring** of your methods. An experienced clinician can show you how to hold your hands just so; it is always easier to demonstrate than to explain.

3. Although there are many individual styles and methods of conducting the general screening exam, a good physician will choose one examination sequence and stick to it. Most people prefer to work in a head-to-foot order, with exceptions made as necessary for convenience and completeness. Most physicians stand at the patient's right side. As each part of the body is examined, it is usually best to follow an orderly sequence of **inspection, palpation, percussion,** and **auscultation** (except in the abdomen, where auscultation precedes palpation and percussion). This routine will help ensure thoroughness, and also will aid in putting the patient at ease by minimizing the unexpected.

4. The physical examination should always be conducted and assessed in the context of the patient's clinical history. The range of what is normal varies from patient to patient, and physical findings cannot be gathered and interpreted in a vacuum. Think in advance about **what you expect to find** in any given part of the exam. What kind of peripheral neurologic exam might you expect of a long-term diabetic? Are there other physical exam findings that might help you to gauge the progress of the disease?

5. Do not be alarmed if, during the first few weeks, the complete exam takes you much longer than expected; first concentrate on learning each subsection, then work on stringing all the parts together smoothly. Do not be afraid to **repeat** parts of the exam if the findings are equivocal. Realize, however, that the diagnostic success of your exam depends on the cooperation of the patient, and that it is tedious and uncomfortable to be poked and maneuvered for hours at a time. It is often useful to repeat parts of the physical exam after looking at the results of the

physical diagnostic tests; a patient whose chest x-ray shows some lobar consolidation provides a good opportunity to fine tune your auscultatory abilities.

6. **Practice** your exam techniques when you are away from the bedside. Take the time to familiarize yourself with your equipment, so that you will not, for example, fumble around with an inside-out blood pressure cuff. Practice on other medical students to get a good idea of the normal range.

7. Realize that the physical exam provides a perfect **opportunity to question** the patient concerning review of systems (ROS) topics you may have forgotten or you may be unclear about. It is often quite natural to introduce your next step with a general question concerning the organ system being examined (e.g., begin the otoscopic exam with, "So you've had no difficulties with earaches or infections?").

8. Each exam you do is **tailored to the patient** involved and directed by his or her problems. You will learn to run rapidly through the organ systems that you do not suspect to be involved and quickly decide whether findings are within normal limits. This takes practice, but it is certainly possible to do a brief, general screening physical in 10 minutes, once you are familiar with and can conduct easily the various parts of the exam.

9. A knowledge of **surface anatomy** is important in performing the physical examination. Note the relation of the internal organs in **Figs. 7-10** and **7-11** to the thoracic cage depicted in **Fig. 7-12**.

B. **Specific points concerning the physical exam.** There are six traditionally difficult or problematic sections of the physical examination: the funduscopic exam, the cardiac exam, the neurologic exam, the rectal exam, the pelvic exam, and the breast exam. Each of these is discussed specifically below.

1. The **funduscopic exam** is very difficult to master. Work first on getting the **"red reflex."** If you have a cat at your house, practice by looking into its eyes, since the cat's pupil remains relatively dilated. If you are around when a patient's eyes are pharmacologically dilated for some reason, ask to be permitted to examine his or her eyes as well.

Once you can elicit the red reflex easily, concentrate on **visualizing the disc** and then trace its perimeter. Dial up or down 1 or 2 diopters in each direction on the funduscope after you have visualized an edge of the disc, and try to get a sense of how the disc relates to the retinal surface. Remember, the beautiful textbook pictures of fundi are generated with a special ophthalmoscope that allows visualization of much more of the fundus than your handheld model.

Finally, begin to follow the course of the **vessels** from the fundus outward into the four quadrants. Do not subject your patient to too long an exam; divide it into two parts if necessary. Note where veins and arteries cross; look for nicking and other abnormalities. The funduscopic exam takes months to learn and years to master. In some patients it is impossible to visualize the fundi without dilating their pupils. (The oph-

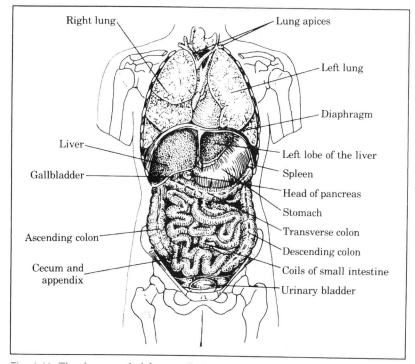

Fig. 7-10. The thorax and abdomen. (Redrawn from R. S. Snell, *Clinical Anatomy for Medical Students*, 2nd ed. Boston: Little, Brown, 1981.)

thalmologist usually insists on dilating a patient before performing an exam.)

2. The **cardiac exam** is made up of several parts. Of these, auscultation of the heart usually takes the longest time to master.

   a. The first goal of auscultation of the heart is **distinguishing systole from diastole**. This aim may sound simplistic, but it is not. Here are a few hints to make the distinction easier.

      (1) Begin auscultating with the stethoscope held on the apex with one hand while your other hand gently feels the carotid pulse; the first heart sound just precedes the carotid pulsation. This often can help you distinguish S_1 (and, therefore, systole).

      (2) In the absence of valvular pathology, the **intensity** of S_1 is greater than that of S_2 at the apex of the heart, while the intensity of S_2 is greater than that of S_1 at the base. (Listen at the aortic and pulmonic areas for the two components of S_2 and at the mitral area or PMI for S_1.)

      (3) Although more subtle, the **pitch** of S_1 is discernibly lower than that of S_2 in most patients. Remember, high-frequency sounds

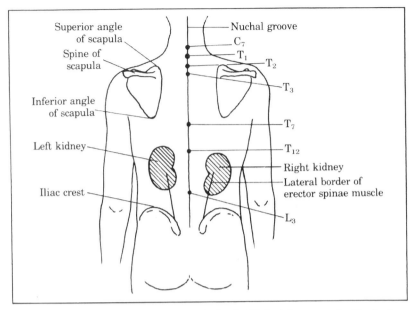

Fig. 7-11. The back. (Redrawn from R. S. Snell, *Clinical Anatomy for Medical Students,* 2ⁿᵈ ed. Boston: Little, Brown, 1981.)

are best heard with the diaphragm of your stethoscope, while low-frequency sounds are better appreciated with the bell.

(4) Remember that the PMI correlates with systole. This means that S_1 just precedes the onset of the apical impulse, which you may both see and feel with your hand and your stethoscope.

b. "Inching." Once you are oriented to systole and diastole, you can begin a systematic exam. It is helpful to base this assessment on an initial, routine path of movement of the stethoscope from the aortic to the pulmonic area and down the left sternal border (tricuspid area) to the mitral area (**Fig. 7-8**).

(1) Develop a specific sequence at each step in this path, in which the components of the cardiac cycle are systematically sought.

(2) Thus, at each stop along the inching "path," **listen selectively** to: S_1, S_2, other heart sounds, and murmurs. It is crucial to learn to listen selectively to each of these components. Concentrate on each item individually in the above list, starting with S_1, at each step of the way. Inching will be lengthy, even tedious at first, but it will soon become routine, and it is the best way to "hear" heart sounds effectively.

c. Maneuvering and murmur analysis. Although a thorough description of murmur analysis is beyond the scope of this section, there are several basic points to remember from the start. Examine the patient first

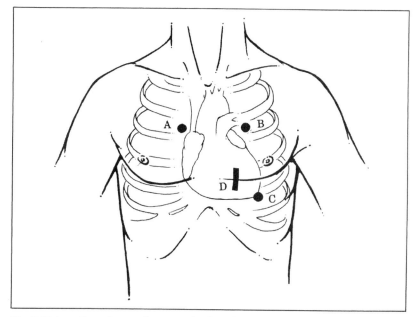

Fig. 7.12. Locations for cardiac auscultation. A. Aortic valve; second right interspace. B. Pulmonic valve; second left interspace. C. Mitral valve; apex. D. Tricuspid valve; lower left sternal border. (Modified from R. Judge and G. Zuidema, *Methods of Clinical Examination: A Physiologic Approach*, 3rd ed. Boston: Little, Brown, 1974.)

in the **supine position**, then the **lateral decubitus position**, and then the **sitting position**. The murmur of aortic insufficiency is often appreciated only with the patient sitting up and leaning slightly forward. Murmurs at the apex are best heard with the patient in the left lateral decubitus position, which brings the heart closer to your stethoscope.

It is possible to alter the character of murmurs heard by maneuvering your patient in certain ways. Maneuvering is the physiologic alteration of venous return, peripheral arterial resistance, or cardiac output. For instance, the **handgrip** increases peripheral arterial resistance, which in turn decreases the gradient across the aortic valve in systole or increases the degree of mitral regurgitation. Therefore, an aortic systolic ejection murmur can sometimes be heard to decrease in intensity with the patient doing the handgrip maneuver, while that of mitral regurgitation may increase. See **Table 7-3** for a list of common murmurs.

3. The **neurologic exam** has five main parts: the mental status, motor, sensory, cranial nerve, and reflex exams. Because a thorough neurologic exam has so many specific parts, confusion often results, largely because the neurologic exam is approached in a shotgun manner during a typical physical exam sequence.

TABLE 7–3 Effect of some physical maneuvers on cardiovascular dynamics and heart sounds

Maneuver	Peripheral resistance (afterload)	Left ventricular volume (preload)	Murmur of aortic stenosis	Murmur of hypertrophic obstructive cardiomyopathy	Murmur of mitral regurgitation	Click murmur of mitral valve prolapse	Murmur of mitral stenosis	Murmur of aortic insufficiency and Austin Flint
Supine with passive leg raising	— or ↑	↑	↑	↓	—	↓	↑	—
Sitting or standing	↓	↓	—	↑	—	↑	—	↑ or —
Prompt squatting	↑	↑	— (early) ↓ (late)	↓	↑	↓	↓	↑
Isometric exercise (e.g., handgrip)	↑	↑	↓	↓	↑	↓	↓	↑
Valsalva maneuver	↓	↓	↓	↑ or ↓ or —	↓	↑	↓	↓
Exercise	↓	↑	↑	↓	—	↑	↑	↑
Amyl nitrate	↓	↓	↑	↑	↓	↑	↑	↓

↑ = increased; ↓ = decreased; — = no change; → = later in systole; ← = earlier in systole.
Reproduced with permission from Judge RD, Zuidema GD, Fitzgerald FT. *Clinical Diagnosis*, 5th ed. Boston: Little, Brown, 1989.

Most patients will only require a screening neurologic exam. When it is warranted, however, consider performing on appropriate patients a more complete neurologic exam, separate from and in addition to the usual screening physical exam. With the neurologic examination as your specific (and only) task, it is much easier to organize your thoughts and your work-up.

4. The **rectal exam** is sometimes difficult simply because it is unpleasant for both the patient and physician; it is not hard to learn or to execute, however. (It does take practice to learn how to palpate the prostate and judge its size and firmness, but this becomes much easier over time.)

   Relax yourself and your patient, be firm and gentle, and be sure to guaiac the small bit of stool that is invariably on your glove after the exam. In men, especially older men, practice defining the lobes of the prostate, assess its texture, and search for focal areas of induration. The normal prostate should have the consistency of the tip of your nose; a harder nodule may be pathologic. In women the rectal exam is part of the pelvic exam in many cases, and it is especially important when defining the extent of gynecologic tumor and for the stool guaiac.

   Do not be tentative about doing a rectal exam; it is a brief exam but a very important one. On the other hand, when first learning, you will often examine patients who have already had several rectal exams. It is prudent to check the chart ahead of time to see how many such exams have been done, and to defer if one has already been performed that day.

5. The **pelvic exam** is often considered separately for two reasons: it requires a special setup, and it is an examination that is extremely sensitive and personal.

   a. A male should never perform a pelvic examination without a **female chaperone** (nurse or physician) present.

   b. The exam is best learned by spending a concentrated period of time doing **several pelvic examinations each day**, for example through going on an obstetrics-gynecology rotation or by arranging to work for several consecutive days in an outpatient gynecology clinic.

   c. Traditionally, the most difficult part of the exam is the **speculum insertion**. The speculum exam should be observed several times and then practiced, paying special attention to warming and moistening the speculum before its insertion, the angle at which the speculum is introduced, and opening the speculum after it is fully inserted.

6. The **breast exam**. Like the blood pressure measurement, the breast examination is one of the few parts of the physical exam that will frequently yield crucial information prompting major medical interventions in the entirely asymptomatic patient. Nearly one of nine American women will develop breast cancer, and every medical student should be familiar with its signs.

   a. **Inspection**. The patient should be disrobed to the waist and both breasts should be inspected concurrently to allow comparison. Pay particular attention to symmetry of the left and right breasts. Though it is quite common for one breast to be somewhat larger than the other, the asymmetry should not include major differences in the appearance or texture of the skin or the nipples, nor should there be lumpy irregularities in the normally smooth breast contours.

(1) Local areas of erythema and swelling may be due to tumor, inflammation, or merely to tight clothing, and should be carefully scrutinized. While breast cancer with lymphatic engorgement may produce only subtle changes (peau d'orange, best seen with a tangentially directed flashlight), direct skin invasion often produces an angry red cellulitic appearance that is unmistakable. Except in the nursing mother, any nipple discharge should be regarded as suspicious.

(2) Skin retraction is one of the most subtle findings in this part of the exam. It is often best appreciated in the arms-over-the-head and hands-against-hips maneuvers.

(3) A small, innocuous-looking bulge in the upper outer quadrant that moves up into the axilla when the arms are raised is a classic early finding in breast carcinoma.

b. **Palpation**. Though many different sequences of breast palpation are used, all are thorough, systematic, and bimanual. One good technique for the novice involves starting at the nipple and following a clockwise spiral pattern around the breast and into the axilla. The fingertips are used alternately to compress and push the breast tissue toward the other hand. The palms of the hand are less sensitive and do not play a major role in this technique. If a suspicious area is felt, it is localized under the examiner's fingertips with the patient's arms down. The arms are then slowly raised over the head to allow an assessment of mobility of the lesion.

(1) In addition to a careful breast exam, it is critical to investigate thoroughly the possibility of associated lymphadenopathy in the axillary and supraclavicular regions in all patients.

(2) The axilla must be deeply palpated with the patient's arm draped across the chest to accomplish maximal relaxation of the pectoral muscles. Once again, asymmetry between the left and right breast may be the only clue to an abnormal finding.

c. **Recording the exam**. Accurate recording of the breast exam is absolutely crucial and may spare the patient unnecessary surgery at some point in the future. It is usually best to accompany a verbal description with diagrams and precise polar coordinates (e.g., "a 2-cm by 3-cm freely mobile mass located in the 3 o'clock position, 2.5 cm from the areolar edge"). For premenopausal patients, the exact position in the menstrual cycle at the time of the exam should also be noted.

d. **Benign processes**, including chronic cystic mastitis and fibroadenomas, are common in the breast, and the vast majority of breast masses are not malignant. However, serial breast exams with mammographic correlation provide the best means of detecting this very common malignancy in its early stages.

REFERENCES

Bickley LS. *Bates' Guide to Physical Examination and History Taking*. 8th ed. Philadelphia: Lippincott Williams & Wilkins, 2003, pp. 157–158, 196-197, 593–594.

Braunwald E, Fauci AS, Kasper DL, et al. *Harrison's Principles of Internal Medicine*. 15th ed. New York: McGraw-Hill, 2001.

DeGowin RL. DeGowin and DeGowin's Diagnostic Examination. 6th ed. New York: McGraw-Hill, 1994.

McGee S. *Evidence-based Physical Diagnosis*. Philadelphia: W.B. Saunders, 2001.

Novey DW. *Rapid Access Guide to Physical Examination*. 2nd ed. St. Louis: Mosby, 1998, pp. 454–455.

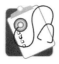

CHAPTER **8**

Pediatric History and Physical Exam

There are three issues which must be understood and addressed in the care of adolescent-young adult patients. First, the history must be given by the patient alone. Parents may, of course, make their contribution, but not initially. Second, the physical examination is not complete unless the sexual maturation stage is noted and recorded. Third, the patient must be informed at the close of the evaluation what the diagnostic possibilities are, what tests and studies are necessary and why, and what treatment is planned, giving the responsibility to the patient, not the parents, for carrying out the therapy. Following these simple guidelines will open up the opportunity for you to talk about and counsel in the more sensitive areas of behavior, sexuality, education, career decisions, drugs, and alcohol. Care for your adolescent patients—don't delegate and triage!

Robert P. Masland, Jr., M.D., FAAP

Dr. Masland is an Associate Professor of Pediatrics at Harvard Medical School, where he serves on the Committee on Admission of Students at Harvard Medical School, and a member of the faculty at Children's Hospital Boston.

The toughest pediatric patients to examine are young toddlers aged 9 months to 2 1/2 years. Even the most experienced and skilled physicians will usually be met by a screaming child who continues to scream even if the child is repeatedly examined by the same person.

In this age group I have always found it helpful to begin the examination with the child in a parent's lap, on a chair rather than on the examining table. A brief period might be spent trying to find ways to, at best, entertain the child and, at least, let them know you won't hurt them. The exam should begin with the heart since this may be the only opportunity to examine the child while he/she is not (yet) crying. After the cardiac exam, the physical assessment can be continued in any order as long as it remains systematic. As much of the exam as possible should be performed in the caretaker's lap, including abdominal and otoscopic examinations.

Michael Shannon, M.D., MPH, FAAP

Dr. Shannon is Associate Chief of Emergency Services at Children's Hospital Boston and Associate Professor of Pediatrics at Harvard Medical School. He also serves as Clinical Director of the Pediatric Environmental Health Center and is the author of Clinical Management of Poisoning and Drug Overdose. *He is past president of the American College of Medical Toxicology.*

In this chapter we will describe how to conduct those parts of the physical examination of infants and children that require a different approach or technique from those used in the physical examination of adults. When assessing an infant or a child, always consider where the patient is on the continuum of growth and development. In general it is helpful to think of the pediatric population as having four developmental levels: infancy (the first year), early childhood (ages 1–4), late childhood (ages 5–12), and adolescence (ages 13–20).

I. The pediatric history. When conducting the history establish a **rapport with both the parents and the patient**. All too often the examiner focuses on the parents and neglects the child, or vice verse.

   A. General approach. When taking a history from an adolescent, be sure to **set some time aside to talk to the patient alone**. This gives the patient an opportunity to discuss problems or issues that he or she may not feel comfortable discussing in front of the parent or guardian. When approaching a child, avoid being too obtrusive or overbearing. Gently approach the child at his or her level, kneeling down (if necessary) to speak with them to avoid standing over them. Toddlers often have a fear of separation, and it is best to interact with this age group while the child sits on the parent's lap. Allow the child some time to warm up to the examiner, letting them play with your stethoscope or a toy in the examining room.

   B. Past medical history. The amount of detail here depends on the nature of the problem and the age of the child. In general, the younger the child the more pertinent perinatal events become.

   1. Antenatal. Health of the mother during pregnancy including prenatal care, diet history and weight gain, infections during pregnancy including sexually transmitted diseases, Rh typing, medications, cigarette use, and alcohol intake.

   2. Natal. Anesthesia used, labor description including whether it was a vaginal delivery or Cesarean section, Apgar scores, birth weight, and gestational age.

   3. Neonatal. Color, cyanosis, anemia, jaundice, muscle tone, convulsions, fever, congenital or acquired abnormalities, difficulties sucking, difficulties feeding or rashes.

   4. Developmental. Developmental assessment is done utilizing the **Denver Developmental Screening Test**, which evaluates the child's expected level of development based on age. You are looking to see that the child is at the appropriate stage of development based on age and that they have successfully mastered the previous stages of development.

   5. Nutrition. For infants you should assess and record the type, amount, and frequency of feedings, documenting whether breast milk or formula. Record vitamin supplements and when solid food was introduced to the diet. A record of the number of feedings to wet and soiled diapers needs to be established to assess adequate nutrition.

   6. Illness. Contagious diseases, fevers, rashes, communicable childhood diseases and the age at which these illnesses occurred must be recorded.

   7. Immunizations. A record of the required immunizations with the age of the patient at the time of the immunizations must be recorded.

8. **Surgeries.** Type of surgery and why required, outcome of the surgery, and the age of the child at the time of surgery.

9. **Social history.** Who is the child's primary care giver? Does the child attend day care? Does the child have any other siblings and do they live in the same household? Do both parents live with the child and what is the level of participation in the upbringing by the parents?

10. **Family history.** The assessment of possible inherited disorders or traits is the goal of this line of questioning.

II. The pediatric physical exam. The following is a step-by-step outline of the pediatric physical exam, highlighting what to look for in children that is different from adults.

A. **General Appearance.** How the child is dressed. Is it appropriate for the climate? Are the clothes clean? Is the child well groomed and clean? Does the child look sick?

B. **Vital signs.** Temperature, pulse, respiratory rate, blood pressure, height or length, weight, and head circumference (for infants). Place the height, weight, and head circumference in percentiles for age.

1. **Temperature.** For infants and children younger than 5 years, rectal temperatures should be used almost exclusively because accurate oral and tympanic readings are hard to obtain. Activity, apprehension, and fear may elevate the temperature.

2. **Heart rate.** Obtain the heart rate in infants by observing the pulsations of the anterior fontanelle, by palpating the carotid or femoral arteries, or by direct auscultation of the heart. The heart rate in infants and children is quite labile and more sensitive to the effects of illness, exercise, and emotion than in adults.

3. **Respiratory rate.** In infancy and early childhood, diaphragmatic breathing is predominant over thoracic excursion; therefore you can more easily ascertain the respiratory rate by observing and counting the abdominal excursions.

4. **Blood pressure.** Always remember to use a blood pressure cuff that is appropriate to the patient's size, as using a cuff too large will give you a false reading. The point at which the first sound becomes **muffled** rather than disappears is recorded as the diastolic pressure in children, unlike adults. At times, especially in early infancy, the heart sounds are not audible, due to a narrow or deeply placed brachial artery; in such instances palpate the radial artery at the wrist to determine the blood pressure. The point at which the pulse is first felt is recorded as the systolic pressure. This is approximately 10 mm Hg lower than the systolic pressure determined by auscultation. The diastolic pressure cannot be determined by using the radial pulse method.

C. **Skin.** Color, texture, cyanosis, erythema, rash, edema, hemangiomas, and nevi, Mongolian blue spots, pigmentation (whether hyperpigmented or hypopigmented), turgor, and elasticity. The soles and the palms are often bluish and cold in early infancy (**acrocyanosis**); this is of no significance. Use natural daylight rather than artificial daylight when evaluating for the presence of **jaundice** at any age.

D. HEENT

1. **Head.** Size, shape, symmetry of face and skull, molding, hydrocephalus, and fontanelles. Lightly palpate the fontanelles for fullness while the child is quietly sitting in the upright position.

2. **Eyes.** Photophobia, visual acuity, muscular control, nystagmus. The assessment of vision of an infant or newborn is based on the presence of visual reflexes: direct and consensual pupillary constriction in response to light, blinking in response to bright light and to movement of an object quickly toward the eyes, and red reflex to rule out retinoblastoma.

3. **Ears.** Pinna, canals, tympanic membranes (landmarks, perforation, inflammation, discharge, bulging). A crying child typically has a red tympanic membrane; do not confuse this with an infection. Using an otoscope, gently place the speculum into the external canal and gently pull on the external ear to bring the tympanic membrane into view. Look for the cone of light as an indication of visualization of the membrane. Elicit auditory acuity of a child by observing for the blink of the eyes (**acoustic blink reflex**) in response to a loud snapping of the fingers or clapping of the hands at a distance of 12 inches from the ear. **Pneumatic otoscopy** should be part of every otoscopic exam; it is accomplished by observing the tympanic membrane as the pressure in the external auditory canal is increased or decreased by insufflating a rubber squeeze bulb.

4. **Nose.** Exterior, mucosa, patency, discharge, and bleeding. Most infants are nose breathers, so when checking patency of the nares do not occlude both at the same time.

5. **Mouth.** Lips, teeth, mucosa, palate, and tongue.

6. **Throat.** Tonsils (size, symmetry, inflammation, exudates, and crypts), evidence of a post-nasal drip, voice (hoarseness, stridor, grunting).

   a. Young children may have to be restrained to allow you to fully examine the throat. Eliciting a gag reflex may be necessary if the oropharynx is to be adequately seen.

   b. Permit the child to handle the tongue blade and nasal speculum, to help him or her overcome a fear of instruments. A child's head may be restrained by having the parent hold the child's arms firmly over their head while the child is lying on their back on the examining table.

   c. If the child can sit up, have the parent hold the child erect on their lap with the child's back against the parent's chest. The parent then gently holds the child's head turned to one side against the parent's chest.

E. **Neck.** Thyroid, neck stiffness, and lymph nodes (location, size, sensitivity, mobility, and consistency). Lymph node enlargement occurs much more readily in the child than in the adult. Small inguinal lymph nodes are palpable in almost all healthy children.

F. **Thorax.** Shape and symmetry, retractions, paradoxical breathing.

G. Lungs. Type of breathing, expansion, flatness or dullness to percussion, fremitus, resonance, breath and voice sounds, crackles, wheezing.

    1. Expiration is more prolonged in infants and children than in adults.

    2. The stethoscope may be a very threatening instrument to a young child. Allow the child to warm up to the stethoscope by letting him or her to play with it first (listen to the parent's lungs to assure them it is not painful).

H. Heart. Carefully check for murmurs and extra beats. Auscultation is much more difficult in the child compared to the adult since the heart rate is faster in the child. Nevertheless, the examination is the same as in the adult.

I. Abdomen. Size and contour, visible peristalsis, respiratory movements, umbilicus, tenderness, rigidity, and shifting dullness, hepatosplenomegaly.

J. Genitalia

    1. Male. Hypospadias, phimosis, adherent foreskin, cryptorchidism, hydrocele, hernia size and shape of testes and penis, and testicular torsion. Testicular retractibility can be overcome by having the child sit in a cross-legged squatting position on the examining table, as illustrated in **Fig. 8-1.** A diagnosis of undescended testicle should not be made until you have palpated the inguinal canal and scrotum with the patient in this position.

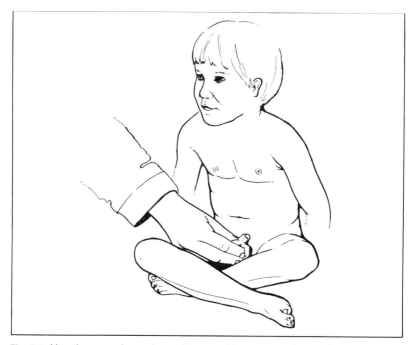

Fig. 8-1. Use the cross-legged squatting position to examine testicular retractibility. (Redrawn from Bates BA. *A Guide to Physical Examination and History Taking*, 5th ed. Philadelphia: Lippincott, 1991.)

2. **Female**. Imperforate vagina, vaginal discharge, clitoral hypertrophy, pubertal changes. Digital or speculum examination is rarely done until after puberty, but the vagina and cervix often can be visualized with the infant in a knee-to-chest position. The examination of the genitalia in a child in early or late childhood can be made easier for you and more comfortable for the child by using the child's own hands to spread the labia majora, as shown in **Fig. 8-2**. This will both distract and reassure her.

K. **Rectum**. Imperforate anus, pinworms. In infants, digital examination is done only for a specific indication or complaint. Use the gloved little finger, slowly insert into the rectum to assess for muscle tone, character of stool, and presence of any masses.

L. **Extremities**

1. **General**. Deformities, bowleggedness, knock-knees, paralysis, muscle weakness.

2. **Joints**. Swelling, erythema, pain, limitations, rheumatic nodules, hip dislocations or fractures, clavicular fractures. To detect congenital dislocation of the hip in the infant, use the Ortolani test (**Fig. 8-3**). Place the baby in the supine position with the legs pointing toward you. Flex the legs to right angles at the hips and knees, placing your middle fingers over the greater trochanter of each femur and your thumbs over the lesser trochanter. Abduct (push in) and adduct (push out) each hip, one

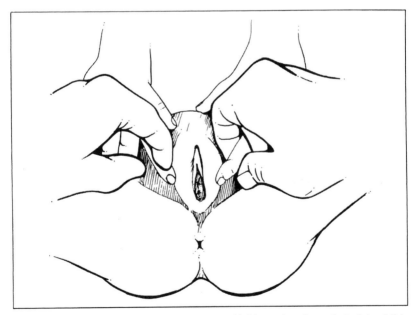

Fig. 8-2. Use the child's own hands to spread labia majora in early to late childhood, prior to puberty. (Redrawn from Bates BA. *A Guide to Physical Examination and History Taking*, 5th ed. Philadelphia: Lippincott, 1991.)

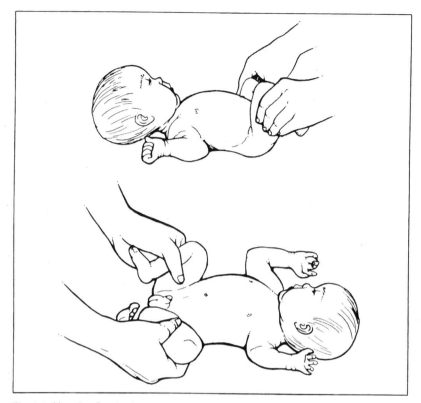

Fig. 8-3. Use the Ortolani test to check for congenital hip dislocation. (Redrawn from Bates BA. *A Guide to Physical Examination and History Taking*, 5th ed. Philadelphia: Lippincott, 1991.)

at a time, while stabilizing the other hip by putting the lateral aspect of the knee you wish to stabilize against the examining table. If there is congenital dislocation, you will hear a click and feel movement of the femoral head, as it lies in the posterior acetabulum.

3. **Hands and feet.** Extra digits, clubbing, simian creases, splinter hemorrhages, koilonychia.

M. **Neurological exam.** Reflexes, gait, ataxia, strabismus, nystagmus, muscle strength, sensation, developmental delay. The Babinski response and clonus are normal for the first year of life.

N. **Spine and back.** Posture, curvatures, rigidity, webbed neck, spina bifida, pilonidal dimple or cyst, Mongolian spot.

III. **Immunization schedules for the pediatric patient.** Recommended childhood and adolescent immunization schedules are updated frequently by the American Academy of Pediatrics and approved by the Advisory Committee on Immunization Practices of the Centers for Disease Control (CDC) in

Atlanta, Georgia. These recommendations are distributed yearly by the National Immunization Program.

A. Practical points for the pediatric physical exam

1. **Approaching the child.** Time should be spent in becoming acquainted with the child and allowing the child to become acquainted with you. A friendly manner, quiet voice, and a slow and easy approach will help to facilitate the examination. If however, you are not able to establish a friendly feeling between the child and yourself, and if you feel it is important that the examination be performed at that time, you should proceed with the physical examination in an orderly, systematic manner in the hope that the child will then accept the inevitable.

2. **Observation of the patient.** Although the very young child may not be able to speak, one may still gather a lot of information by observing the child. Much useful information can be gained by observing how the parent and child interact and how the patient relates to the examiner. The neurologic examination of a toddler may often consist mostly of, or even solely of, watching the child play, run, jump, and so on. Spend time watching the child and thinking about what you see.

3. **Developmental assessment.** It is best to perform the developmental assessment before subjecting the child to upsetting parts of the examination. It is important to observe what the child can and cannot do.

4. **Holding the child for the examination**

    a. **Younger than 6 months:** Examining table usually is well tolerated. **Never walk away and leave the child unattended.**

    b. **6 months to 3–4 years:** Often the examination may be carried out while the child is held in the caregiver's lap, over his or her shoulder, or with the caregiver standing at the head of the table while holding the child's hands.

5. **Removal of clothing.** Clothing should be removed gradually, in order that the child will not be chilled and to prevent the development of resistance in a shy child. To save time and to avoid creating unpleasant associations with the physician in the child's mind, undressing the child and taking his or her temperature are best performed by the parent or caregiver. The physician should respect the marked degree of modesty that may be exhibited by some children. Underpants may be left on during the examination and removed only when necessary.

6. **Sequence of exam.** Heart and lungs should be examined first; **ears, throat, and any other areas that will be sensitive or painful should always be examined last.**

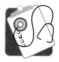

CHAPTER **9**

Biostatistics and Lab Results

> Nothing is more important to the care of the patient than the personal attention of a competent and conscientious physician. There is no substitute for the information a physician can obtain from a careful history and physical examination. This information should guide all diagnostic and therapeutic efforts. Without it, laboratory tests cannot be used effectively, therapeutic plans lack direction, and serious errors in management are likely to occur. The greatest mistake in the practice of internal medicine these days is the tendency to let indiscriminate laboratory testing and diagnostic procedures replace the common sense of the doctor.
>
> *Arnold S. Relman, M.D., MACP*
>
> *A graduate of Columbia University College of Physicians and Surgeons, Dr. Relman completed his residency in Internal Medicine at Yale-New Haven Hospital. In 1977 he was appointed Professor of Medicine at Harvard Medical School, Senior Physician at the Brigham and Women's Hospital and Editor of the* New England Journal of Medicine, *where he became Editor-in-Chief Emeritus in 1991.*

One of the most important skills that you will need to learn is how to "work up" a patient. This involves interviewing and examining a new patient, and then determining what steps need to be taken to diagnose and treat the patient's illness. While many attempts have been made to develop computer systems to help clinicians make diagnostic decisions, such approaches have achieved only limited success and the clinician remains at the forefront in utilizing selected diagnostic tools to practice his or her art. One of the primary tools for diagnosis, as well as for following the course of disease, is the laboratory test.

This chapter will discuss some of the things you need to keep in mind when deciding when to order tests, what tests to order and how to interpret their results. Though some of this is quite complex, the bottom line is simple: **Always know why you are ordering a test, and what you will do with each possible result, before you order it.** This will serve your patient, by reducing false-positive results and inconvenience, as well as society, by cutting down on wasteful medical spending.

I. Ordering tests

A. Routine tests. In the past, most patients admitted to a hospital were given a battery of routine tests, and then, presented with this data, a clinician would make a diagnosis. Many studies have found little use for such "routine" tests. Some years ago, for instance, Durbridge and colleagues randomly selected 1,500 patients to either receive a battery of 50 tests on admission, or to get only the needed ones. They found no difference in mortality, morbidity, length of stay, or any other clinical parameter between those who got the routine battery of tests and those who did not, but they did see higher costs and lower patient satisfaction in the routine-test group.

B. **Scientific method.** Good clinicians use a variant of the scientific method in deciding when to order tests. As you take a history and examine the patient, you should be generating a list of hypotheses as to what may be wrong. Further questions and physical exam findings may narrow this list of hypotheses, called the **differential diagnosis.** Next, you should order only those tests needed to either confirm or rule out these hypotheses; use the results to narrow your list further or to generate new hypotheses. The reiterative method will lead most efficiently to the proper diagnosis.

C. **Consequences.** In addition to considering the chances of getting a false positive or a false negative result when ordering a test (see p. 91), you should think about the consequences of each. The consequences of a false positive HIV test for an individual, for instance, could be huge, including loss of insurance and job, much anguish, and so on. In testing blood in a blood bank, on the other hand, the consequences of a false positive may be small (i.e., you throw away one unit of blood), while the consequences of a false negative may be huge (i.e., a recipient might get infected).

D. **Costs.** In an era of limited medical resources, you should keep in mind the cost of the laboratory tests you are ordering. Although many patients are insured and do not face the full cost of the work-ups you order, we all collectively pay for them through our insurance premiums, co-payments, and our taxes. Being able to conduct cost-effective work-ups will be a much-valued skill for you in the future, and you should get into the habit of thinking about this aspect of medicine early in your career.

E. **Disease prevention and screening**. In addition to working up a patient and determining the specific reason(s) for his or her chief complaint, it is worth remembering that the patient admitted to a hospital may not be an individual who regularly visits a primary physician for health promotion and disease prevention. During your patient's hospital stay, you should consider discussing with your health care team the benefit of offering your patient the opportunity to be screened (e.g., cholesterol level, colonoscopy, etc.) for various conditions and diseases while still hospitalized. Upon discharge from the hospital, it would be appropriate to remind your patient of appropriate ways of promoting health (e.g., quitting smoking, avoiding excessive alcohol consumption, etc.)

II. Interpreting tests

A. **Lab tests and probability.** Lab tests, like most things in life, are not perfect. The best they can do is influence what we think is the probability of a certain (or given) outcome. Before ordering a test, we have some notion of how likely it is that a person has a given disease (called the **pre-test** probability), and the test simply raises or lowers that likelihood (the **post-test** probability).

For instance, suppose a 45-year-old man comes to you with chest pain. After taking a good history and physical examination, you conclude (as we will demonstrate in some detail) that there is a 64% chance that he is having a heart attack. To test this hypothesis, you check his serum creatine phosphokinase-MB (CK-MB), which usually begins to rise 4.8 hours after the onset of symptoms with myocardial infarctions (serum troponin, elevated about 3.8 hours after the onset of symptoms, is most useful in patients who do not have raised CK-MB levels or ST-segment elevation but have an electrocardiogram suggestive of ischemia). If the test is positive (the patient has a serum CK-MB above a certain cutoff value), you raise the probability that he is having a heart attack to 93%, while if the CK-MB is below the cutoff value, you drop the probability to 12%. The basic point of this example is this: **A positive test does not guarantee the patient has the disease, and a negative test does not ensure absence of disease.**

B. **False and true results.** Let us describe this in more detail, using the example of serum CK-MB levels and myocardial infarction. Suppose we did a study in which we measured the CK-MB of 360 men who had chest pain, and then also used another test to definitively diagnose whether they indeed had suffered a heart attack. (Such a definitive test is called a **gold standard**, as it is the basis of comparison for all other tests.) The results of the test are summarized as shown:

	MI	No MI	Total
Test positive (CK-MB ≥80)	215 (a)	16 (b)	231 (a + b)
Test negative (CK-MB <80)	15 (c)	114 (d)	129 (c + d)
Total	230 (a + c)	130 (b + d)	360 (a + b + c + d)

1. **True positives** (a): those who tested positive and really had an MI.
2. **False positives** (b): those who tested positive but did not have an MI.
3. **True negatives** (d): those who tested negative and had no MI.
4. **False negatives** (c): those who tested negative but really did have an MI.

C. **Test characteristics.** How good a test is depends on its rates of false positives and false negatives. Ideally, one would like to have none of either, but in most cases there is a trade-off between them. Thus, as you change the cutoff value of the test, you change the ratio of false positives to false negatives. If we made the CK-MB cutoff value very high (e.g., called the test positive only if CK-MB ≥200), we would have almost no false positives, but we would get many false negatives. If we made the cutoff value low, on the other hand, we would get very few false negatives, but many false positives. We can quantify these characteristics of a test by two measures: the **sensitivity** and the **specificity**.

1. **Sensitivity** (a/[a + c]) tells how well the test does among those with disease; that is, of those who really had a heart attack, how many did we find with our test? In this case, the sensitivity is 215/(215 + 15) = 93%.

2. **Specificity** (d/[b + d]) tells how the test does in the world of the non-diseased; that is, of those without **MI**, how many tested negative? In this case, the specificity is 114/(114 + 16) = 88%.

D. **Predictive values.** These two statistics tell us how good a test is, but in reality we do not know if a person really has the disease or not (if we did, we wouldn't have to do a test at all). What we really want to know is this:

If a test result is positive or negative, what is the probability that the patient either has or does not have the disease?

1. **Positive predictive value** (a/[a + b]) tells us what proportion of those with positive test results really have the disease. Here, if you have a positive test, your probability of having an MI was 215/(215 + 16) = 93%.

2. **Negative predictive value** (d/[c + d]) tells us what proportion of those with negative test results really did not have an MI. In this case, if you had a negative CK-MB test, your probability of not having an MI was 114/(114 + 15) = 88%.

E. **Back to probabilities.** Now we can go back to the statements we made earlier in the chapter. The pretest probability of MI in this situation is also called the:

1. **Prevalence** ([a + c]/[a + b + c + d]), which is the proportion of people in the test group (i.e., men with chest pain) who had an MI. Here, this is 230/360 = 64%.

2. Now we see that a positive test makes the **post-test probability** 93% (the **positive** predictive value), while a negative test makes it 12% (100 minus the **negative** predictive value).

F. **Prevalence and probability.** Note that the positive and negative predictive values of a test are very dependent on the pre-test probability or prevalence of disease. This is an especially important issue in **HIV testing**. The usual initial screening test used for HIV disease is called the ELISA (see Chap. 27), which has a sensitivity of 99.5% and a specificity of 99.2%. (The most commonly used confirmatory test for the presence of HIV virus, when the ELISA test is positive, is the Western blot assay.)

1. **Positive predictive value.** Even with such good test characteristics, the positive predictive value of the ELISA test varies greatly with the pretest probability of disease. For instance, if we know that the prevalence of HIV in gay men in San Francisco is 50%, then the positive predictive value of the test in this group is 99.2%. (This calculation uses Bayes' theorem, which is beyond the scope of this book. You should review or learn it if you do not already know it; see the references at the end of this volume for help. The general idea involves creating grids like the one on p. 91.) On the other hand, if the prevalence of HIV in male army recruits is only 0.16%, the positive predictive value of the test in members of that group is only 16.6%.

2. **Interpreting test results.** Thus, how you interpret a test, even one with extremely high specificity and sensitivity, depends greatly on what you think the pretest probability of the disease is. In gay men in San Francisco, a positive HIV test is more than 99% likely to indicate they are infected with the HIV virus, while in male army recruits, a positive test indicates a less than 17% probability of their having HIV, because there are many more false positives than true positives in this group.

G. In the next few chapters we will discuss several major categories of lab tests. For each category, we will look at the indications for ordering the tests, the basis for interpreting their results, and useful tips for a beginning student. While reading each section, you should keep in mind the concepts discussed in this chapter. Ordering the proper tests and interpreting them correctly is truly one of the hallmarks of an excellent clinician.

REFERENCES

Braunwald E, Fauci AS, Kasper DL, et al. *Harrison's Principles of Internal Medicine.* 15th ed. New York: McGraw Hill, 2001, pp. 13, 1876.

Durbridge TC, Edwards F, Edwards RG, et al. An Evaluation of Multiphasic Screening on Admission to Hospital. *Med J of Australia* 1976;1:703.

Khan F, Sachs HJ, Pechet L, et al. *Guide to Diagnostic Testing.* Philadelphia: Lippincott Williams & Wilkins, 2002, pp. 33–36.

CHAPTER **10**

Hematologic Tests

> The practice of medicine is an art, based on science. With this great increase in our knowledge of the laws governing the processes of life, has been a corresponding, not less remarkable, advance in all that relates to life in disorder, that is, disease.
>
> *Sir William Osler, M.D. (1849–1919)*

After studying medicine at McGill University, Montreal, Osler moved to Philadelphia to become the Chair of Clinical Medicine at the University of Pennsylvania. Appointed Professor of Medicine at the newly opened Johns Hopkins University and first Physician-in-Chief in the Johns Hopkins Hospital, Osler wrote The Principles and Practice of Medicine, *an authoritative textbook, in 1892. In 1905, he was appointed Regius Professor of Medicine at Oxford University. He is hailed as the most influential physician in modern history.*

I. Overview of hematologic tests

A. Reasons for ordering general hematologic tests.
Many laboratory tests that physicians previously ordered routinely for patients are now restricted in their utilization because of specific practices of many managed care companies. Depending on the health maintenance organization (HMO) or preferred provider organization (PPO) the patient subscribes to, reimbursement from these companies for such tests may only be available for certain patient groups or for certain specific indications.

Hematologic tests are generally the least restricted and provide useful information on four general categories of disease processes:

1. **Hematopoietic problems,** such as anemia and leukemia, both of which involve an alteration in the number and function of the blood cells.

2. **Systemic diseases,** especially renal and liver disease, which alter the hematologic environment, causing morphologic and functional changes in the blood cells.

3. **Infection,** which often results in increased total leukocyte count. Depending on whether this increase is predominantly toward early myeloid forms ("shift to the left") or toward lymphoid forms, one can draw a general conclusion about the nature of the insult.

4. **Hemostatic problems,** which often manifest themselves through a prolonged clotting time on one or more of the clotting screens.

B. Specific hematologic tests

1. **Complete blood count (CBC) and red cell indices.** In most hospitals, the CBC is a mechanized spectrophotometric analysis of an anticoagulated specimen of the peripheral blood. It results in a reasonably accurate estimate of the number, size, and hemoglobin content of the erythrocytes. The reported results include the **hematocrit** (Hct), the **red blood cell count** (RBC) and **white blood cell count** (WBC), the **hemoglobin concentration** (Hgb), and the red cell morphologic indices **mean corpuscular volume** (MCV), **mean corpuscular hemoglobin** (MCH), **mean corpuscular hemoglobin concentration** (MCHC), and **red blood cell distribution width** (RDW). See Table 10–1 for normal values.

2. **Differential white cell count.** The differential (commonly called the "diff"), either done by machine or manually by a technician, is a quantitation of the proportions of different types of leukocytes in the smear of the patient's peripheral blood. It is reported as the percent of total leukocytes made up by each individual type of white cell.

3. **Blood smear analysis** involves an inspection, under high magnification, of the size and appearance of the red and white cells.

4. **Platelet count and clotting indices** are mechanized tests that screen for hemostatic problems. The usual battery of hemostatic tests includes, in addition to a platelet count, a **prothrombin time** (PT) and an **activated partial thromboplastin time** (aPTT, usually referred to simply as the PTT). Other clotting-factor tests may be ordered if the results of the initial screening battery are abnormal, or if a specific defect is suspected. Because commercial assays vary in sensitivity, the same plasma sample may yield many PT values depending on the thromboplastin used. The INR **(international normalized ratio)** represents a normalization of these values using an international reference (for example, the desired INR for effective prevention of deep vein thrombosis is 2.0–3.0)

5. **Erythrocyte sedimentation rate** (ESR) is a non-specific test that is loosely correlated with the serum levels of fibrinogen and globulin. It is especially useful in screening for malignancy, connective tissue disorders, and infection, and in following the course of chronic inflammatory disease states.

C. Analyzing and interpreting results of hematologic tests

1. **Complete blood count (CBC) and indices**

   a. The **hematocrit** and the **red blood cell count** are reflections of the concentration of erythrocytes in the blood. Although the hematocrit will usually indicate whether or not the patient has some degree of anemia, you must analyze it together with the hemoglobin concentration and the red cell indices to determine the class of anemia (e.g., hypochromic microcytic versus normochromic normocytic) and to gain insight into the etiology of the anemia.

Table 10-1. Complete blood count (CBC): Normal values and ranges

Hct:	Men: 47 ± 7.0
	Women: 42 ± 5.0
Hgb:	Men: 14–18 gm/100 ml
	Women: 12–16 gm/100 ml
MCV:	85–100 μm3; MCH: 28–31 pg; MCHC: 30–35%
RBC:	Diameter: 7.3–7.5 μ
	Men: 4.2–5.4 × 10⁶ cells/mm³
	Women: 3.6–5.0 × 10⁶ cells/mm³
	Reticulocytes: 0.5–1.5%
WBC:	Total: 4–11 × 10³ cells/mm³
	Diff
	PMN: 40–75%
	Lymphocytes: 15–45%
	Eosinophils: 1–6%
	Basophils: 0–2%
	Monocytes: 1–10%
Platelets:	145–375 × 10³/mm³
PT:	Depends on lab; usually ~ 12–14 sec. Always given with control; should be within 2 secs of control.
aPTT:	Depends on lab; usually 25–45 sec. Always given with control; should be within 4 secs of control.
ESR:	Wintrobe
	Men: 0–5 mm/hr
	Women: 0–15 mm/hr
	Westergren
	Men: 0–15 mm/hr
	Women: 0–20 mm/hr

b. The **red cell indices** represent average values for the size and hemoglobin content of the red cells. The RDW, by contrast, is calculated by automated counters and is essentially a mathematical representation of anisocytosis (i.e., variation in red blood cell size); increases suggest a mixed population of cells. The red cell indices are calculated as follows:

$$MCV = \frac{Hct\ (\%) \times 10}{RBC\ (millions/mm^3)}$$

Normal range is 85–100 μm³.

$$MCH = \frac{Hgb\ (gm/100\ ml) \times 10}{RBC\ (millions/mm^3)}$$

Normal range is 28–31 pg.

$$MCHC = \frac{Hgb\ (gm/100\ ml)}{Hct\ (\%)}$$

Normal range is 30–35%.

Fig. 10–1 represents an approach to the differential diagnosis of anemia based on the red cell indices and the reticulocyte count.

c. The **total white blood cell count** is useful both as a diagnostic tool and in following the course of diseases. Shown below are the most common types of processes associated with decreased and increased WBC values.

  (1) Processes consistent with **WBC decrease:**

    (a) Infections, especially overwhelming bacterial infection, septicemia, and so on.

    (b) Viral infections: infectious mononucleosis, hepatitis, influenza.

    (c) Drugs, for example, sulfonamides, antibiotics.

    (d) Radiation and cytotoxic chemotherapy.

    (e) Hematologic diseases: pernicious and aplastic anemia.

  (2) Processes consistent with **WBC increase:**

    (a) Acute infections: pneumonia, meningitis, rheumatic fever, septicemia.

    (b) Intoxications: uremia, acidosis, eclampsia, chemical poisoning, drugs (e.g., prednisone).

    (c) Leukemia.

2. **Differential white blood cell count.** This reflects the response of the bone marrow hematopoietic feedback systems to physiologic and pathologic processes. Although the differential is usually too nonspecific to suggest an exact diagnosis, it is a fairly convenient way of following the course of many types of diseases, especially infections and neoplastic processes. For these two types of disease, it is also useful to analyze the maturity of the various leukocyte types. In general, high numbers of immature cells in the peripheral blood reflect either a "push on the marrow" to produce these cells in large quantities (e.g., a common manifestation of a bacterial pneumonia is a "shift to the left," with high numbers of immature granulocytes [bands] seen on the diff) or a developmental arrest suggesting primary hematologic disease. The following images show the disease processes associated with increases and decreases in the proportions of the various specific leukocyte types reported on the diff.

a. **Granulocytes**

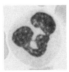

(polymorphonuclear [PMN])
Increase consistent with bacterial infections (endocarditis, pneumonia, septicemia), granulocytic leukemia, burns, eclampsia, RBC destruction, diabetic ketoacidosis, uremia, steroids, pancreatitis.
Decrease consistent with drugs, viral infections, bone marrow invasion or aplasia, dialysis, hypoadrenalism, hypopituitarism, severe bacterial infections, mononucleosis, low B_{12} or folate.

b. **Lymphocytes**

Increase consistent with viral infections (influenza, chicken pox, mononucleosis, infectious hepatitis, and other viral infections), tuberculosis (TB), lymphocytic leukemias.

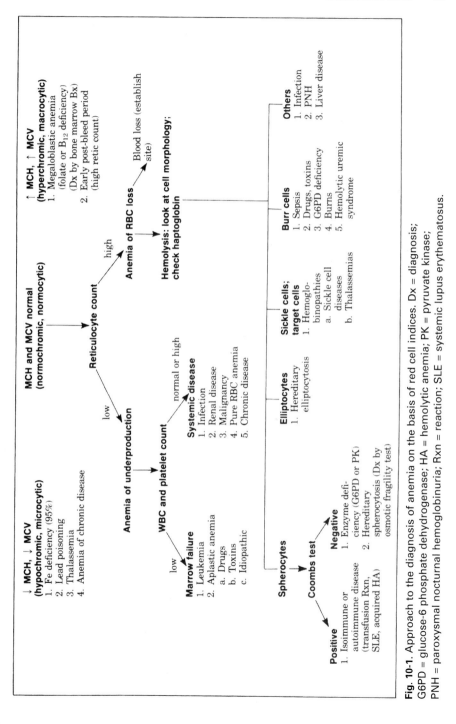

Fig. 10-1. Approach to the diagnosis of anemia on the basis of red cell indices. Dx = diagnosis; G6PD = glucose-6 phosphate dehydrogenase; HA = hemolytic anemia; PK = pyruvate kinase; PNH = paroxysmal nocturnal hemoglobinuria; Rxn = reaction; SLE = systemic lupus erythematosus.

c. **Monocytes**
   Increase consistent with monocytic leukemia, TB, myeloproliferative disorders, Hodgkin's disease (HD), lipid storage diseases,
   subacute bacterial endocarditis (SBE), collagen vascular disease
   (rheumatoid arthritis [RA], systemic lupus erythematosus [SLE]),
   chronic infection or inflammation, ulcerative colitis.

d. **Eosinophils**
   Increase consistent with allergic disorders (asthma, hay fever), parasitic infection, collagen vascular disease, pernicious anemia, Addison's disease, neoplasm, pulmonary disease.
   Decrease consistent with hypercortisolism, infections, burns, stress,
   trauma.

e. **Basophils**
   Increase consistent with chronic myelogenous leukemia (CML),
   polycythemia, myeloid metaplasia, hypothyroidism, infection.

3. **Blood smear analysis.** While the WBC differential is concerned primarily with the association between disease processes and the **proportions** of various leukocytes seen in the blood, the blood smear analysis
   is concerned primarily with the association between disease processes
   and red and white blood cell **morphology.** Since the morphology of
   blood cells is a function of both **intracellular events** and **extracellular
   environment,** analysis of the peripheral smear is a simple and powerful
   screening test for assessing systemic disease as well as cellular metabolic pathology.

   Table 10-2 shows the most significant abnormalities commonly noted in
   red cells and leukocytes (together with the pathophysiologic basis for
   these abnormalities) and the common differential diagnoses associated
   with them.

4. **Platelet count and clotting indices.** The platelet count and clotting
   indices are reflections of the state of the patient's hemostatic systems.
   Fig. 10-2 reviews the classic model of the coagulation cascade and
   illustrates which factors are measured by the **PT** and **aPTT.** Recent
   evidence shows that the actual workings of coagulation are more complex than this simple cascade model, with positive and negative feedback loops between many of the factors.

   a. **Platelet counts are increased** with malignancy, myeloproliferative
      diseases, post-surgery or post-splenectomy states, collagen vascular
      disorders (rheumatoid arthritis), Fe^{2+} deficiency anemia, bleeding,
      acute infection, primary thrombocytosis, CML, polycythemia vera,
      trauma, thrombocytosis. **Note** that the platelet is an acute phase
      reactant.

   b. **Platelet counts are decreased** with idiopathic thrombocytopenic
      purpura (ITP), marrow invasion or aplasia, hypersplenism, cytotoxic
      therapy, DIC, mononucleosis, viral infections, thrombotic thrombo-
      cytopenic purpura (TTP).

5. **Erythrocyte sedimentation rate.** Because it is so nonspecific, the ESR
   is most useful in deciding between sets of disease states that may have
   similar presentations but different degrees of inflammatory reaction and

Table 10-2. Abnormalities of red cells and white cells

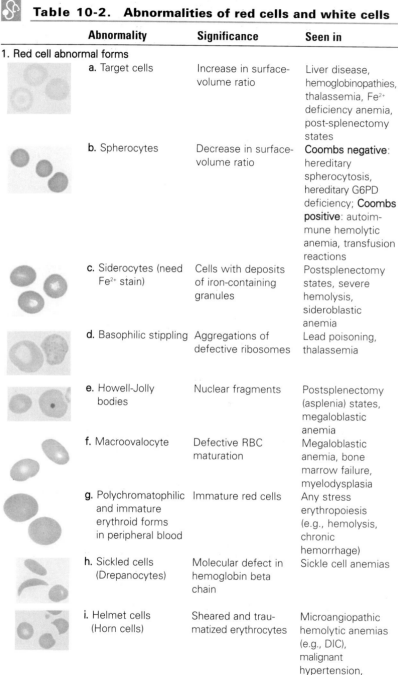

	Abnormality	Significance	Seen in
1. Red cell abnormal forms			
	a. Target cells	Increase in surface-volume ratio	Liver disease, hemoglobinopathies, thalassemia, Fe^{2+} deficiency anemia, post-splenectomy states
	b. Spherocytes	Decrease in surface-volume ratio	**Coombs negative:** hereditary spherocytosis, hereditary G6PD deficiency; **Coombs positive:** autoimmune hemolytic anemia, transfusion reactions
	c. Siderocytes (need Fe^{2+} stain)	Cells with deposits of iron-containing granules	Postsplenectomy states, severe hemolysis, sideroblastic anemia
	d. Basophilic stippling	Aggregations of defective ribosomes	Lead poisoning, thalassemia
	e. Howell-Jolly bodies	Nuclear fragments	Postsplenectomy (asplenia) states, megaloblastic anemia
	f. Macroovalocyte	Defective RBC maturation	Megaloblastic anemia, bone marrow failure, myelodysplasia
	g. Polychromatophilic and immature erythroid forms in peripheral blood	Immature red cells	Any stress erythropoiesis (e.g., hemolysis, chronic hemorrhage)
	h. Sickled cells (Drepanocytes)	Molecular defect in hemoglobin beta chain	Sickle cell anemias
	i. Helmet cells (Horn cells)	Sheared and traumatized erythrocytes	Microangiopathic hemolytic anemias (e.g., DIC), malignant hypertension, uremia, burns

Table 10-2. Abnormalities of red cells and white cells

	Abnormality	Significance	Seen in
	j. Teardrop cells (Dacryocytes)	Deformed RBC membrane	Marrow infiltration, myeloproliferative syndromes, extramedullary hematopoiesis
	k. Reticulocytes (need special stain)	RNA network visible in very young RBC	Any state of high erythropoietic activity, e.g., post-bleed, post-Fe^{2+} treatment for anemia
2. White cell abnormal forms			
	a. Toxic granules in PMN	Reaction to sepsis	Infection or inflammatory disease
	b. Dohle bodies in PMN	Ribosome-containing immature granules	Infection, burns
	c. Hypersegmented PMN	Abnormality of nuclear division or chromatin	Folate or B_{12} deficiency, marrow failure
	d. Auer rods (in myeloblasts)	Clumped granule material	AML, AMoL
	e. Atypical lymphocytes (vacuolated cytoplasm; elongated nucleus; nucleoli)	Activated T cells or lymphoblasts	Infectious mononucleosis, viral infections, immunologic reactions
	f. Bacteria in PMN	Phagocytosed bacteria	Severe infection

antibody formation. For instance, the ESR may be useful in deciding between rheumatoid arthritis (increased) and degenerative joint disease (normal).

    a. Increased ESR values are seen with acute MI, infection, rheumatic fever, malignancy, myeloma, collagen vascular diseases (RA, SLE), pregnancy, tuberculosis, active hepatitis, inflammatory necrosis.

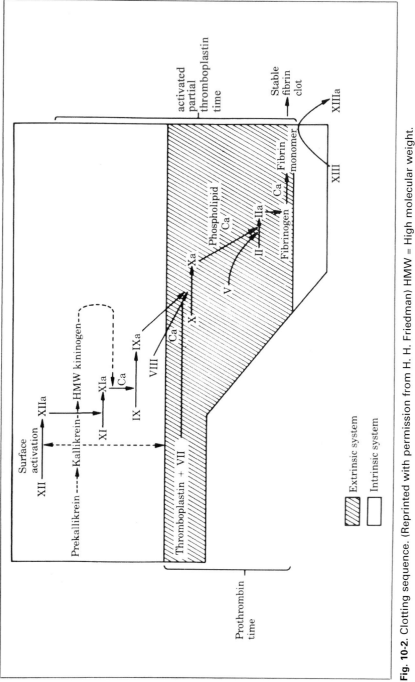

Fig. 10-2. Clotting sequence. (Reprinted with permission from H. H. Friedman) HMW = High molecular weight.

A very high ESR (more than 100 mm/hr) may suggest temporal arteritis or polymyalgia rheumatica, osteomyelitis, endocarditis, malignancy, or an abscess.

b. **Decreased ESR values are seen** with sickle cell anemia, polycythemia, congestive heart failure (CHF), diabetes insipidus (DI), and trichinosis.

II. Practical points concerning hematologic tests

A. Complete blood count (CBC) and indices

1. Remember that the red cell indices are mechanically calculated as the average of a great many cells. **Look at the smear** yourself, or order a peripheral smear to be performed by the hospital laboratory, to confirm that the erythrocytes are morphologically homogeneous. Multiple erythrocyte populations with mathematically compensatory abnormalities may result in falsely normal results.

2. You can get a good estimate of the hematocrit by multiplying the hemoglobin by three (e.g., a Hgb of 10 predicts a Hct of 30). Also note that, because the MCHC depends on these interlinked Hgb and Hct values, it will almost always be approximately 33 (and is therefore relatively useless).

3. When discussing a patient's problems, always state the **type of anemia** (e.g., microcytic hypochromic). Strictly speaking, anemia is not a disease; it is a family of diseases. You must specify the nature of the anemia. This will help the listener narrow down the various etiologies of the specific type of anemia.

4. Remember that the most common etiology of anemia is **iron deficiency**, which results in microcytic hypochromic erythrocytes. This is a very common finding, especially among menstruating women.

5. **Bleeding** can produce either a normochromic normocytic or hyperchromic macrocytic picture. In a patient with a normal hematocrit who becomes anemic over the course of a few hours, always think about an acute bleed.

6. In working up an anemia of unknown etiology, always guaiac the stool to help rule out **gastrointestinal bleeding.**

B. Differential white cell count

1. The differential is a relatively expensive test and is probably overordered in most hospitals. You can sometimes perform your own minidifferential simply by requesting to look at the smear and quickly scanning the field for **PMN band forms**. If the smear shows more than a few percent bands, the sample is probably left-shifted.

2. Remember to look at the **eosinophil count** in patients with allergic disorders. A high eosinophil count may be seen in parasitic infections, allergic conditions, asthma, and Addison's desease. (A mnemonic for remembering which problems are associated with high eosinophil levels: **worms, wheezes, weird diseases.**)

C. Blood smear analysis

1. Make friends with the **technicians** in the hematology lab. You should

try to look at each smear you order (or at least the interesting ones) with the technicians—it is a great way to learn more about your patients' diseases.

2. Learn to scan the microscopic field with an eye to four parameters: (1) **cell size,** (2) **cell shape,** (3) **nuclear shape,** and (4) **cytoplasmic inclusions.** As in all lab tests, you should think about the patient's clinical history while looking at the smear. (Is there a history of liver disease? If so, does the peripheral smear show acanthocytosis?) Ask yourself not only, "What do I see?" but also, "What do I not see?"

D. Platelet count and clotting indices

1. Specific factor deficiency tests are expensive and should not be ordered routinely. Remember that abnormalities on clotting screens are more commonly due to **systemic disease** (e.g., liver failure) than to congenital factor deficiencies.

2. Because the platelets are important in the **primary hemostatic reaction** but play virtually no role in clotting, a hemophiliac with normal platelet levels will usually have a normal bleeding time.

E. Erythrocyte sedimentation rate. There are three different ways to test the ESR: the Wintrobe and Landsberg, the Westergren, and the zeta methods. The normal values differ for each method, as well as for men and women. Always check what the technicians in your hospital lab consider a normal ESR.

REFERENCES

Anderson SC and Paulsen KB. *Atlas of Hematology.* Philadelphia: Lippincott Williams & Wilkins, 2003.

Friedman HH. *Problem-Oriented Medical Diagnosis.* 5ᵗʰ ed. Boston: Little, Brown, 1989.

Matthews AM. *Pocket Labs: Laboratory Medicine Study Cards.* Philadelphia: Lippincott Williams & Wilkins, 2001, pp. 3, 20.

McGovern JP and Roland CG, eds. *The Collected Essays of Sir William Osler, Volume II: The Educational Essays.* New York: Gryphon Editions, 1985, p. 36.

CHAPTER **11**

Serum Chemistry Tests

Time can be a physician's ally and a legitimate diagnostic test. The desire to reach a rapid diagnosis is often medically and economically justifiable. But in many instances, when the answer is not readily revealed, the pressure to find the diagnosis need not force the clinician to obtain more and more tests and to engage in ever more invasive procedures. Time allows a disease process to "declare itself" (or go away). The physician working in close communication with the patient can use time with little risk.

Thomas P. Stossel, M.D.

A graduate of Harvard Medical School, Dr. Stossel was Chief of the Division of Hematology and Medical Oncology in the Department of Medicine at Massachusetts General Hospital prior to establishing the Division of Experimental Medicine at the Brigham and Women's Hospital in 1991. A former President of the American Society of Hematology, he is Co-Director of the Division of Hematology and Oncology in the Department of Medicine at the Brigham and the American Cancer Society Professor of Medicine at Harvard Medical School.

I. Outline of serum chemistry tests

A. Indications for ordering serum chemistry tests. Serum chemistry tests have become an important part of modern medical management. In general, they are ordered for four reasons:

1. To aid in medical **diagnosis.**

2. To allow the physician to **follow the course** of a problem or treatment regimen.

3. To monitor **fluid and electrolyte balance.**

4. To **screen for occult disease.**

   Chemistry tests are usually run in batteries of 6 to 20, which are run at the same time on a single machine. One such battery is the BMP, the basic metabolic panel, which consists of a set of electrolytes (Na, K, Cl, HCO_3), a measure of renal function—BUN (blood urea nitrogen) and serum creatinine—and serum glucose. Though many clinicians routinely order these batteries both on admission and at times during a patient's hospitalization, you should always ask yourself why you are ordering each test, and what you would do with abnormal results.

   This chapter covers 22 of the most important serum tests, providing short lists of common diseases associated with abnormal values for these tests, and some essential points related to their interpretation. Further clinical points related to serum chemistries in general are included in sec. II of this chapter.

B. **Interpreting serum chemistry tests.** The following lists of physiologic and pathologic conditions associated with lab abnormalities include only some of the more common serum chemistry correlates. For a more complete treatment of the general subject, see Khan's *Guide to Diagnostic Testing*. The numbers in parentheses indicate normal ranges for these tests.

1. **Sodium** (136–145 mEq/L)

   a. **Increase:** dehydration, diabetes insipidus (DI), Cushing's syndrome, hyperaldosteronism.

   b. **Decrease:** congestive heart failure (CHF), diuretic use, syndrome of inappropriate antidiuretic hormone (SIADH).

   c. **Note:**

      (1) Hyperlipidemia and hyperglycemia are causes of spurious hyponatremia. For each 100 mg/dl increase in blood glucose above normal, you should correct the serum sodium by adding 1.6 mEq/L. For example, in a patient with a glucose of 700 and sodium of 130, the corrected sodium would be $130 + (1.6 \times 6) = 140$.

      (2) Most hyponatremia is secondary to free water retention (in excess of retained sodium) rather than to sodium loss.

2. **Potassium** (3.5–5.2 mEq/L)

   a. **Increase:** renal failure, acidosis, iatrogenic cause, mineralocorticoid deficiency.

   b. **Decrease:** metabolic alkalosis, diuretic use, mineralocorticoid excess.

   c. **Note:**

      (1) RBC hemolysis in blood sample acquisition, as sometimes occurs in blood collection through small gauge catheters, can spuriously increase serum potassium.

      (2) Thrombocytosis (increased platelet count) spuriously elevates serum potassium.

      (3) Alterations in serum potassium may produce electrocardiogram (ECG) changes, including peaked T waves, wide QRS, and loss of P wave in hyperkalemia; and flattening of T wave and presence of U waves in hypokalemia.

3. **Chloride** (96–108 mEq/L)

   a. **Increase:** dehydration, non-anion gap metabolic acidosis, hyperalimentation, mineralocorticoid deficiency.

   b. **Decrease:** diuretic use, CHF, SIADH, compensated respiratory acidosis, vomiting.

   c. **Note:**

(1) Hypochloremia is the most common cause of metabolic alkalosis.

(2) The laboratory method for measuring chloride is a nonspecific test for halides; hence, bromides and iodides may spuriously elevate serum chloride.

4. **Bicarbonate** (24–30 mEq/L). The serum bicarbonate level can be a **crucial gauge of disease severity,** as in sepsis, and as a marker of disease presence (a decrease in serum bicarbonate from metabolic acidosis is part of the triad of findings, along with hyperglycemia and ketone production, seen in diabetic ketoacidosis).

   a. **Increase:** dehydration ("concentration alkalosis"), compensated respiratory acidosis.

   b. **Decrease:** metabolic acidosis of any cause, compensated respiratory alkalosis.

5. **Anion gap** (10–12 mEq). The anion gap represents unmeasured anions and is calculated as the difference, in milliequivalents, between serum sodium and the sum of serum chloride and bicarbonate.

   a. **Increase:** renal failure/uremia, lactic acidosis, ketoacidosis, salicylate toxicity, ethylene glycol ingestion, methanol ingestion.

   b. **Decrease:** multiple myeloma, bromide ingestion, polycythemia vera, disseminated intravascular coagulation (DIC), pregnancy.

   c. **Note:**

      (1) Use of the anion gap helps to distinguish between two types of metabolic acidosis: hyperchloremic metabolic acidosis (the type associated with a *normal* anion gap) and high-anion gap metabolic acidosis.

      (2) The anion gap is technically described as the difference, in milliequivalents, between the sum of the positively-charged electrolytes (sodium plus potassium) and the sum of the negatively-charged electrolytes (chloride plus bicarbonate), but most people ignore the potassium because its contribution to the total result is relatively negligible. From a practical standpoint, either method may be used.

6. **BUN** (6–26 mg/dl)

   a. **Increase:** renal failure of all types, accelerated protein catabolism (e.g., gastrointestinal [GI] bleed), dehydration.

   b. **Decrease:** liver damage, protein deficiency states.

7. **Creatinine** (0.7–1.3 mg/dl). Affected by muscle mass and turnover as well as renal function.

   a. **Increase:** renal failure, muscle disease, increased muscle mass.

   b. **Decrease:** rarely clinically significant.

   c. **Note:**

      (1) Creatinine is a more specific indicator of renal disease than BUN.

(2) The BUN-creatinine ratio is sometimes helpful in distinguishing prerenal azotemia (>20) from intrinsic renal disease producing azotemia (<20).

(3) Hemodialysis of patients with chronic renal failure (CRF) usually normalizes BUN; creatinine, however, may not change at all with dialysis.

8. **Glucose** (fasting, 65–110 mg/dl)

   a. **Increase:** diabetes mellitus (DM), pregnancy, stress, pancreatic disease, impaired fasting glucose (a precursor of DM).

   b. **Decrease:** reactive hypoglycemia, pancreatic islet-cell tumors, starvation, liver disease.

   c. **Note:**

   (1) Measuring the fasting blood sugar (FBS) is the fastest and most convenient method to document the level of glucose in emergency situations and to determine the need to make adjustments in dosages of insulin and other diabetic medications in hospitalized patients. Having patients keep a diary of fasting blood sugar values they record over days and weeks in the outpatient setting is likewise helpful in making such adjustments.

   (2) Be careful of **spuriously high readings** from blood drawn from a site above an IV line containing dextrose.

9. **Calcium** (9.0–11.0 mg/dl)

   a. **Increase:** malignancies, primary hyperparathyroidism.

   b. **Decrease:** hypoparathyroidism, CRF, malabsorption syndromes, vitamin D deficiency, hypoalbuminemia.

   c. **Note:**

   (1) Free ionized calcium is the physiologically important form of the cation; hence, correction must be made for the concentration of the major calcium-binding protein, albumin. (Correction = 0.8 mg/1.0 mg change in albumin.) A patient, for instance, with a calcium level of 8.0 mg/dl and an albumin level of 3.0 mg/dl (1.0 mg/dl less than the normal value of albumin, generally rounded to 4.0 mg/dl) actually has a corrected calcium level of 8.8 mg/dl.

   (2) Changes in serum calcium are reflected in the ECG. An increase in calcium shortens the Q–T interval while a decrease in serum calcium lengthens the Q–T interval.

10. **Phosphorus** (2.5–4.2 mg/dl)

    a. **Increase:** CRF, hypoparathyroidism, vitamin D excess, bone disease.

    b. **Decrease:** alcoholism, nutritional deficiency states, hyperparathyroidism, diabetes, gout, antacid use.

    c. **Note:** Hypophosphatemia can decrease myocardial contractility and effective tissue oxygenation (through decreased production of 2,3-DPG).

11. **Albumin** (3.5–5.5 gm/dl)

    a. **Increase:** rarely clinically significant.

    b. **Decrease:** chronic disease, nutritional deficiency states, protein-losing enteropathy.

12. **Total protein** (6.0–8.5 gm/dl)

    a. **Increase:** multiple myeloma.

    b. **Decrease:** chronic disease, protein-losing enteropathy.

    c. **Note:** The difference between the levels of total protein and albumin is the amount of globulin.

13. **Amylase** (5–75 IU/L)

    a. **Increase:** pancreatitis, mumps, parotitis, duodenal ulcer, ectopic pregnancy, diabetic ketoacidosis, biliary tract disease, peritonitis, macroamylasemia.

    b. **Decrease:** pancreatic destruction.

    c. **Note:**

       (1) Almost any intra-abdominal process can elevate serum amylase.

       (2) Salivary gland amylase and pancreatic amylase are different isozymes and can be distinguished by electrophoretic analysis.

       (3) The amylase-to-creatinine clearance ratio may be useful in distinguishing macroamylasemia (<1%) and other causes of increased amylase from pancreatitis (>5%).

       (4) An increase in lipase, when amylase is elevated, suggests pancreatitis unless proven otherwise.

14. **Uric acid** (1.5–8.0 mg/dl)

    a. **Increase:** gout, asymptomatic hyperuricemia, renal failure, cancer with rapid tumor cell turnover, use of thiazide diuretics.

    b. **Decrease:** allopurinol use, uricosuric-agent use, Hodgkin's disease, Wilson's disease, aspirin ingestion.

    c. **Note:** The greatest acute risk in elevated uric acid is the development of uric acid nephropathy, particularly in patients receiving chemotherapy. This can be avoided by adequate hydration, allopurinol therapy, and urinary alkalinization.

15. **Cholesterol** [desirable total cholesterol 140–200; see p. 112]

    a. **Increase:** hypercholesterolemia, hyperlipidemia, biliary tract obstruction, pancreatitis, hypothyroidism.

    b. **Decrease:** starvation, chronic disease, hyperthyroidism.

    c. **Note:**

       (1) Cholesterol levels increase postprandially.

       (2) Elevated total cholesterol levels are a risk factor for coronary heart disease (CHD), and thus this is an important screening test for the general population. Other related risk factors for CHD include elevated low-density lipoproteins (LDLs) and triglyc-

erides, as well as low high-density lipoprotein (HDL) cholesterol.

(3) In persons with high total cholesterol, fasting triglycerides and
HDL levels should be measured, and then the LDL fraction calculated using Friedewald's formula (total cholesterol = [HDL +
LDL + triglycerides]/5). An LDL level under 100 is considered
desirable. Patients with either high cholesterol, or borderline-
high values in addition to other risk factors for heart disease
should consider lifestyle changes and/or have pharmacologic
intervention implemented.

16. **Bilirubin** (total 0.2–1.0 mg/dl; direct <0.2 mg/dl; indirect <0.8 mg/dl)

    a. **Increase: direct (conjugated) hyperbilirubinemia** (biliary obstruc-
    tion, hepatitis), **indirect (unconjugated) hyperbilirubinemia**
    (hemolysis, Gilbert's syndrome).

    b. **Decrease:** rarely clinically significant.

    c. **Note:** The most prevalent cause of mild, asymptomatic unconjugated
    hyperbilirubinemia is Gilbert's syndrome.

17. **Alkaline phosphatase** (30–115 units/L)

    a. **Increase:** biliary tract obstruction, bone disease (especially Paget's
    disease), women in their third trimester of pregnancy.

    b. **Decrease:** rarely clinically significant.

    c. **Note:**

    (1) Heat fractionation helps distinguish alkaline phosphatase of
    hepatic origin from that of bone origin ("bone burns"). Elec-
    trophoretic analysis of isozymes is useful but less widely avail-
    able.

    (2) The finding of an elevated alkaline phosphatase but a normal 5'-
    nucleotidase or gamma-glutamyltransferase (GGT) level should
    prompt an evaluation for bone diseases.

18. **AST** (8–20 U/L), and **ALT** (8–20 U/L). Aspartate aminotransferase
(AST) was previously known as serum glutamic-oxaloacetic transaminase (SGOT), and alanine aminotransferase (ALT) was known as serum
glutamic-pyruvic transaminase (SGPT). Generally, changes in these two
enzymes parallel each other.

    a. **Increase:** myocardial infarction (MI), alcohol-related liver injury,
    chronic hepatitis B and C, autoimmune hepatitis, hepatic steatosis,
    celiac sprue, other hepatocellular diseases, CHF, muscle disease,
    hemolysis, medications.

    b. **Decrease:** rarely clinically significant.

    c. **Note:**

    (1) Increased AST levels can help in diagnosis of MI, when used in
    the context of other abnormal chemistries, for example, an ele-
    vated creatine phosphokinase-MB fraction (CPK-MB). See
    Chap. 19 for further discussion.

(2) Elevations of AST, ALT, and lactate dehydrogenase (LDH) suggest hepatocellular disease, whereas elevations of alkaline phosphatase and bilirubin suggest obstructive liver disease.

(3) ALT is more elevated than AST in viral hepatitis, and AST is elevated more than ALT (usually by a ratio greater than 2:1, especially when AST and ALT are each greater than 100 U/L) in alcoholic hepatitis.

19. **LDH** (lactate dehydrogenase; 45–100 units/L)

   a. **Increase:** MI, CHF, hepatitis, pulmonary embolus, muscle disease, neoplasia, hemolysis.

   b. **Decrease:** rarely clinically significant.

   c. **Note:** There are five isozymes of LDH, which can be electrophoretically fractionated. This fractionation may be useful in distinguishing LDH elevations of myocardial origin (isoenzymes I and II) from that of other sources. An LDH_1–LDH_2 ratio greater than 1 may be used to help predict recent MI (within the past 3–5 days); LDH_5 is greater than LDH_4 in liver diseases. LDH fractionation is not commonly performed today in the setting of an acute coronary syndrome, its usefulness having been supplanted by the introduction of more sensitive and specific cardiac markers (e.g., troponin, myoglobin), though the value of total LDH is still commonly reported and of use in gauging the extent of an MI.

20. **CPK** (creatine phosphokinase; in women 50–60 IU/L, in men 50–180 IU/L). This cardiac enzyme is also often abbreviated as **CK**.

   a. **Increase:** MI, striated muscle necrosis, cerebrovascular accident, hypothyroidism.

   b. **Decrease:** rarely clinically significant.

   c. **Note:**

   (1) Isozyme fractionation of CPK produces three bands: MM (striated muscle), MB (cardiac muscle), and BB (brain). The MB band (normally less than 6 percent) is elevated in an acute MI, but other sources of MB-band CPK include tongue and diaphragm. The BB band is elevated in cerebrovascular accidents only if the blood-brain barrier is interrupted. See Chap. 19 for a diagram of the time course of elevation after MI.

   (2) CPK is increased in hypothyroidism and renal failure because of decreased renal clearance.

21. **Troponin I** (values vary with each assay) and **troponin T** (0.1 to 0.2 ng/ml). Troponin I and T are regulatory proteins found in skeletal and cardiac muscle. Cardiac isoforms are specific for troponin I and T, and are completely specific to the myocardium in adults.

   a. **Increase**: MI, unstable angina, CHF.

   b. **Note:**

   (1) The rate of change of troponin is more important than the absolute value. An increase without a rate change is seen more often with unstable angina and CHF.

(2) Troponin rises about 3.8 hours after the onset of symptoms (compared with 4.8 hours for CPK-MB) in an MI and peaks at about 12 hours. Because it remains elevated for about 10 days before it normalizes, unlike CPK-MB, troponin is helpful in assessing the meaning of cardiac symptoms that last for longer than a few hours or days.

(3) The absence of increased troponin levels does not by itself rule out an MI.

22. **Myoglobin** (values vary, depending on the lab) is another cardiac marker that doubles within 2 hours of presentation with an acute MI and peaks at about 4 hours. Serial measurements of myoglobin are more sensitive than CPK-MB for MI, but they are less specific.

II. Practical points concerning the serum chemistries

A. Ordering serum chemistry tests

1. At many hospitals, you can **order just one test**, even though tests are done as automated batteries. If all you really care about is the potassium concentration, try ordering just that test rather than a full electrolyte panel. Also, because lab tests are generally done as automated batteries, you often can call the lab and get results of lab tests not originally requested.

2. Learn to think of serum chemistry tests in **groups**:

   a. The electrolytes (Na, K, Cl, HCO_3).

   b. Kidney function tests (BUN, creatinine). Also helpful in assessing fluid status.

   c. Liver function tests (AST, ALT, albumin, total protein, bilirubin, alkaline phosphatase). Since some of these tests are actually a measure of damage to the liver cell membrane, some people consider **albumin/protein, cholesterol**, and the **prothrombin time** as "true" markers of liver function.

   d. Acute MI enzymes (troponin, myoglobin, CPK-MB, AST, LDH). Some physicians order a C-reactive protein (CRP), a non-specific test of inflammation, in the work-up of a suspected acute MI. In 2003, myeloperoxidase elevation was proposed as a novel marker of plaque vulnerability in persons presenting to the emergency department with chest pain.

   e. Metabolic bone disease tests (Ca, P, alkaline phosphatase).

3. **Know the status** of each lab test that you have ordered (i.e., keep track of whether it has been officially ordered, drawn, received in the lab, and finished). Know the results for patients you are following; remember that you may call the lab to learn the results if they have not yet made it back to the ward or to the patient's chart in the outpatient setting. A big part of learning to be an effective and efficient clinical clerk is knowing how to keep track of the progress of your patient's work-up.

4. Note that the electrolytes, BUN, creatinine, and glucose are often recorded quickly using a "standardized" lattice pattern:

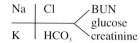

B. Interpreting serum chemistry tests

1. While it is easy to learn a simple collection of common variations in serum chemistries and their causes, it is not very practical. On the wards, you usually will not be faced with an isolated abnormal lab value (except for alkaline phosphatase or glucose); more often you will be confronted with a group of abnormal values derived from all the tests done in your test battery. For this reason, it is more helpful to learn to recognize **common clinical patterns of abnormal routine serum chemistries**, such as those shown below. Note that in these examples the combination of values helps suggest a more limited and directed diagnosis than would any single abnormal value.

165	120	50		135	100	80
		100				100
5.0	30	1.5		7.0	10	10.5

   Dehydration   **Renal failure**

124	80	60		150	120	40
		100				480
3.0	35	1.0		5.0	10	1.5

   Excessive diuretic use   **Diabetic ketoacidosis**

2. Remember that **lab, or measurement, error** is a common explanation for abnormal serum chemistry results. A wise clinician will try to repeat a lab test or confirm an abnormal result by some other test (e.g., an ECG can sometimes help confirm a very high serum potassium) before acting on a lab result that does not seem appropriate for the clinical picture.

3. When prescribing any **medication**, keep in mind which lab tests you would expect to be altered by the administration of the drug. Watch these test results carefully over the following few days, and use them to assess the efficacy or toxicity of your regimen. For example, diuretics commonly lead to hypokalemia.

REFERENCES

Brennan ML, Penn MS, Lente FV, et al. Prognostic value myeloperoxidase in patients with chest pain. *N Engl J Med*: 349(17):1595–1604, October 23, 2003.

Khan F, Sachs HJ, Pechet L, et al. *Guide to Diagnostic Testing.* Philadephia: Lippincott Williams & Wilkins, 2002, pp. 33–35.

CHAPTER **12**

Urinalysis

For the patient with renal disease, the evaluation of the *urinary sediment* is not a laboratory procedure but rather an integral part of the physical examination to be performed by the physician, like listening to the chest or palpating the abdomen. Only then can the physician appreciate the often inconspicuous admixtures of cells and casts that define parenchymal disease: *red cell casts* indicating proliferative glomerular disease, *hyaline casts* indicating proteinuria, *white cell casts* indicating interstitial disease, *broad casts* indicating tubular atrophy, *waxy casts* indicating nephron death.

Warren E. Grupe, M.D.

Dr. Grupe has held full-time faculty appointments at the Schools of Medicine at Case-Western Reserve University, State University of New York (SUNY) at Syracuse, and Harvard University. Author of 161 publications in the medical literature, he is a recipient of the Jacob Ehrenzeller Award from Pennsylvania Hospital. He is currently the Director of the International Center for the Health Sciences in Charlottesville, Virginia and Clinical Professor of Pediatrics at the University of Virginia.

I. Indications for the urinalysis

A. The urinalysis (U/A) is useful for patients with diseases of the urinary tract or certain metabolic diseases, such as diabetes mellitus (DM) (Table 12-1). Because urinary tract infections are so common, serial urinalyses are also done on patients with sepsis or fever of unknown origin.

B. An **admission urinalysis** will be done on most patients. This urine sample may have been collected and sent to the hospital lab before the patient arrives on the hospital floor.

Table 12-1. Parts of the urinalysis

- Specific gravity
- Appearance
- pH*
- Protein*
- Glucose*
- Ketones*
- Blood*
- Sediment analysis
- Gram stain for bacteria (see colorplates)

There are nine basic parts to a complete urinalysis. A test marked with an asterisk (*) is done by dipstick. In instances in which urinary tract infection is suspected, a bacterial **culture and sensitivity** (abbreviated "C and S") screen is added to the above list.

II. Interpreting the urinalysis

A. Specific gravity

1. **Normal range** 1.001–1.035, with urine isotonic to plasma (285–295 mOsm) 1.010–1.012. The specific gravity (SG) is used as an indirect measure of the kidney's ability to concentrate the urine. If a first morning specimen is SG 1.025 or greater, it is generally taken as evidence of adequate concentrating ability.

2. **Elevated in:** dehydration, excessive fluid loss (vomiting, diarrhea, fever), DM, congestive heart failure (CHF), syndrome of inappropriate antidiuretic hormone (SIADH), adrenal insufficiency, decreased fluid intake.

3. **False elevations** of SG may occur with iodinated contrast material, excessive glucose, and massive proteinuria.

4. **Decreased in:** diabetes insipidus (DI), renal disease (glomerulonephritis or pyelonephritis), excessive fluid intake or IV hydration.

B. Appearance.
Urine is often described as "straw" or "yellow" in appearance. Following are common causes of **abnormal color or turbidity:**

Red-brown: hemoglobin, myoglobin, bile pigments, blood, food dyes
Yellow-red: pyridium, vegetable or phenolphthalein cathartics
Blue or green: beets, methylene blue in IV
Dark or black: porphyrins, melanin
Turbid: frequently secondary to urates or phosphates (benign), RBCs, WBCs
Foamy: protein, bile acids

C. pH

1. **Normal range** of urine pH is **4.5–8.5.**

2. **Elevated in:** bacteriuria, renal failure with inability to form ammonia, presence of certain drugs (antibiotics, sodium bicarbonate, acetazolamide).

3. **Decreased in:** acidosis (metabolic or respiratory), presence of certain drugs (ammonium chloride, methenamine mandelate), DM, starvation, diarrhea.

D. Protein

1. **A normal amount** of urine protein is less than 150 mg/day, below the level at which albumin can be generally detected in the urine by dipstick testing. Persistent and/or marked proteinuria is a highly significant finding.

2. **Protein is elevated in** renal disease (glomerular, tubular, interstitial), CHF, hypertension, neoplasms of the renal pelvis and bladder, multiple myeloma, Waldenström's macroglobulinemia.

   a. Protein in urine may be either **normal** serum proteins (indicating glomerular permeability or renal tubular disorders) or **abnormal** serum proteins (suggesting possible plasma cell dyscrasia). In multiple myeloma, Bence Jones (BJ) proteins will give a negative dipstick result about 50 percent of the time.

   b. Since protein is also seen in urine after vigorous exercise or immediately after sexual intercourse with ejaculation (in men), rule out these conditions before embarking on an expensive work-up, particularly in the outpatient setting. In this case, if circumstances permit, repeat the test and have the patient avoid exercise or sex on the day of the planned urinalysis.

E. Glucose

1. A **normal** result is no detectable glucose (negative dipstick).

2. The dipstick is extremely sensitive and specific for glucose, since the reaction relies on the enzyme glucose oxidase. However, the results are qualitative. Other causes of glucose in the urine are renal glycosuria (decreased renal threshold for glucose) and glucose intolerance. In situations where a quantitative assessment of urine glucose is desirable (for example, to monitor how much glucose your patient with diabetes is spilling—an indirect way of assessing the efficacy of insulin therapy), use the Clinitest tablets and follow bottle directions for dilution.

F. Ketones

The dipstick (and the Acetest tablets that are sometimes used) measure only acetoacetic acid and acetone (*not* beta-hydroxybutyrate). Recall that ketosis is seen in cases of **diabetic ketoacidosis, alcoholic ketoacidosis**, and **starvation.**

G. Blood.
Hematuria is virtually always significant, except in a patient with a recent history of catheterization. (See Table 12-2 for a discussion of RBCs in urine.)

Table 12-2.   Cell types in the urine sediment

Cell type	Normal range	Clinical points
RBC	0–3/HPF	Cystitis is the most frequent cause of hematuria, although slight hematuria often occurs secondary to exertion, trauma, or febrile illness.
		Tumors, kidney stones, and glomerulonephritis are also common causes of elevated RBCs.
WBC	0–5/HPF	Polymorphonuclear leukocytes are the most common form of WBCs observed. If seen, and routine cultures × 2 are negative, send culture to be tested for tubercle bacilli.
Epithelial	0–2/HPF	Epithelial cells increase with tubular damage or heavy proteinuria.
Bacteria		Presence of bacteria correlates well with culture growth of $\geq 10^5$ organisms (i.e., indicates presence of urinary tract infection).
		Send specimen for culture and sensitivity ("C and S") if suspicious.
		If culture comes back with between 10^4 and 10^5 organisms of a single type, reculture it; you must culture specimen at least twice to obtain >90% chance of documenting infection.

HPF = high-power field; 40× magnification.

H. Sediment analysis

1. **Cells in the urine sediment**

   a. **Cell counts.** The number of RBCs, WBCs, epithelial cells, and bacterial cells are reported as present in a typical high-power field (HPF) under microscopy.

   b. **Interpretation of cellular sediment.** Table 12–2 lists cell types found in urine sediment and their significance.

2. **Casts in the urine sediment** are often difficult to interpret. Remember that no casts are pathognomonic for a specific renal parenchymal change, and that they may be absent in any of a number of nephropathies.

   Casts are so named because they are casts of the nephron. They are distinguished from other debris by **smooth, parallel sides** (which may show the trapezoidal narrowing of the collecting system). Table 12-3 lists the various types of casts found in the urine and their clinical significance. These casts are illustrated in Fig. 12-1.

3. **Crystals in the urine sediment** are due to precipated chemicals and cellular debris. Some of the more common types of crystals are illustrated in Fig. 12–1. Their interpretation depends on the clinical presentation involved.

III. Ordering and evaluating the urinalysis

A. Beware of assuming that urine samples indicate urinary tract disease if they are entirely normal except for **large numbers of red blood cells**. Menstruating women often contaminate their urine sample accidentally, and Foley

Table 12-3. Casts in urine sediment

Cast type	Clinical points
Hyaline (translucent albumin) cast	The majority of casts seen in normal urine are hyaline. Since their refractile index is close to that of water, they are difficult to see unless light is reduced. A few hyaline casts/HPF may be normal.
WBC cast	Laboratories use acetic acid to prove that these are not RBC casts (acetic acid will lyse RBCs). WBC casts indicate inflammation in kidney parenchyma (often pyelonephritis).
RBC cast	They are most consistent with glomerular inflammation or ischemic injury.
Granular-waxy cast	Granular casts are so named because of their granular appearance under microscope. They are thought to be degenerating cellular casts, usually epithelial in origin.
Broad cast	Broad casts probably originate in the wide collecting duct. They are formed when flow rate is low. They often have ominous prognostic significance.

HPF = high-power field.

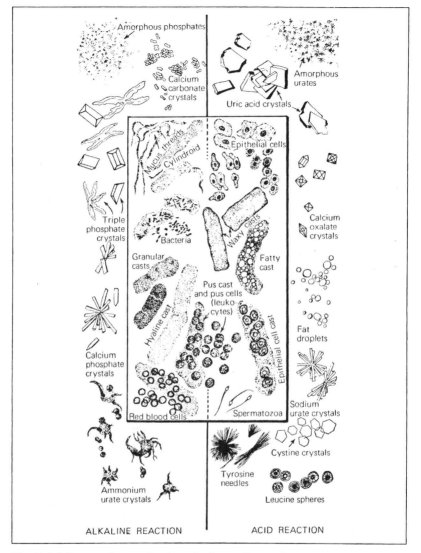

Fig. 12-1. Microscopic examination of urine sediment. (Reprinted with permission from M. A. Krupp et al., *Physician's Handbook* [19th ed.]. Los Altos, Calif.: Lange, 1979.)

catheters commonly cause hematuria, while individuals seeking narcotics may deliberately mix blood into their urine to feign a kidney stone and receive pain medication. If you are suspicious about a urine sample, supervise its collection yourself.

B. Surgical patients or any patients who have had urethral instrumentation often develop urinary tract infections.

CHAPTER 13

Electrocardiography

I. Outline of electrocardiography

A. Indications for ordering an electrocardiogram (ECG). Many patients you work up will need an ECG.

1. In the patient with cardiac disease, the ECG will add to your growing understanding of the altered cardiovascular system, complementing the history and physical exam.

2. In the noncardiac patient, the ECG screens for occult cardiac abnormalities and helps ensure the absence of acute disease.

3. In both cardiac and noncardiac patients, the ECG provides a baseline picture of the heart and its conducting system with which future changes in cardiac status may be compared.

B. Patterns analyzed in electrocardiographic analysis. The best way to analyze the ECG, especially at first, is to systematically look at:

1. Rate and rhythm

2. Axis

3. P-R, QRS, and Q-T intervals

4. QRS morphology

5. S-T segment and T wave changes

6. Comparison with previous tracings

Table 13-1 is a quick checklist for analyzing the ECG.

C. Analyzing and interpreting the electrocardiogram

1. **Rate and rhythm**

a. Every ECG should be inspected to determine the heart's rate and rhythm. Rhythm is often not easily deciphered until the other basic patterns are considered. Decide first whether the ECG shows a normal sinus rhythm (look for a distinct P wave preceding every QRS complex) or an arrhythmia.

b. **Determining rates**

(1) **Regular rate.** Recall that you can learn the rate quickly from the R-R interval. For a normal tracing (2.5 cm/sec or 5 large spaces marked by the heavier black line), an R-R interval of:

1 large box = rate 300
2 large boxes = rate 150
3 large boxes = rate 100
4 large boxes = rate 75
5 large boxes = rate 60

TABLE 13–1. Quick checklist for the ECG

1. **Rate** (bradycardia? tachycardia? regular or irregular?)
2. **Axis** (RAD? LAD?)
3. **P wave morphology** (constant? saw-toothed? notched?)
4. **P-R interval** (<0.12? 0.12-0.20? >0.20?)
5. **QRS interval** (0.08-0.10? >0.10?)
6. **Q-T interval** (within range 0.32-0.40?)
7. **QRS morphology** (shape? height? depth? Q waves?)
8. **S-T segment** (elevated or depressed?)
9. **T wave** (upright or inverted? peaked or flattened?)
10. **Rhythm**
    a. Regular or irregular
    b. P/QRS relationship (1 : 1? extra P waves? extra QRS?)
    c. Reconsider P wave and QRS morphologies
11. **Previous tracing** (change in any lead? How recent?)

RAD = right axis deviation; LAD = left axis deviation.

6 large boxes = rate 50

For example, look at the first two ECGs in Table 13-4. In the first tracing, the adjacent R peaks are between 5 and 6 large boxes apart, giving a rate between 50 and 60. In the second, the RR interval spans between 2 to 3 large boxes, giving a rate between 100 and 150.

(2) Irregular or slow rate. Note the small black marks at the very top of the ECG paper. At normal chart speed, these marks fall 3 seconds apart, therefore, to find the rate of an irregular or slow rhythm, count out the number of beats in 2 consecutive 3-second spaces and multiply by 10.

(3) Always **check the atrial and ventricular rates separately.** Usually they will be the same; if they are not, a second- or third-degree heart block may be present.

2. **Axis.** Determine the axis for every cardiogram you read. To do this quickly, look at limb leads I, II, and aV$_F$, noting whether the major direction of the QRS complex's deflection is positive or negative. Now recall the axis diagrams, as shown in Fig. 13-1. There are only three possibilities for axis that you need consider (+ represents upright QRS complex; – represents negative QRS complex deflection): normal axis, left axis deviation, and right axis deviation..

If right axis deviation (RAD) is present, you must exclude right ventricular hypertrophy (RVH). If left axis deviation (LAD) is present, you must consider that left anterior fascicular block (LAFB)—also referred

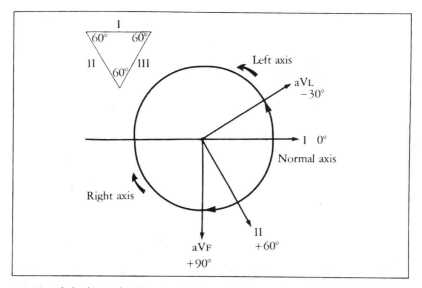

Fig. 13-1. Axis determination. Leads I, II, and III form a hypothetic equilateral triangle, with 60-degree angles as shown. Depolarization moving toward the left arm, parallel to lead I, is designated 0 degrees. Lead aVF, perpendicular to I, is thus labeled 90 degrees, and II is designated 60 degrees. Since aVL is perpendicular to II, forming a 90-degree angle, it is designated −30 degrees. (Reprinted with permission from G. H. Mudge, Jr.)

to as a left anterior hemiblock (LAHB)—or left ventricular hypertrophy (LVH) is present. **If the axis is normal, it does not contribute significantly to the differential diagnosis, unless it has changed significantly from prior tracings.**

   3. **Intervals.** Measure three intervals and record them:

      a. Interval P-R: measure onset of P wave to onset of QRS complex.

        (1) Normal range: 0.12–0.20 sec.

        (2) Physiologic correlate: time spent between sinoatrial (SA) node depolarization to the initiation of ventricular depolarization, including conduction through the atrioventricular (AV) node.

        (3) If the P-R interval is > 0.2 sec or is variable, a type of heart block is present. If it is < 0.12 sec, this variant may be normal or it may be due either to a rhythm whose atrial focus is quite close to the AV node or to a preexcitation syndrome such as the Wolff-Parkinson-White or Lown-Ganong-Levine syndromes.

      b. Interval QRS: measure onset to end of QRS.

      (1) Normal range: 0.08–0.10 sec.

(2) **Physiologic correlate:** time required for the spread of the electrical impulse through the ventricular muscle.

(3) The abnormal QRS duration is important in two instances. First, it will be prolonged in intraventricular conduction defects (IVCD), as outlined in Table 13-2. Second, in arrhythmia analysis a wide QRS may indicate aberrant conduction of a supraventricular impulse or a ventricular ectopic focus (see the footnote to Table 13-4).

c. **Q-T Interval:** measure onset of QRS to end of T wave.

   (1) **Normal range:** rate dependent, but usually 0.32–0.40 sec.

   (2) **Physiologic correlate:** time required for complete depolarization and repolarization.

   (3) The Q-T interval varies with heart rate. The corrected Q-T interval is $(Q\text{-}T)_c = Q\text{-}T$ (measured) $\div$ (R-R interval)$^{1/2}$ and equals 0.42 sec. Usually the uncorrected Q-T interval is 0.32–0.40 sec. Instances to be aware of that will significantly alter the Q-T interval include:

Quinidine	↑ Q-T	by increasing T wave duration
Hypocalcemia	↑ Q-T	by increasing length of S-T segment
Hypokalemia	↑ Q-T	by prolonging T wave with U wave formation
Hypercalcemia	↓ Q-T	by decreasing length of S-T segment

4. **QRS morphology.** The QRS complex is the most important configuration of the ECG. In addition to the duration of the QRS interval, carefully analyze its morphology with respect to:

   a. **General shape.** Are there notches? Is the upstroke jagged or smooth? This is helpful in differential diagnosis of IVCD.

TABLE 13–2. Intraventricular conduction defects (IVCDs)

IVCD	QRS duration	V₁ morphology	V₆ morphology
Right bundle branch block (RBBB)	≥0.12 sec	R' in V₁	Deep S in V₆
Left bundle branch block (LBBB)*	≥0.12 sec	Wide S in V₁	Large R in V₆ often with jagged up-stroke or R'
Left anterior fascicular block (LAFB)	Diagnosis suggested by presence of axis ≤ -30 degrees		
Left posterior fascicular block (LPFB)	Diagnosed by **newly** developed rightward shift in axis in the appropriate clinical setting (e.g., shift from +80 to +160 degrees in setting of an acute posterior MI or by extreme rightward axis)		

*In the presence of LBBB, no other conclusions may be read from the QRS morphology: hypertrophy, ischemia, and infarction are not reliably interpretable because of the abnormal pathway to ventricular depolarization.

b. **Height of R waves and depth of S waves,** especially in leads I, II, V$_2$, V$_5$. Helpful in determining presence of ventricular hypertrophy.

c. **Presence of Q waves,** which are defined as an initial downward deflection in the QRS lasting > 0.4 sec (1 small box) or 25 percent of the height of the associated R wave. This is a criterion for Q wave myocardial infarction.

5. **S-T segment and T wave changes.** One of the mistakes made by beginning electrocardiographers is to focus on the S-T and T wave changes without fully interpreting the QRS complex. The S-T segment and T wave should be analyzed once the QRS complex is evaluated. The S-T segment is most helpful in determining the presence of ischemic changes (see Table 13–3 and Fig. 13–2). Remember that it may vary in normal individuals and is easily affected by drugs (especially digitalis) and electrolyte imbalance. Determine:

   a. **Whether S-T segment is elevated or depressed.** Note elevation ≥ 1 mm or depression ≥ 0.5 mm; clinical correlates of ischemia; any drugs patient may be taking.

   b. **Relation of T wave to S-T segment.** Elevated S-T segment with T wave incorporated into S-T elevation is suggestive of ischemia; T wave that remains discernible from S-T segment elevation is more consistent with a normal variant (early repolarization).

   c. **The T wave** is often a labile entity, and changes in its morphology can be difficult to interpret. However, the presence of T wave inversion is often associated with three clinical situations: myocardial ischemia, digitalis, and strain (a pattern associated with ventricular hypertrophy). Determine whether the T wave is:

      (1) **Upright or inverted.** Note changes in leads I, II, and V$_4$–V$_6$, where T waves are usually upright.

      (2) **Peaked or flattened.** Note T waves can peak in the presence of hyperkalemia (increased potassium); T waves flatten as potassium decreases below normal range; T waves also alter their morphology as ischemic damage to the myocardium occurs.

6. **Comparison with previous tracings.** It is important to compare the ECG with previous tracings on record. The six basics of ECG analysis mentioned on p. 123 (see also Table 13-2) should be compared in detail and any changes noted in the write-up. If there is no significant change, that fact should be specifically mentioned.

7. **Arrhythmias.** Although the teaching of arrhythmia analysis is beyond the scope of this book, you can move a long way toward diagnosis by making this crucial distinction first: **is the rhythm in question regular or irregular?** Note the following diagnostic possibilities for these categories.

Regular rhythm	**Irregular rhythm**
Sinus tachycardia	Multifocal atrial tachycardia (MAT)
Paroxysmal atrial tachycardia (PAT)	Atrial fibrillation
	Regular rhythm with variable block
PAT with block	
Atrial flutter	
Ventricular tachycardia	

TABLE 13–3. ECG criteria for atrial abnormalities and ventricular hypertrophy

	P wave morphology		Major limb lead	Major precordial criteria	S-T and T wave changes
	II	V₂			
Left atrial abnormality	See Fig. 13-2	See Fig. 13-2	–	–	None
Right atrial abnormality	See Fig. 13-2	See Fig. 13-2	–	–	None
LVH (with or without strain)	–	–	R in I + S in III ≥ 20 mm	R in V₅ or V₆ + S in V₁ or V₂ ≥ 35 mm	S-T segment unchanged; T wave may be taller (without strain); S-T segment depressed; T wave inverted in leads V₄-V₆ (with strain)
RVH (with or without strain)	R/S ratio ≥ 1.0 in V₁	R/S ratio ≤ 1.0 in V₆	Right axis deviation (≥ + 90 degrees)		S-T segment unchanged; T wave may be taller (without strain); S-T segment depressed; T wave inverted in leads V₁, V₂ (with strain)

LVH = left ventricular hypertrophy; RVH = right ventricular hypertrophy.

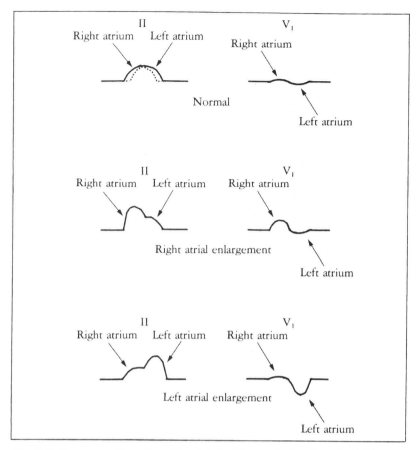

Fig. 13-2. P wave configuration. (Reprinted with permission from G. H. Mudge, Jr.)

Once you have determined the category in which the rhythm in question belongs, there are several ways to analyze the rhythm further. For instance, the response to carotid sinus pressure (see below), the P wave morphology, and the QRS morphology may all be helpful. Further information regarding the analysis of several of the more common arrhythmias is presented in Table 13-4.

II. Practical points concerning electrocardiography

    A. Performing the electrocardiographic test. Within the first few weeks of your clinical rotations, learn how to perform a **12-lead ECG.** The key here is to aim for consistency in lead placement and a flat baseline. Remember to obtain a rhythm strip. The rhythm strip is usually done with lead V_2 or lead II.

TABLE 13–4 . Arrythmias

Rhythms	Atrial rate	Ventricular rate	P wave morphology	CSP response	QRS morphology	Clinical points
Regular rhythms						
Sinus bradycardia	<60	<60	Normal	(Not used)	Normal	Often normal variant, especially in athletes. May accompany obstructive jaundice with ↑ serum bilirubin; ↑ intracranial pressure; digitalis; or acute inferior MIs. Most common cause is probably use of beta blocking drugs.
Sinus tachycardia	>100	>100	Normal	Gradual slowing; change to tachycardia when CSP released	Normal	Especially associated with fever, infections, hemorrhage, hyperthyroidism.

	Rate	P wave	Response	QRS	Comments
Paroxysmal atrial tachycardia	140–220	Usually obscured by preceding T wave. Theoretically abnormal (focus other than SA node)	No change or abrupt termination of arrhythmia	Normal	May see S-T segment depression associated with PAT.
PAT with block	140–220	Fixed fraction of the atrial rate (e.g., $\frac{1}{2}$). Abnormal morphology	No change or ↑ in degree of block (e.g., from $\frac{1}{2}$ to $\frac{1}{4}$)	Normal	May indicate digitalis toxicity.

TABLE 13–4. Arrythmias (continued)

Rhythms	Atrial rate	Ventricular rate	P wave morphology	CSP response	QRS morphology	Clinical points
Atrial flutter	220-320 (300–320 most common)	Fixed fraction of atrial rate (e.g., 1/2 or 1/4, so called 2:1 or 4:1 block)	Saw-toothed "flutter" waves	Usually no change or ↑ in block	Normal	Look for flutter waves in II, III, aVF, V₁, and V₂
Junctional tachycardia	>75	>75	**None** often; may be present in close proximity to QRS (either preceding or following); see Clinical points	No change or termination	Normal	Must exclude digitalis toxicity. Look for inverted P waves (from retrograde conduction) in II, III, and aVF. P waves may arrive at atria after QRS is inscribed and thus follow QRS on ECG.

Ventricular tachycardia	P waves rarely seen (occasionally retrograde P waves appear	140–280	Rare	No change. If retrograde P waves present, CSP may block them out ("V-A" block)	Wide, irregular	Converts at low DC cardioversion energies (≦10 watt-seconds 90 percent of the time).

Ventricular flutter	None seen	>300	None	No help	Bizarre shape, ↑ duration	Ventricular tachycardia with faster rate. An ominous rhythm that may progress to ventricular fibrillation and death.

TABLE 13–4. Arrythmias (continued)

Rhythms	Atrial rate	Ventricular rate	P wave morphology	CSP response	QRS morphology	Clinical points
irregular rhythms						
Multifocal atrial tachycardia (MAT)	>100	>100	≥3 different P wave morphologies	No change or transient slowing	Normal	Present in patients with COPD or pulmonary processes. Often must treat the primary process (not the arrhythmia).
Atrial fibrillation	None seen (flat or undulating baseline between Q waves)	40–300 (variable)	None	Usually no change; occasionally ↑ block	Normal	May be confused with atrial flutter. Classically associated with mitral stenosis and chronic mitral regurgitation; also present in CHF and coronary artery disease.

Regular rhythm with variable block (not pictured)	140–220	Varying fraction of atrial rate (e.g., 2 : 1 block alternating with 4 : 1 block)	Abnormal	See PAT with block and Atrial flutter, above	Normal	This is **not an irregularly irregular rhythm** like atrial fibrillation.

Note: A widened QRS may be due to either (1) conduction of an impulse that originates in the atria but encounters refractory conduction tissue in the ventricular His-Purkinje system **(aberrant conduction)** or (2) an impulse that originates in ventricular tissue **(ventricular ectopic activity).** In either case the widened QRS is due to electrical spread **directly** through ventricular muscle (outside the conducting system). Both mechanisms will lead to QRS interval prolongation, and making the distinction between them is often difficult. At this point it is sufficient to know that these two possibilities exist.

CSP = carotid sinus pressure; PAT = paroxysmal atrial tachycardia; COPD = chronic obstructive pulmonary disease; CHF = congestive heart failure.

B. Patterns analyzed in electrocardiographic analysis

1. It is important to become comfortable enough with ECGs to be able to peruse them quickly and to detect abnormal features. The key task at this point is to pay attention to the basics of analysis and to begin to train yourself to **recognize patterns**—that is, to "eyeball" the tracing, first taking in the overall picture, and then delving into the details of the tracing.

2. It is crucial to analyze the ECG within the **clinical setting**. This point may seem trivial, but it is in fact the most important consideration in ECG interpretation. The ECG has meaning for you as a clinician only in the context of the patient for whom you are caring.

C. Analyzing and interpreting the electrocardiogram

1. In preparation for learning ECG analysis, refamiliarize yourself with the anatomy and physiology of the **His-Purkinje system**. Also relearn the course and distribution of the **coronary arteries** if you have forgotten them.

2. Review a normal 12-lead ECG with particular attention to limb lead II and precordial lead V_2. Analyze the normal tracing step by step, in the manner detailed on p. 123 as a "warm-up" for the wards.

D. Using carotid sinus pressure (CSP). This is a useful technique that employs the physiologic response of increased vagal tone to the AV node by stimulating the afferent limb of the carotid reflex. Two warnings, however, should always be remembered. First, it is important to avoid CSP in patients who have a history of transient ischemic attack (TIA) or stroke or who have known carotid disease on exam. Second, performing this technique can have complications even if you are cautious; it **must** be done in the presence of an experienced house officer and with continuous ECG monitoring.

REFERENCES

Mudge G. *Manual of Electrocardiography*, 2nd ed. Boston: Little, Brown, 1986.

CHAPTER **14**

Chest, Abdomen, and Head Radiology

L ife is short. Art is long. Opportunity fugitive. Experience delusive. Judgment difficult. It is the duty of the physician not only to do that which immediately belongs to him, but likewise to secure the cooperation of the sick, of those who are in attendance, and of all the external agents.

Hippocrates (460 B.C. –356 B.C.)

Universally acknowledged as the father of medicine, Hippocrates was given credit in Athens for bringing the plague under control. The Hippocratic method of care has been described as follows: observe all, study the patient rather than the disease, evaluate honestly and assist nature. Only a few Hippocratic treatises were translated into Latin in the early Middle Ages until the wave of translations from the Arabic brought new texts. The Renaissance saw a revival of the Hippocratic approach to patient care and, as time went on, his fame increased. While many of his writings—collected as the Hippocratic Corpus—*are not considered a product of his alone, the* Aphorisms of Hippocrates, *from which this quotation is taken, is considered genuine.*

I. **Indications for ordering chest roentgenographs.** Chest radiology is a vital tool in the work-up of pulmonary, cardiovascular, and systemic medical problems and is the radiologic examination you will likely be ordering and reviewing most often. It is estimated that between 5% and 15% of the abnormalities on a chest roentgenogram are missed by radiologists and, since you have the advantage of knowing the patient's full history and other data, it behooves you to carefully review all films that are ordered on your patient.

There are many indications for ordering chest radiographs. In addition to providing valuable information about adjacent structures such as the gastrointestinal (GI) tract, the thyroid gland, or the bony structures of the thorax, a chest film series (which usually includes both posteroanterior [PA] and lateral views) is ordered for the following indications:

A. **Admission chest x-rays** used to be a standard part of the admission test battery at virtually all hospitals. Today, however, many experienced clinicians believe that doing routine chest x-rays (CXRs) on every patient is not beneficial, wastes scarce resources, and exposes many patients to unnecessary radiation. Always ask yourself why you are ordering an x-ray and what you will do with the results, before you order it.

B. **Sepsis and fever** work-ups almost always include a chest x-ray, even if there are no obvious respiratory symptoms.

C. **Cardiovascular** pathologic processes are often accompanied by changes in the cardiac silhouette, the appearance of the great vessels, or the pattern of pulmonary vascular distribution.

D. **Pulmonary disease** processes as diverse as infection and neoplasm may be indistinguishable on the basis of the physical exam, and the CXR interpreted in the context of the clinical history is often the *sine qua non* of pulmonary diagnosis.

E. **Chest pain**, whenever thought to be due to musculoskeletal processes, routinely involves a chest x-ray as part of the diagnostic work-up. The CXR is especially indicated in patients with "atypical chest pain" syndromes, where one must decide between cardiovascular or noncardiovascular etiologies.

F. **Systemic diseases** often result in roentgenologic changes that, while rarely pathognomonic, are useful in diagnosis.

G. All of the pathologic processes mentioned in **B–F** can be followed with **serial chest x-ray studies**, although the radiologic picture may "lag behind" the clinical exam as a process resolves.

H. **Interventional procedures** such as thoracenteses and central line placements are often concluded with a CXR to assess the efficacy of the procedure (e.g., what is the position of a central line?) and to rule out complications (e.g., is there a pneumothorax?).

II. **General approach to chest x-ray interpretation.** Before reading any x-ray be sure that the film is, in fact, your patient's since it is not unheard of for films to sometimes be erroneously placed in another patient's folder. Always check the "R" (right) or "L" (left) markers; ignoring this may someday cause you to miss diagnosing a case of dextrocardia or, even worse, send a surgeon to investigate a suspicious lesion on the wrong side. Because many critically ill patients have multiple studies performed the same day, be sure to check the time stamped on the film.

Unlike many lab tests that can be successfully interpreted without any knowledge of the actual test methodology, the interpretation of all radiologic studies requires that the interpreter understand some basic radiologic principles. Most of these principles are intuitively obvious and follow from the concept that roentgenographs are actually **transilluminations of body structures**, similar to the transillumination of the cheek produced with a flashlight when one is investigating an oral lesion. On a properly exposed radiograph, the thoracic vertebrae should be barely discernible through the image of the heart.

A. **Radiologic densities and images.** The x-ray is a two-dimensional composite shadow produced by transmission of x-ray photons through three-dimensional structures that differ in their ability to attenuate the photons. It gives two types of information: shape and density. There are several important corollaries to this concept.

1. All shapes except a sphere will show dramatic changes in their **shadow profiles,** depending on how the objects are positioned and rotated in front of the x-ray beam. An object that looks circular on both the PA and lateral views is almost certainly spherical.

2. An object will have a distinct **silhouette border** only if it differs significantly in density from the objects around it (the **silhouette sign**; see p. 143). For the purposes of this chapter, there are **four basic**

densities: (1) air, (2) fat, (3) tissue-fluid, and (4) bone. Because it is the most dense, bone will cause high levels of photon attenuation (and hence low photon transmission) and will appear to be the whitest on the x-ray. Conversely, the air in the lungs will allow high photon transmission and will show up as black or dark gray.

3. A single image on the x-ray may involve the superimposition of multiple shadows. One must learn to use the PA and lateral views together to break down composite shadows into shapes of individual objects.

B. **Systematic roentgenographic interpretation.** Like the physical exam, x-ray interpretation is best done in a systematic and methodical manner, following the same sequence of analysis every time. Although the more experienced interpreter may develop a "gestalt" from a cursory reading of a film, making an almost instant diagnosis after observing the integrated pattern for a few seconds (much like the snap diagnosis that an experienced clinician may be able to make), the novice reader of roentgenographs should choose a certain sequence of analysis and stick to it. View the film first from about 6 feet; then move in closer to inspect in fine detail. One useful method is to begin with the least prominent information on the film and gradually move toward the most prominent findings. For example, such an analysis sequence might be (1) introductory background information, (2) bones, (3) pulmonary vasculature, (4) pulmonary parenchyma and lung fields, and (5) cardiac silhouette and mediastinum. Each of these areas will be discussed. Fig. 14-1 shows reproductions of a normal PA and lateral chest x-ray with a trace drawing of the heart.

1. **Introductory background information.** Much information about the context of an x-ray study can be found on the film or the film folder.

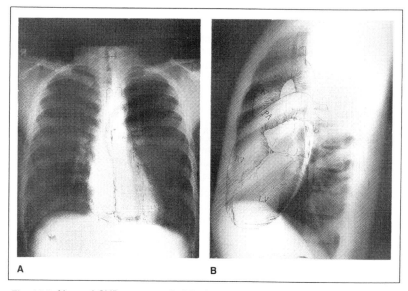

A   B

Fig. 14-1. Normal CXR patterns. **A.** PA view. **B.** Lateral view.

Always check this information first to ensure that you are looking at the correct CXR and that you understand the technique of the study. In particular, note:

a. **Date of study.** Check the film itself, not just the envelope.

b. **PA or anteroposterior (AP) projection.** Standard films are PA, while portable films are AP. AP views make the heart appear enlarged and thus make true cardiac size difficult to assess.

c. **Supine or upright patient position.** Check stomach bubble position. Supine position causes increased prominence of pulmonary vasculature.

d. **Patient rotation.** Check the clavicles for symmetry. If the patient is rotated, the film will be harder to interpret and to compare with other studies.

e. **Film penetration.** An underpenetrated film makes pulmonary vasculature more prominent.

f. **Dates of previous CXR studies.** Are old films available for comparison?

2. **Bone radiology in the chest x-ray.** Most CXR studies are not ordered to investigate the thoracic bones, but it is important to make a habit of looking at the bones every time you analyze a CXR, both because the bones themselves may provide valuable diagnostic information about a patient's condition (especially in cases of systemic disease) and because the bones provide a kind of grid or coordinate system, which will be useful in the identification, comparison, and description of the soft tissue.

An investigation of the bones often begins with the clavicles, whose symmetry allows an assessment of patient rotation. It then proceeds to the shoulders, where one checks the appearance and relationships of the various elements of each joint and the general symmetry of the two shoulder joints. Although an appreciation for the texture and the limits of normal in the appearance of the skeletal system is difficult to acquire, the novice may make many diagnoses by paying special attention to any cortical breaks, fissures, "moth-eaten" areas, or areas that seem to have increased or decreased radiolucency when compared with the other bones and with the mirror-image area on the other side of the body.

Finally, every rib may be individually located, mentally numbered, and visually inspected along the length of its spiral course. Once again, the clinical history is of paramount importance. A patient complaining of localized chest pain should have a very careful CXR rib analysis to rule out skeletal pathology, while the asymptomatic patient needs only a quick scan.

3. **Pulmonary vasculature.** One of the most important clinical questions encountered in chest radiology in adult patients is whether or not a patient has congestive heart failure (CHF). Although the pulmonary vascular pattern is useful in assessing other types of cardiopulmonary pathology, it is in the clinical setting of heart failure that the novice reader of roentgenographs will most often be concerned with these patterns. In addition to the appearance of the heart itself, three features of the pulmonary vasculature's appearance are important in making this diagnosis:

(1) the pattern of vascular prominence and redistribution, (2) the existence of pulmonary edema, and (3) the finding of pleural effusion.

a. **Vascular patterns.** The vasculature is most prominent in the medial lower lung (75 percent of total perfusion is normally to the lower lobes, due to the mass of lung parenchyma and to gravitational effects).

The ratio of upper to lower vasculature is approximately 1 to 3 in the normal CXR. Vascular prominence can represent engorgement of arteries, veins, lymphatics, or all three. In general, pulmonary arteries run vertically, while pulmonary veins empty lower and course horizontally. Lymphatics are normally not visible. Although it is often difficult to decide between the arteries and veins on the basis of the x-ray alone, it is useful to remember that the backup or regurgitation of blood from the left ventricle to the lungs (consistent with [c/w] mitral stenosis, CHF, myocardial infarction, mitral regurgitation) will lead to venous prominence, while arterial engorgement will result from increased right-sided flow, as in left-to-right shunts (c/w patent ductus arteriosus, septal defects, etc.).

b. **Pulmonary edema.** Pulmonary edema is the result of pulmonic vascular congestion to the point that the oncotic pressure of the blood is no longer able to maintain the integrity of the vascular system. The resulting edema (fluid) is taken up by the pulmonary lymphatics, which increase in radiologic prominence due to the increased flow.

When the edema becomes severe, it is associated with **horizontal linear densities** known as **Kerley's lines.** Probably the most important of these are **Kerley's B lines**, which are assumed to represent engorgement of interlobular septa and are often observed in cases of CHF as well as tumor, fibrosis, and so forth (Fig. 14-2).

c. **Pleural effusion.** The costophrenic angles should be sharp and free of fluid on the normal CXR. If the patient has made a good inspiratory effort, the diaphragm should be visible at the level of rib 10 or 11. You may see that findings suggestive of cardiomegaly or bibasilar consolidation on films taken with suboptimal inspiration miracu-

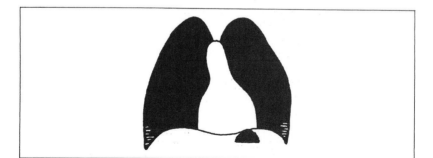

Fig. 14-2. Kerley's B lines. Small linear densities often found at the lung periphery, Kerley's B lines are assumed to represent engorgement of lymphatics due to pulmonary edema.

lously disappear when the films are retaken with the patient taking a full inspiratory effort.

Because pleural fluid collects in the costophrenic recess, in the upright patient it first fills up the deeper **posterior** part of the recess; practically, this means that the **lateral view** will show evidence of an effusion before the PA view will. A caveat here: fluid may accumulate between the lung pleura and the diaphragm. In this case, the subpulmonic effusion may be difficult to distinguish from an elevated diaphragm or a consolidated left lower lobe. Repeating the lung exam after looking at the x-ray often helps to resolve this confusion.

4. **Segmental bronchial anatomy.** There are three lobes in the right lung and two in the left. Each lobe is divided into anatomic segments supplied

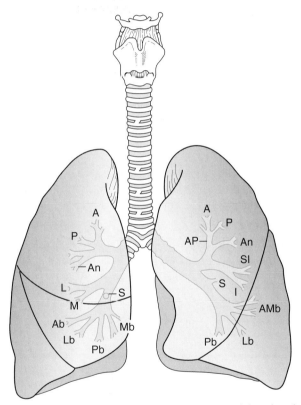

Fig. 14-3. Segmental bronchial anatomy. Right upper lobe: *A,* apical; *P,* posterior; *An,* anterior. Right middle lobe: *L,* lateral; *M,* medial. Right lower lobe: *S,* superior; *Ab,* anterior basal; *Mb,* medial basal. Left upper lobe: *AP,* apical-posterior; *A,* apical; *P,* posterior; *An,* anterior; *Sl,* superior lingular; *I,* inferior lingular. Left lower lobe: *S,* superior; *AMb,* anterior-medial basal; *Lb,* lateral basal; *Pb,* posterior basal. (Reprinted with permission from Daffner RH: Clinical Radiology: The Esssentials, 2/e, Baltimore, MD, 1999, page 94.)

by its own bronchus and blood vessels (Fig. 14-3). A general knowledge of the location of these segments is helpful in localizing disease.

III. Pulmonary parenchyma and lung field infiltrates. While vascular problems present radiographically as linear densities, the roentgenographic changes that suggest disease in the pulmonary air-space compartment involve space-occupying, often "patchy" densities. Such findings are called **infiltrates**, and are associated with many types of disease processes, notably infections, neoplasms, and hemorrhage. The patient's clinical history and physical exam are very important in the interpretation of infiltrates; an infiltrate without a history of fever might suggest a hemorrhage or neoplasm, whereas a clinical history suggesting infection would place pneumonia much higher on the differential list.

   A. Infiltrate localization. The first step in analyzing an infiltrate is to attempt to determine exactly where it is. For the novice, there are three basic ways to locate an infiltrate.

   1. Using the PA and lateral views together, an attempt is made to identify the three-dimensional location of the infiltrate. This is especially important in the analysis of small densities that may seem to represent coin lesions on the PA view but, when sought on the lateral, often turn out to signify either superficial structures (e.g., nipples, buttons) or collections of interlobular fluid **(pseudotumors).** Nipple markers are often placed on the patient by radiology technicians to avoid the nipple being interpreted as representing a lesion in the lung parenchyma.

   2. If an infiltrate is large enough to occupy a significant part of a lobe, it may result in the disappearance of the silhouette of an adjacent structure. This phenomenon is called the **silhouette sign**, and is actually nothing more than an application of the general principle that distinct outlines are visible on the x-ray only when there is a difference in density between adjacent structures. When lung tissue is replaced by blood, pus, or tumor, the radiographic outlines of the mediastinal or diaphragmatic organs superimposed on these infiltrated areas will disappear. By paying attention to exactly which outlines are obscured by the infiltrate, and by using both the PA and lateral films, one can usually establish which lobes are involved and gain insight into the etiology and extent of the infiltrate.

   Fig. 14-4 illustrates the x-ray changes associated with consolidation in each of the pulmonary lobes. Note, for instance, that involvement of the right lower lobe, which is posterior, will lighten but will not totally obscure the right heart outline because the heart is anteriorly placed. By contrast, a right middle lobe infiltrate often obliterates the right side of the cardiac shadow.

   3. The presence of some degree of **mediastinal shift** is a third key to deciding where a lesion is located. The mediastinum is normally a set of roughly midline structures. Note that these appear superimposed on the vertebral column in the normal PA film in Fig. 14-1. Consider especially the positions of the column of air in the trachea, the aortic arch, and the right heart border; these serve as reference points to the upper, middle, and lower mediastinum.

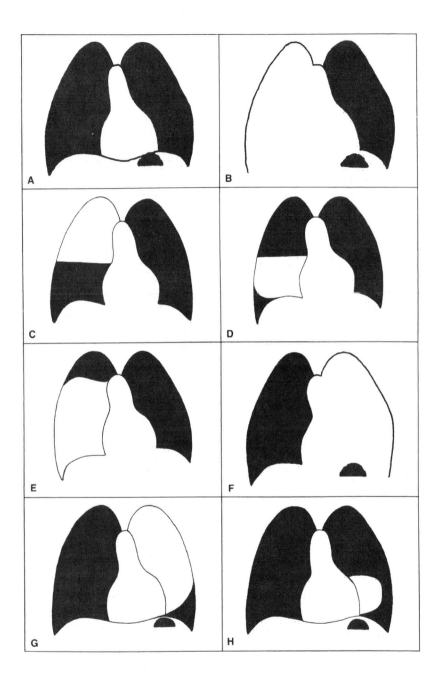

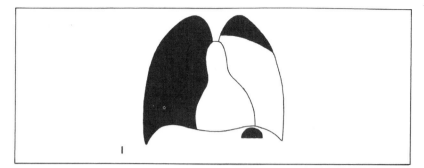

Fig. 14-4. CXR patterns produced by lobar consolidations such as those caused by pneumonia or tumor. Note the disappearance of various parts of the cardiac and diaphragmatic borders due to the increased density of the consolidated lung tissue. This loss of density contrast borders is called the *silhouette sign*. **A.** Normal CXR. **B.** Total R lung consolidation with obliteration of the R heart border. **C.** R upper lobe consolidation. **D.** R middle lobe consolidation. **E.** R lower lobe consolidation. **F.** Total L lung consolidation with obliteration of the L heart border. **G.** L upper lobe consolidation. **H.** L upper lobe lingular consolidation with disappearance of the L heart border. **I.** L lower lobe consolidation; L heart border still faintly visible due to air in lingula.

If the mediastinal structures appear to bow to one side, this may suggest either a **vacuum effect** caused by lung collapse or a **mass effect** caused by neoplasm, exudate, or hyperinflation. Once again, the specific pulmonary lobes affected may be deduced from the mediastinal borders that are shifted. For instance, if only the right lower lobe is collapsed, the cardiac border will shift to the right while the trachea and the aortic arch may remain in their usual positions. **The mediastinum will be shifted toward the side of lung collapse and away from the side of lung overexpansion** (e.g., as in emphysematous change) and thoracic masses (e.g., as in pleural effusions, tumors). Shifts in the positions of the major and minor pulmonary fissures may be used in the same way. These are probably somewhat more revealing, although slightly more difficult to recognize.

B. Infiltrate identification. The radiologic differential diagnosis of pulmonary infiltrates is difficult and is dependent on the hints given by the clinical history. Often the most useful approach is to think in terms of broad categories of disease (e.g., infectious, neoplastic, collagen vascular, hemorrhagic) and then to use the clinical history to determine the most likely specific diagnosis. For instance, a right lower lobe infiltrate may suggest pneumonia, while the production of thick sputum with gram-positive diplococci would make the diagnosis of pneumococcal pneumonia virtually certain.

One very important question in the identification of a lung-field density is whether the density is simply a collection of fluid located outside the alveoli or whether there is actual **consolidation** of the air spaces. A useful sign to look for is the presence of the **air bronchogram** pattern, which basically is nothing more than the air in the bronchial tree made visible by increased density of the surrounding structures. Normally, the bronchi are not well seen because there is not enough contrast in radiologic density; they consist of a tubelike arrangement of air spaces surrounded by a very thin wrapping of tissue. However, under conditions of lobar consolidation, due to tumor or pneumonia, the radiologic density surrounding these air spaces is much greater, and the contrast makes the bronchial markings visible.

Table 14-1 summarizes some of the classic findings useful in the differential diagnosis of pulmonary infiltrate.

IV. **Cardiac silhouette.** An analysis of the cardiac silhouette on the chest roentgenograph extends the information acquired during the physical exam. For example, a soft S_3 coupled with an enlarged ventricle on CXR strongly suggests the possibility of congestive heart failure.

The key to interpreting a patient's cardiovascular status via the CXR lies in the recognition of **specific chamber abnormalities**. Deciding that "the heart looks abnormal" is much less useful than deciding that there is dilatation of the left atrium and straightening of the left heart border, suggestive of mitral valve disease.

A. **Components of the cardiac silhouette.** The borders of the cardiac shadow can be broken down into a series of nine overlapping arcs (Fig. 14-5). The right atrium forms the right heart border. The systematic analysis of the cardiac shadow involves breaking the shadow down into these arcs and determining which, if any, are abnormal. Once you memorize the information in Fig. 14-5, it will be much easier to apply knowledge of cardiovascular pathophysiology to the interpretation of the chest film.

B. **Cardiothoracic ratio.** A specific example of the use of cardiac chamber appearance in radiologic diagnosis is the cardiothoracic ratio. This concept, illustrated in Fig. 14-6, is based on the rule of thumb that, in the PA exposure, the extreme right and left borders of the cardiac outline (segment A-B) should be no farther apart than one-half the width of the chest at its widest point (segment C-D).

Because an enlarged left ventricle is most often the cause of an enlarged cardiothoracic ratio, this rule is most useful in the diagnosis of heart failure associated with ventricular dilatation or hypertrophy.

See Table 14-1 for a summary of some of the common CXR findings associated with specific cardiovascular problems.

V. **Ordering the chest roentgenograph**

A. The **requisition form** for a CXR usually includes a space for you to provide **clinical information** to be used in the radiologist's interpretation of the film. It is very important that you provide the radiologist with two types of information:

1. The clinical history that relates to your **specific questions** (e.g., "55-year-old male with long smoking history, recent weight loss, and chronic fever; rule out cancer.").

2. Clinical details relating to known **x-ray findings** that might otherwise confuse the radiologist (e.g., "Patient has history of pulmonary radiation treatment 2 years prior to admission.").

Table 14-1. Summary of roentgenographic findings associated with disease processes of various organ systems

Disease process	Roentgenographic findings
Cardiovascular*	
1. Atrial septal defect	RA and RV prominence with normal LA; prominent lung vascularity
2. Tricuspid regurgitation	RA enlargement; cardiac enlargement
3. Tricuspid stenosis	RA enlargement
4. Pulmonic regurgitation	No good CXR findings
5. Pulmonic stenosis	May be normal; otherwise, RV and outflow prominence; PA poststenotic dilatation
6. Pulmonary hypertension	RA and RV enlargement; prominent central pulmonary vessels near hilum; rapid tapering; avascular peripheral lung fields
7. Mitral regurgitation	LA and LV enlargement; mitral valve calcification; pulmonary congestion if chronic
8. Mitral stenosis	LA enlargement; prominent pulmonary venous system; mitral calcification; Kerley's B lines
9. Aortic regurgitation	LV enlargement; more prominent if chronic aortic dilatation
10. Aortic stenosis	Calcified aortic valve. LV enlargement; prominent ascending aorta
11. Hypertension	LV hypertrophy; prominent tortuous aorta
12. Congestive heart failure	LV enlargement and pulmonary congestion; Kerley's B lines
13. Constrictive pericarditis	Small or slightly enlarged heart; pericardial calcification
14. Coarctation of aorta	Notching of lower rib borders
Pulmonary infiltrates: infectious	
1. Viral pneumonia	Nodular infiltrate; diffuse involvement
2. Pneumococcal pneumonia	Lobar or bronchopneumonic infiltrates and consolidation; air bronchograms; pleural effusion
3. Tuberculosis	Apical infiltrate; parenchymal calcification
4. Granulomas (due to tuberculosis, histoplasmosis, coccidioidomycosis, etc.)	Fibrosis; calcifications; satellite densities
Neoplasms	
1. Bronchogenic carcinoma	Solitary lesions without calcifications
2. Bronchoalveolar cell cancer	Segmental distribution; can mimic infiltrate
3. Metastatic cancer	Often multiple lesions
4. Hodgkin's disease, lymphoma, leukemia	Parenchymal infiltrate; hilar node enlargement; mediastinal widening

Continues

Table 14–1. Summary of roentgenographic findings associated with disease processes of various organ systems (Continued)

Disease process	Roentgenographic findings
Pulmonary	
1. Foreign body	Foreign body may be obvious on CXR; may cause "check valve" hyperinflation
2. Atelectasis	Plate-like densities
3. Bronchiectasis	Basilar patchy densities
4. Emphysema	Over-expanded lungs; low diaphragms; increased radiolucency of lungs; heart may seem small
5. Interstitial lung disease (due to inhalants, drugs, collagen vascular disease, etc.)	Diffuse infiltrate
6. Pneumothorax	Visceral pleural line visible on x-ray

*Cardiac enlargement is usually a late finding in cardiovascular diseases.
LA = left atrium; LV = left ventricle; PA = posteroanterior; RA = right atrium; RV = right ventricle.

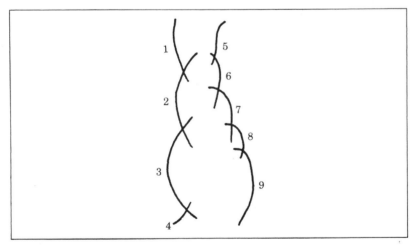

Fig. 14-5. The normal mediastinal profiles are all vascular and resolve into a series of nine intersecting arcs: (1) superior vena cava; (2) ascending aorta; (3) right atrium; (4) inferior vena cava and cardiac fat pad; (5) left subclavian vein and artery, left common carotid artery; (6) aortic arch; (7) pulmonary artery; (8) left atrium; (9) left ventricle. (Reprinted with permission from L. Squire and R. A. Novelline, *Fundamentals of Radiology.* 4th ed. Cambridge, MA: Harvard University Press, 1988.

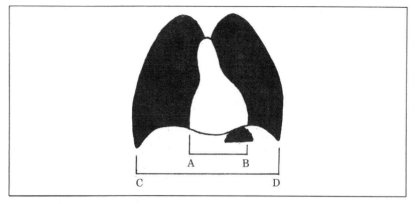

Fig. 14-6. Cardiothoracic ratio. In a routine PA CXR, the width of the cardiac shadow (segment A-B) should be no more than half the width of the thoracic cavity (segment C-D). This is a rough rule of thumb, and it should be used together with an analysis of the cardiac chamber configuration to obtain a reasonable estimate of heart size.

The better your clinical summary, the better your radiology reports will be.

B. Every radiology department has its own set of **protocols** for working up specific problems. It is worth your while to talk to a radiologist about the department's preferences (e.g., "Should this suspicious CXR be followed by magnetic resonance imaging [MRI] or by a computed tomography [CT] scan of the chest?"). Try to use the radiologist as a diagnostic consultant as well as a film interpreter. In the process you will learn a lot of medicine.

VI. General approach to chest x-ray interpretation

A. Before attempting to interpret chest x-rays, you should review the gross anatomy of the **thorax** concentrating especially on:

1. The relations of the internal organs in the thorax, especially the mediastinal structures around the T_4 level (e.g., determine the relation of the heart to the tracheal bifurcation and the esophagus).

2. The exact position of the heart and its chamber in the thorax. Think about possible pathophysiologic changes in the shape of the heart. For instance, where on the cardiac margin would you see the protruding atrium in an instance of left atrial dilatation? What diseases might cause this change?

3. The lobes of the lungs and the approximate positions of the pulmonary fissures. Which fissures would you expect to see from the PA perspective? Which from the lateral?

B. **Commonsense principles** are of the utmost importance in attempting to learn CXR interpretation. Keep the following general principles in mind:

1. With certain obvious exceptions, the human body is a bilaterally symmetric structure. Consequently, an area on one of the lungs that appears to demonstrate vascular prominence may be profitably compared to the mirror-image area on the other lung (bearing in mind, of course, that the lungs themselves are not perfectly symmetric).

2. **Changes** in serial x-ray studies are of the utmost importance, especially if the changes occur around the time that the patient's clinical history changes. Try to review the patient's x-ray files to find when the films first began to deviate from normal. To develop the ability to recognize changes, you will have to study many normal films and pay careful attention to serial films taken on your patients. For hospitalized patients who receive a film daily, take the time every so often to compare that day's film with one taken a week earlier; changes may be more obvious.

3. Although it is often a good teaching exercise to try to interpret an x-ray before you read the clinical history, you should always think about your patient's films in relation to their clinical conditions. Could you hear crackles in the patient whose chest films suggest pulmonary edema? Was there the sudden onset of pleuritic pain or dyspnea just before the patient's films began to show a segmental lower lobe infiltrate consistent with a pulmonary embolus? You should constantly recheck old films as the clinical story evolves; often an old x-ray finding can be reinterpreted in light of new information. You should learn to use the x-rays to sharpen your physical examination skills; the **listen-look-listen** method (listen to the lungs; look at the x-ray; listen to the lungs again) is an excellent self-teaching device.

4. **Pathophysiologic processes** that are very different clinically may look very similar on the x-ray (for instance, bronchoalveolar cell carcinoma may appear identical on x-ray to lobar pneumonia). Therefore, the vocabulary with which you speak of and think about the roentgenograph should be that of radiologic appearance ("nodule," "opacity," "infiltrate") and not diagnosis ("tumor," "granuloma," "pneumonia"). First describe what you see; then attempt to interpret it in light of the facts of the case. The essence of radiology is **shrewd pattern recognition** coupled with a keen knowledge of radiologic differential diagnosis.

5. **Straight lines** usually belong in the province of physics, not biology. Differentiate between discrete lines, such as a fibrotic strand, and a straight interface, such as a pleural effusion. If you see an anomalous straight line cutting across a film, consider the possibility that it is caused by fluid collecting under the force of gravity or by something extrinsic to the thorax. Tilting the patient often causes a change in the fluid level, which may help in your interpretation. The gas-fluid interface in the stomach (stomach bubble) helps determine if the patient was standing up or lying down when the film was taken.

6. **Displaced organs** and anatomic structures generally suggest that something is either pushing or pulling them out of normal position, even though the deforming agent or process may not be visible on the x-ray. (A 16-year-old girl with a history of Hodgkin's disease, whose chest film shows progressively increased splaying of the carina, would therefore be investigated carefully for possible relapse.)

VII. Chest x-ray interpretation. As a student doing core clinical rotations, you will be confronted with two different scenarios during which you will be asked to interpret the CXR.

   A. Reviewing your patients' roentgenographs before you have obtained an "official" interpretation from a radiologist should be a routine part of your work-up, just like interpreting the ECG. Though you may wish to consult a radiologist before deciding on further diagnostic or treatment plans, you should formulate your own opinion of the CXR findings before asking for an expert opinion. Moreover, radiologists are often excellent teachers and will spend much more time with a student who seems to have some idea of basic radiologic principles than with one who simply puts a CXR on the viewbox and asks, "Is this normal?" Table 14-2 is a quick checklist for the review of a CXR.

   B. When presenting roentgenographs as part of formal case presentations, it is best to **be systematic and complete**. Many radiologists use the following algorithm:

   1. Describe what you see in very general terms.

   2. Describe the pertinent findings that you do **not** see.

   3. Give the radiologic differential diagnosis.

   4. Now use the clinical history to defend your top diagnosis or group of diagnoses.

   5. Finally, suggest what further studies should be done to arrive at a definitive diagnosis.

Table 14–2.   Quick checklist for the CXR

PA views
1. Clavicles (rotation?)
2. Bones (lesions?)
3. Breasts, soft tissue
4. Costophrenic angles (inspiratory effort? pleural effusion?)
5. Lung markings (engorgement? redistribution? hydrothorax or pneumothorax?)
6. Lung fields (coin lesions? consolidation? hilar adenopathy?)
7. Mediastinal shift
8. Cardiac shadow (cardiothoracic ratio? pericardial effusion?)
9. Specific cardiac chamber profiles (dilatation or hypertrophy? aortic profile?)

Lateral views
1. Right and left diaphragm outlines
2. Posterior sulci (pleural effusion?)
3. Thoracic vertebrae
4. Hilar markings
5. Trachea (air column position?)
6. Anterior and posterior clear spaces
7. Cardiac shadow (profile? specific chamber enlargement?)

An example of a formal CXR interpretation follows:

There is a patchy wedge-shaped density in the right middle lung field, best seen on the lateral view. The hemidiaphragms are flat and there is some linear scarring at the bases. The heart and great vessels appear normal. There is good inspiratory effort with the diaphragm visible at about rib 11 and good penetration overall. I do **not** see any evidence of pleural effusion, and there are no air bronchograms. The top differential diagnosis would be right middle lobe pneumonia superimposed on a picture of chronic bronchitis versus a tumor. The clinical history of acute-onset cough and green sputum production favors the diagnosis of pneumonia, but in a man with a 75 pack-year smoking history, a tumor must be vigorously excluded. The trial of antibiotics that is presently being undertaken will be informative. Bronchoscopy would probably be the next step in the evaluation of the infiltrate if no response to the antibiotic course is noted.

C. The **spot analysis** of a CXR is a frequent part of teaching rounds. A student will be asked to give an off-the-cuff analysis of a CXR that he or she has never seen before and knows nothing about. The best approach here is to be systematic. *Spend about 20 seconds looking at the CXR without saying anything.* If you want to, you can gain time by saying something such as, "I would have to know a bit of clinical history before being able to make a reasonable statement." (You may not get it, but you can always ask.) The first determination you must make is the organ system or systems involved in the abnormality. Once you have decided on the **type of process** going on, you can then refine your statements by zeroing in on the **exact findings.** A typical student-level spot analysis might be, "These lung fields look congested. There is a moderate degree of pulmonary vascular redistribution bilaterally. I don't see any Kerley's B lines, but there is a small pleural effusion on the right, seen best in the lateral. The heart looks big, and the profile suggests left ventricular dilatation. I don't see any infiltrates or bony lesions. Overall, I would call this a picture of moderate congestive heart failure."

VIII. **General approach to ordering abdominal roentgenographs.** The abdominal radiograph is an important examination for evaluating patients with suspected intra-abdominal disease. Unlike chest radiographs, which provide natural contrast due to the presence of bones, abdominal radiographs are somewhat more difficult to evaluate. Reviewing your anatomy and pathophysiology well is, therefore, an advantage in differentiating and discerning abnormal from normal findings. Understand also the reasons you wish to order abdominal x-rays (AXRs). Numerous radiographs are sometimes ordered in patients with known or suspected bleeding from esophageal varices or peptic ulcers when endoscopic or contrast examination would be more helpful in picking up abnormalities. Pelvic ultrasound is usually the initial imaging study of choice for uterine and adnexal structures. Here are some helpful tips:

A. The standard abdominal radiograph, or **"KUB"** (a film that shows kidneys, ureters, and bladder), consists of a supine view, the so-called **"flat plate"** of the abdomen. This latter term dates to a time when glass plates were used instead of radiographic film and is now considered obsolete, though still widely used, having been replaced by the more descriptive term **"abdominal radiograph."**

B. Most patients suspected of having an acute abdominal pathology will have an **"upright film"** in addition to the KUB film. The purpose of this view is to identify the presence of free intraperitoneal air and to detect the presence of intestinal air-fluid levels. The study is typically made by having the patient stand or sit, or a **left lateral decubitus** (left side down, right side up) film is obtained if the patient can only lie on his or her side (Fig. 14-7). It is prudent to have the patient stay in this position for several minutes to allow any free air to rise over the dome of the liver before the x-ray is taken.

C. As a rule, **portable radiographs** are usually helpful only in detecting gross intra-abdominal abnormalities.

D. Abdominal **CT**, especially with spiral CT technology, can differentiate organ densities better than radiographs, can outline these organs, and can detect subtle abnormalities that may not be visible on plain abdominal radiographs.

E. **Ultrasonography** (US) is most useful for evaluating masses (Fig. 14-8) and aortic aneurysms and detecting diseases of the biliary tract, kidney (i.e., hydronephrosis, renal calculi), adnexal and pelvic structures, and for masses suspected of being cystic, rather than solid, in nature.

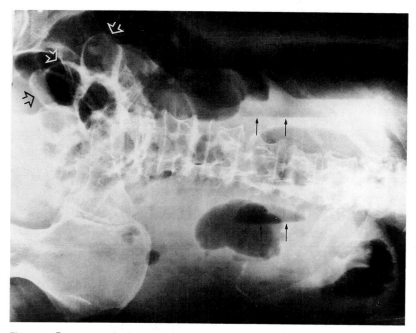

Fig. 14-7. Pneumoperitoneum demonstrated on a lateral decubitus radiograph. There is a large collection of free air along the right flank. Note air on both sides of the bowel wall (open arrows) and the presence of air-fluid levels (small arrows) within the bowel. (Reprinted with permission from Daffner RH: Clinical Radiology: The Esssentials, 2/e, Baltimore, MD, 1999, page 250.)

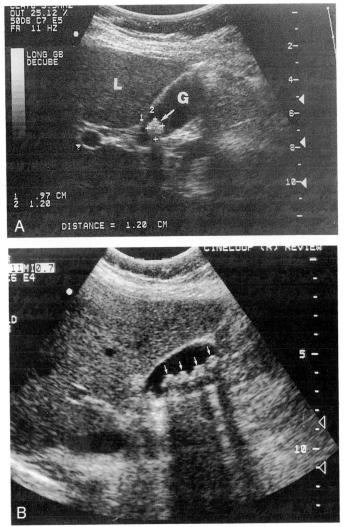

Fig. 14-8. Cholelithiasis. **A**, ultrasound shows a single stone (arrow) measuring 1.2 × 0.97 cm in the dependent portion of the gallbladder. *L*, liver; *G*, gallbladder. **B**, ultrasound showing multiple stones (arrows). (Reprinted with permission from Daffner RH: Clinical Radiology: The Esssentials, 2/e, Baltimore, MD, 1999 page 330.)

F. Under normal circumstances, the **gas patterns** should change over a period of several minutes if successive films are made. This just means there is normal peristaltic activity and absence of this consistency can be a sign of acute abdominal pathology, such as bowel infarction, or the presence of an adynamic ileus, as is seen postoperatively.

G. It is diagnostically helpful to remember that an abdominal radiograph often has the **lower lobes of each lung** visible. While you may not have been thinking of pneumonia or a pleural effusion when you ordered the abdominal radiograph, pulmonary pathology can sometimes present with signs and symptoms related to the abdomen, such as abdominal pain.

IX. **General approach to head radiology.** CT, MRI, digital subtraction angiography (DSA), and positron emission tomography (PET) have been major breakthroughs in the imaging of the brain and spinal cord. The abnormal findings on any of these examinations are often subtle and frequently frustrating for the novice student, resident, or even attending physician. Here are some general tips:

A. As CT and MRI become the prime investigative tools for cranial imaging, there is a diminishing role for plain **skull radiography**: penetrating injury, sinus disease, destructive lesions, metabolic bone disease, congenital anomalies, and postoperative changes. The occipitomental (Waters) projection used in skull radiographs is used primarily to study the facial bones and

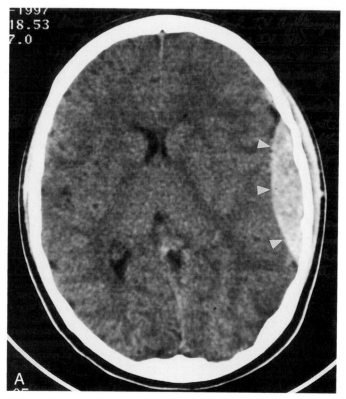

Fig. 14-9. Acute epidural hematoma. Note the classic lentiform shape of the hematoma. (Reprinted with permission from Daffner RH: Clinical Radiology: The Esssentials, 2/e, Baltimore, MD, 1999 page 513.)

sinuses. **Facial radiographs** are still used for suspected trauma. Three-dimensional CT examination is particularly useful to the surgeon planning facial bony reconstruction.

B. A **CT examination** of the brain is usually performed as the initial study for evaluation of patients with suspected intracranial abnormalities. This examination is generally performed first without and then with intravenous contrast enhancement to demonstrate vascular structures or abnormalities, certain types of hematomas, or enhancement of lesions.

1. **Epidural hematomas** are usually the result of fractures that involve one of the meningeal arteries and characteristically have a lentiform shape (Fig. 14-9).

2. **Subdural hematomas** result from injury, often trivial, to the meningeal veins and in the acute stage conform to the contour of the brain and have a crescentic shape. The shape becomes lentiform when the hematoma becomes chronic (Fig. 14-10).

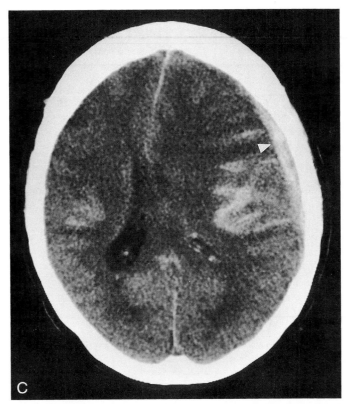

Fig. 14-10. Acute subdural hematoma. This image demonstrates a significant midline shift from an intracerebral hemorrhage as well as a subdural hematoma (arrowhead). (Reprinted with permission from Daffner RH: Clinical Radiology: The Esssentials, 2/e, Baltimore, MD, 1999, page 527.)

C. Cranial MRI is the primary investigative tool for suspected intracranial abnormalities, such as tumors and multiple sclerosis. MR imaging is a noninvasive radiographic technique that does not use ionizing radiation and, therefore, without significant health hazard. MR imaging uses a pulsed radiofrequency (RF) beam in the presence of a high magnetic field to produce high-quality images of the body in any plane. There are two main magnetic relaxation times (T1 and T2) utilized that reflect quantitative alterations in MR signal strength due to interactions of the nuclei being studied and their surrounding chemical and physical environment: the resulting radiographs are referred to as T1- and T2-weighted images.

Magnetic resonance angiography (MRA) is now commonly performed for evaluating carotid, vertebral, and cerebral arteries.

REFERENCES

Coar T. *The Aphorisms of Hippocrates: with a translation into Latin and English.* New York: The Classics of Medicine Library. 1982, p. 1.

Daffner RH. *Clinical Radiology: The Essentials.* 2nded. Philadelphia: Lippincott Williams & Wilkins, 1999.

Krone KD, Weiner SA. How to Read Chest X-Rays. *Hospital Medicine,* July, 1992, pp. 79–101.

Rosenow EC. Radiography I Primary Care: Honing your skills in interpreting chest films. *Consultant,* October, 1994, pp. 1415–1426.

Squire L, Novelline RA. *Fundamentals of Radiology.* 4thed. Cambridge, Mass: Harvard University Press, 1988.

CHAPTER **15**

Arterial Blood Gases and Acid-Base Disorders

> A mong the various diagnostic possibilities pertaining to any seriously ill
> patient, *the curable ones* ought to be pursued first and most vigorously,
> whatever the diagnostic probabilities.
>
> *Alexander S. Nadas, M.D. (1913–2000)*
>
> *After completing medical school in his native Budapest, Dr. Nadas served as a rotat-
> ing intern in Cleveland, followed by a residency in pediatrics at Massachusetts
> Memorial Hospital, Boston. He earned a second M.D. degree from Wayne University
> and was invited by Charles Janeway, M.D., Chief of Pediatrics at Boston Children's
> Hospital to develop a program in pediatric cardiology, the first such program in the
> United States. The Alexander Nadas Professorship in Pediatric Cardiology at Harvard
> Medical School was created in his honor at the time of his retirement in 1984. He is
> considered a founder of the field of pediatric cardiology.*

I. **Indications for testing arterial blood gas.** The arterial blood gas (ABG) is a
   test used to assess acid-base status and the ability of the cardiopulmonary system to oxygenate blood. Because a sample of arterial blood is somewhat difficult to collect and painful for the patient, an ABG is obtained only when there
   is reason to believe that hypoxemia, hypocapnia, hypercapnia, or a pH disturbance is present, or when there has been a serious alteration in the patient's cardiac or ventilatory status. Common clinical situations in which these disturbances are encountered include:

   A. Suspected **myocardial infarction** or **cardiac arrest.**

   B. **Respiratory distress** secondary to asthma or chronic obstructive pul-
      monary disease.

   C. **Stroke** with altered level of consciousness.

   D. **Right-to-left circulatory shunt.**

   E. **Suspected acid-base disturbance.**

   F. **Poisoning** or **trauma** with cardiopulmonary depression.

II. **Normal blood gas values.** The results of an ABG are given as pH, PO_2,
    PCO_2, HCO_3^-, base difference (excess or deficit), and percent oxygen satura-
    tion. pH, PCO_2, HCO_3^-, and base difference give information about acid-base
    homeostasis, while PO_2 and O_2 saturation give information on blood oxygena-
    tion.

    A. Partial pressure of oxygen (**PO_2: normal 80–100 mm Hg**).

    B. Oxygen saturation (**SaO_2: normal > 95 percent**).

C. Partial pressure of CO2 (**PCO$_2$: normal 35–45 mm Hg**).

D. CO$_2$ content (**[HCO$_3^-$]: normal 22–26 mEq/L**).

E. Arterial pH (**pH: normal 7.40**).

F. All of these tests are usually performed together with an automated blood gas analyzer. The analyzer directly measures the pH, PCO$_2$, PO$_2$, and SaO$_2$, and calculates the HCO$_3^-$ from the Henderson-Hasselbalch equation:

$$pH = pKa + \frac{\log [HCO_3^-] \text{ in mEq/L}}{0.03 \times PCO_2 \text{ in mm Hg}}$$

III. Defining acid-base disorders

A. The basics of acid-base disorders

1. Acid-base disorders can be divided into two types: **acidosis (pH < 7.40)** and **alkalosis (pH > 7.40)**. Acid-base disturbances occur due to abnormalities in the respiratory system, the metabolic-renal system, or both.

2. **For any primary disturbance in acid-base homeostasis there is a normal compensatory response.** A primary metabolic disorder leads to a respiratory compensation; a primary respiratory disorder leads to an acute metabolic response, due to the buffering capacity of body fluids, **and** a more chronic compensation, due to alterations in renal function.

3. In a normal patient, the **degree of compensation for a given primary disturbance has been well defined** and can be expressed in terms of the given primary disturbance. Table 15-1 lists the four major categories of primary acid-base disorders, the primary disturbance, the secondary compensatory response, and the expected degree of compensation in terms of the magnitude of the primary disturbance.

B. Simple versus mixed acid-base disorders

1. Most acid-base disorders result from a single primary disturbance and its normal physiologic compensatory response; these are called **simple acid-base disorders**. Fig. 15-1 is a nomogram that allows rapid systematic interpretation of ABG results to define simple acid-base disorders.

2. Sometimes, in particularly ill patients, two or more different primary disturbances may occur simultaneously, resulting in a **mixed acid-base disorder**. The net effect of mixed disorders may be additive (metabolic acidosis and respiratory acidosis) and result in extreme alterations in

TABLE 15–1. Simple acid-base disturbances

Acid-base disorder	Primary abnormality	Secondary response	Expected degree of compensatory response
Metabolic acidosis	↓ [HCO$_3^-$]	↓ PCO$_2$	PCO$_2$ = (1.5 × [HCO$_3^-$]) + 8
Metabolic alkalosis	↑ [HCO$_3^-$]	↑ PCO$_2$	PCO$_2$ = (0.9 × [HCO$_3^-$]) + 9
Respiratory acidosis	↑ PCO$_2$	↑ [HCO$_3^-$]	Δ [HCO$_3^-$] = 0.35 × Δ PCO$_2$
Respiratory alkalosis	↓ PCO$_2$	↓ [HCO$_3^-$]	Δ [HCO$_3^-$] = 0.50 × Δ PCO$_2$

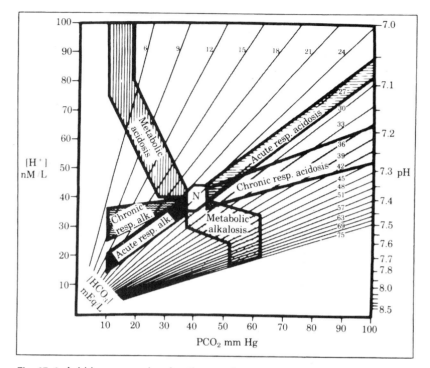

Fig. 15–1. Acid-base map showing the usual compensatory range of pH, PCO_2, and plasma HCO_3^- concentrations in simple acid-base disorders. Values on the vertical axis represent plasma H^+ concentration (left) in nanomoles per liter, or pH (right). Values on the horizontal axis represent PCO_2 in mm Hg. Diagonal lines are isopleths for the plasma HCO_3^- concentration in mEq/L. Clear area in the center of the graph is the range of normal (N). Note that the metabolic component (plasma HCO_3^- concentration) and the respiratory component (arterial blood PCO_2) of the acid-base equation always change in the same direction. (Reprinted by permission from M. Goldberg et al., Computer-based instruction and diagnosis of acid-base disorders: A systemic approach. *J.A.M.A.* 223:269, 1973. Copyright @ 1973, American Medical Association.)

acid-base homeostasis, or may be opposite (respiratory acidosis and metabolic alkalosis) and cancel each other's effects.

    a. Additive mixed acid-base disorder. Consider a patient who has just suffered an acute myocardial infarction and has gone into respiratory arrest. The tissues of the patient are not being perfused, and a metabolic acidosis due to the buildup of lactic acid will develop quickly. Because the lungs of the patient are not functioning, the patient will also retain CO_2, resulting in a respiratory acidosis as well. The patient's disorder is thus a mixed **metabolic acidosis and respira-**

tory acidosis, and the pH of the patient may be extraordinarily low, requiring immediate HCO_3^- treatment and mechanical ventilation.

b. **Nullifying mixed acid-base disorder.** Consider a patient who has emphysema and is being treated for congestive heart failure (CHF) with high-dose diuretics. Due to the emphysema, the patient will suffer from a respiratory acidosis (increased PCO_2), and due to the diuretic, the patient will suffer from a metabolic alkalosis (increased $[HCO_3^-]$). In this case the pH of the patient may be normal, as the two acid-base disturbances cancel each other's effects on pH.

IV. **Arterial blood gas interpretation.** The easiest way to interpret a blood gas result is to ask yourself four questions, first about the primary disturbance, and then about any compensatory mechanisms.

A. **Question 1: Is the primary disturbance an acidosis (pH < 7.40) or an alkalosis (pH > 7.40)?**

B. **Question 2: Is the primary disturbance metabolic or respiratory in nature?** The best way to answer this is to determine **which component, respiratory or metabolic, is altered in the same direction as the pH.** For instance, in the case where the blood gas pH > 7.40 (an alkalosis):

1. If the PCO_2 < 40 mm Hg and $[HCO_3^-]$ < 24 mEq/L, then the acid-base disturbance is a respiratory alkalosis.

2. If the PCO_2 > 40 mm Hg and $[HCO_3^-]$ > 24 mEq L, then the acid-base disturbance is a metabolic alkalosis.

3. If both $[HCO_3^-]$ and PCO_2 are changed in the same direction, then there is a mixed acid-base disorder present. For example, if the PCO_2 < 40 mm Hg and $[HCO_3^-]$ > 24 mEq/L, then the acid-base disorder is a mixed respiratory alkalosis and metabolic alkalosis.

4. Refer to Table 15–1, and make sure you understand this logic.

C. **Question 3: Is the degree of compensation adequate?** Given the primary disturbance identified in question 2, use the equations in Table 15–1 to calculate the expected compensatory response. If this expected response is significantly different from what is observed, then a mixed acid-base disturbance is present. As an alternative to remembering the exact equations for the four acid-base derangements given in Table 15–1, there are two guidelines that follow from the Henderson-Hasselbalch equation that are helpful in discerning simple versus mixed acid-base disorders:

1. A change in PCO_2 equal to 10 mm Hg results in a change in a pH equal to 0.08 units.

2. A pH change of 0.15 results in a change in $[HCO_3^-]$ of 10 mEq/L.

D. **Question 4: What is causing the disorder?** Each type of simple or mixed acid-base disturbance has its own differential diagnosis, as described in sec. **V.** The final step in interpreting a blood gas is to correlate the whole of the patient's clinical presentation with the acid-base disorder you have determined, come up with a diagnosis, and then plan for treatment.

Note: If ABG values do not seem possible, assume there is human or mechanical error and draw a new arterial blood sample.

V. Differential diagnoses of acid-base derangements

A. Metabolic acidosis: pH < 7.40, PCO_2 < 40 mm Hg, $[HCO_3^-]$ < 24 mEq/L. Metabolic acidosis is caused by an increase in acid in body fluids, which results in a decrease in $[HCO_3^-]$ as it attempts to buffer the new acid load, and a compensatory decrease in PCO_2 as the lungs attempt to blow off CO_2. Causes of metabolic acidosis are classified as either an anion gap acidosis or a non-anion gap acidosis.

The **anion gap** = $[Na^+] - ([Cl^-] + [HCO_3^-])$; normal range: 8–12 mEq/L.

1. Anion gap acidosis: anion gap > 12 mEq/L. Caused by a decrease in $[HCO_3^-]$ that results from the buffering of unmeasured acid ion from either endogenous production or exogenous ingestion (normochloremic acidosis).

A useful mnemonic to remember the causes of anion gap acidosis is

SLUMPED:

Salicylates
Lactic acid
Uremia
Methanol
Paraldehyde
Ethylene glycol/Ethanol
Diabetic ketoacidosis

2. Non-anion gap acidosis: anion gap = 8–12 mEq/L. Caused by a decrease in $[HCO_3^-]$. The anion gap is not increased here, because of an increase in chloride (hyperchloremic acidosis).

Fig. 15–2 outlines the causes of anion gap and non-anion gap acidosis.

B. Metabolic alkalosis: pH > 7.40, PCO_2 > 40 mm Hg, $[HCO_3^-]$ > 24 mEq/L. Metabolic alkalosis results from a primary increase in $[HCO_3^-]$ with a compensatory increase in PCO_2.

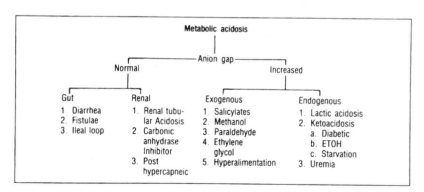

Fig. 15–2. Differential diagnosis of metabolic acidosis. ETOH = ethyl alcohol. (Reproduced with permission from Gomella LG, *Clinician's Pocket Reference.* 7th ed. Norwalk, Conn: Appleton and Lange, 1993.)

There are two mechanisms by which the kidneys retain $[HCO_3^-]$. They can be differentiated by the level of urinary $[Cl^-]$ and the way in which they respond to NaCl treatment.

1. **Chloride-responsive metabolic alkalosis:** urinary $[Cl^-] < 10$ mEq/L. The initial problem is a sustained loss of chloride out of proportion to the loss of sodium (either by renal or gastrointestinal losses). This chloride depletion results in renal sodium conservation leading to a corresponding reabsorption of $[HCO_3^-]$ by the kidney. These disorders **respond to treatment with intravenous NaCl.**

2. **Chloride-resistant metabolic alkalosis:** urinary $[Cl^-] > 10$ mEq/L. Results from direct stimulation of the kidneys to retain bicarbonate, irrespective of electrolyte intake or losses. These disorders **do not respond to treatment with intravenous NaCl.**

3. **Chloride-responsive metabolic acidosis is far more common** than the resistant form. Fig. 15–3 outlines the causes of chloride responsive and resistant metabolic alkalosis.

C. **Respiratory acidosis: pH < 7.40, $PCO_2 > 40$ mm Hg, $[HCO_3^-] > 24$ mEq/L.** Respiratory acidosis results from an increase in PCO_2 with a compensatory elevation in plasma $[HCO_3^-]$. Increased PCO_2 occurs when alveolar ventilation is decreased. Conditions in which respiratory acidosis occurs include:

1. **Neuromuscular abnormalities with ventilatory failure**

   a. Defects in the muscles of respiration (myasthenia gravis, muscular dystrophy)

   b. Depression of respiratory center (due to anesthesia, narcotics, tranquilizers, sedatives, vertebral artery embolism or thrombosis, increased intracranial pressure)

   c. Defects in peripheral nervous system (ALS, poliomyelitis, Guillain-Barré syndrome, botulism, tetanus, organophosphate poisoning, spinal cord injury)

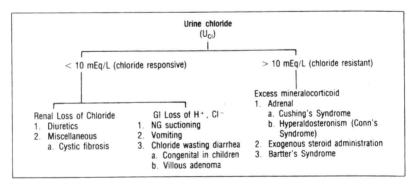

Fig. 15–3. Differential diagnosis of metabolic alkalosis. (Reproduced with permission from Gomella LG, *Clinician's Pocket Reference.* 7th ed. Norwalk, Conn: Appleton and Lange, 1993.)

2. Airway obstruction

a. Chronic (chronic obstructive pulmonary disease [COPD])

b. Acute (due to asthma, foreign body, laryngospasm)

3. Thoracic-pulmonary disorders

a. Thoracic cage disorders (flail chest, rib fractures, pneumothorax, kyphoscoliosis)

b. Pulmonary disease (pneumothorax, severe pulmonary edema, severe pneumonia, interstitial fibrosis)

D. Respiratory alkalosis: pH > 7.40, PCO_2 < 40 mm Hg, $[HCO_3^-]$ < 24 mEq/L. Respiratory alkalosis results from a decrease in PCO_2 with a compensatory decrease in plasma $[HCO_3^-]$. Decreased PCO_2 occurs when alveolar ventilation is increased. Conditions in which respiratory alkalosis occurs include:

1. Central stimulation

a. Hyperventilation syndrome (anxiety, pain, hysteria)

b. Head trauma or cerebrovascular accident (CVA) with neurogenic hyperventilation

c. Tumors

d. Drugs (salicylate, xanthines, progesterone, epinephrine, thyroxin, nicotine)

e. Gram-negative sepsis

f. Hyponatremia

2. Peripheral stimulation

a. Congestive heart failure

b. Interstitial lung disease

c. Hypoxemia (pneumonia, pulmonary embolus, atelectasis, high altitude)

3. Miscellaneous

a. Hepatic encephalopathy

b. Pregnancy

c. Iatrogenic overventilation

VI. Performing the arterial blood gas determination

A. The order of preference for **ABG puncture site** is radial artery, then brachial artery, and finally femoral artery. You should familiarize yourself with the exact location of these arteries and practice palpating them on yourself. Learn to feel for these arteries in a way that lets you "see" their course underneath your fingertips.

B. Allen's test is a procedure for evaluating the collateral circulation in patients in whom arterial puncture might result in severe hypoperfusion of the hand if the collateral circulation were inadequate. First, have the patient make a tight fist to expel the blood from the surface vessels of the palm, and use your finger to occlude either the radial or ulnar artery. Then have the patient open his or her hand and check to see if the blood returns to the palm and fingers (indicated by the return of a pink hue to the surface). If this pink hue is delayed, then you should suspect obstruction to the blood flow in the artery that you did not compress.

C. Take opportunities to practice your arterial puncture technique in non-emergency situations so that you will be able to act quickly, safely, and competently when speed is necessary. Being able to obtain a sample of arterial blood without unduly traumatizing your patient is an important clinical skill.

VII. Interpreting arterial blood gas results

A. Recall that **the oxygen saturation curve for hemoglobin has a steep sigmoid shape** that starts to level off near a PO_2 of 70 mm Hg. This means that a patient may have a PO_2 of 65 mm Hg and still have an O_2 saturation > 90 percent. Conversely, the difference between a PO_2 of 50 mm Hg and a PO_2 of 60 mm Hg is very significant clinically, because it lies on the steep slope of the curve.

B. Always **note whether an ABG was drawn while the patient was receiving oxygen therapy.** This fact is often forgotten in the heat of the moment and obviously affects the PO_2 and oxygen saturation.

C. Always **analyze the ABG results together with the serum electrolytes and the anion gap.** If the patient is acidotic, the anion gap becomes the next step in constructing the differential diagnosis.

D. In analyzing the clinical status of a patient who has undergone an ABG, you must **know what baseline values are normal for your patient.** Many patients with chronic pulmonary disease exist quite happily with a PO_2 of 60 mm Hg, and it would be futile and dangerous to attempt to improve respiratory status much beyond this level.

REFERENCES

Goldberg M, et al. Computer-based instruction and diagnosis of acid-base disorders: a systematic approach. *JAMA* 1973;223:269.

Gomella LG. *Clinician's Pocket Reference.* 7th ed. Norwalk, Conn: Appleton and Lange, 1993.

CHAPTER **16**

The Medical Write-up and Progress Notes

> L ife and death crises actually occupy a reasonably small portion of clinical
> medicine, and an even smaller portion of the patient's concern over the
> quality of life. We must recognize that *when a patient feels a problem is an
> emergency, it is, by definition, an emergency* to the patient, whether or not the
> physician views the problem as life threatening. Even the highest quality of
> scientific medical management will not satisfy the patient unless these
> underlying concerns are answered.
>
> *Harley A. Haynes, M.D.*
>
> *A graduate of Harvard Medical School, Dr. Haynes completed residency training in
> internal medicine and dermatology at the Peter Bent Brigham Hospital and Massa-
> chusetts General Hospital in Boston, followed by additional fellowship training in
> dermatology at the National Institutes of Health. He is Senior Physician and Vice
> Chairman of the Department of Dermatology at the Dana-Farber Cancer Institute,
> Boston, and Professor of Dermatology at Harvard Medical School.*

I. General points concerning the medical write-up

A. Purpose. The medical progress note (write-up) is the official, permanent
account of professional medical care. It not only shapes the style and focus
of its various offshoots (oral case presentations and published case reports)
but also determines what students take seriously in an antecedent activity,
the medical interview. The write-up has three major purposes.

1. **To convey information to consultants**, who are not as familiar with
the case, and to **covering house officers**, who may be asked to make a
decision in the middle of the night concerning a patient with whom they
are not familiar.

2. **To document and clarify the impression and approaches** of the medical team for future medical reference and medicolegal inquiries.

3. To force the writer **to quantify and organize** his or her own impressions in order to gain a better understanding of the case.

The student write-up, for better or worse, has an additional purpose:
to show the student's preceptors how thoroughly the student has
investigated and analyzed the case, and how familiar he or she is
with the differential diagnosis and the various management options
that exist.

B. **Format.** Three major formats are currently in use for teaching hospital write-ups.

1. The first, sometimes called the **comprehensive write-up**, is used typically by first or second year medical students performing a complete history and physical examination on a patient they have been asked to evaluate. An example of this lengthy and exhaustive write-up is reproduced on pages 169–181 taken from a format for patient-write-ups prepared by Sandra Kammerman, M.D. that is required of students at New York University School of Medicine. In addition to the usual elements found on a patient write-up prepared by an attending physician (e.g., chief complaint, history of the present illness, etc.), the comprehensive write-up is unique because it also often contains information you will probably not find elsewhere in the medical record: an overview of the proposed pathogenesis for the presenting complaints as well as a discussion of the patient's presentation.

2. The second, sometimes called the **traditional write-up**, is widely used and is the format most often utilized by third and fourth year medical students asked to write-up a patient's admission. Its outline is shown in the sample write-up on pages 183–188. Its major advantage is that it is issue-oriented and a somewhat streamlined version of the comprehensive write-up: within a general framework, its complexity expands and contracts in relation to the complexity of the medical case. Its major disadvantage is that information may be recorded and organized in a rather haphazard way. Information pertaining to multiple separate medical problems, for instance, may be grouped in a single long paragraph, making future chart review more difficult.

3. The third write-up format is the **problem-oriented medical record (POMR)** and is reproduced in Fig. 16-1 (page 189). It is often used in the outpatient setting but is also often utilized by attending physicians and is a useful format for focused follow-up progress notes in the medical record, after the patient has been admitted to a hospital or after the patient has been seen for the first time in an outpatient setting. Its chief advantage is that it allows pertinent information to be assessed with relative ease, without a detailed recap of the patient's admission information or commentary on medical problems that are not active. A complete description of the problem-oriented system is beyond the scope of this chapter; essentially it involves the recording of all medical data as entries under the headings of specific medical problems in a **SOAP** format (**subjective** information from the patient's medical history, **objective** information obtained after a physical exam and review of laboratory findings, an **assessment** by the examining clinician, and an outline of the clinician's **plan** for managing the patient's care and each of his or her active medical problems).

The problem-oriented system has been used with increasing frequency in recent years in the United States, particularly as medical records have become computerized. Many physicians are also starting to incorporate certain elements of the POMR into a traditional write-up framework (e.g., an "active problem list" is now a standard part of many hospital charts), and hybrids of the two systems are now common. **Students beginning their clinical rotations should check with their preceptors to determine which specific write-up format is preferred for them.**

PROGRESS NOTES

Please date and sign each entry

1/3/04, 9:58 A.M.

Name of Patient: John Jones

Source and Reliability: patient (who appears reliable.)

Chief Complaint

Mr. Jones is a 67-year old male who presented to the ED with "sharp pain in my chest" and night sweats for three days.

History of the Present Illness

Mr. Jones has smoked cigarettes continuously since age 17, for a total of 118 pack-years. At age 25, the patient began working in a shipyard and as a result had extensive asbestos exposure for the next 20 years. He was well until 10 years ago, when he developed a cough almost every morning, productive of about a teaspoon of greenish sputum, without any change over time, or any blood. The sputum production clears over the course of the morning, and in general is worst in the spring. When the patient takes antibiotics for any reason, on average, once a year, he notes that his sputum becomes clearer and decreases in volume.

Over the past six months, the patient lost 25-pounds without either trying to lose weight or a change in his appetite. Two months ago, the patient noted occasional flecks of blood in his sputum, but no change in his chronic cough.

Mary Smith, MS II

→

PROGRESS NOTES

Please date and sign each entry

1/3/04 (continued)

Over the past two weeks, sputum production has increased to 3 teaspoons per day, and includes the afternoons, and now is blood-streaked.

Three days prior to admission the patient noted a sharp pain in his right chest. The pain came on gradually, does not radiate, is worsened by taking a deep breath, dyspnea on exertion, and peripheral edema. He denies fever, but for the last three nights he soaked his sheets with sweat. This morning he saw his private doctor who told him his chest X-ray was abnormal. The doctor also reported that his white blood count was elevated, and recommended that he come to the ED, where he arrived at 1 PM. Because of his abnormal CXR, the ED admitted him directly to the medical service with no further evaluation or treatment.

He has no history of TB, previous hospitalization for pulmonary symptoms or pneumonia, abnormal CXR, asthma, international travel, or trauma to the chest. He is unaware of his PPD status. There is no history of cardiac illness or cancer.

                                        Mary Smith, MSII
                                             ⟶

ED = Emergency Department, CXR = chest radiograph,
PPD = purified protein derivative, TB = tuberculosis

PROGRESS NOTES

Please date and sign each entry

1/3/04 (continued)

Past Medical History

1. Gout – 1975, 1996, brief episodes of pain and swelling in right big toe, effectively treated with allopurinol.
2. Major Depression – 1980, following prolonged illness and death of father. Treated with oral medication (unknown) and psychotherapy for two years. No recurrences.
3. No other history of any major medical illnesses or hospitalizations since childhood. Specifically no history of hypertension, high cholesterol, cancer, STD, diabetes, liver & heart disease.

Past Surgical History

1. Appendectomy – Age 19, uncomplicated
2. Repair of fractured left tibia – Age 26

Allergies

1. Allergic to tetracycline – caused rash on body about 20 years ago.
2. No other known drug or food allergies.

Family History

Father died aged 70, due to cancer of the colon. Mother alive and well at 85. Daughter, age 39 A & W.

Mary Smith, MS II

→

STD = sexually transmitted disease
A&W = alive and well

PROGRESS NOTES

Please date and sign each entry

1/3/04 (continued)

Two siblings, brother 59 A&W, sister 65, HTN on medication. There is no family history of TB, other cancers, premature heart disease, diabetes, or alcoholism.

Social History

Patient retired five years ago after 40 years of work in shipyards and a shoe factory. He lives in Brooklyn with his wife and daughter who is divorced, both of whom accompanied him to the hospital. He is heterosexual with one partner, his wife. He drinks 5 cans of beer a week on average. He denies any illicit or recreational drug use. He receives social security and a pension.

Medications

Allopurinol 300 mg. p.o. daily

Review of Systems

General: denies chills or malaise.
HEENT: denies head trauma, headaches, or dizziness. Has used eyeglasses for past 35 years. Denies other problems with vision. Denies problems with hearing or tinnitus. Denies chronic sinus problems, but suffers from hay fever in the fall. Denies frequent sore throats or dental problems.

Mary Smith, MS II →

HTN = hypertension

PROGRESS NOTES

Please date and sign each entry

1/3/04 (Continued)

Pulmonary: see HPI.

Cardiovascular: Denies hx of congenital heart disease, murmur, rheumatic fever, angina, hypertension, palpitations, MI, abnormal EKG, orthopnea, dyspnea on exertion, edema, heart surgery, PVD angiography, or syncope.

GI: Denies hx of ulcer disease, hepatitis, cholecystitis, upper or lower GI bleeding, or hemorrhoids. Denies nausea, vomiting, change in appetite, diarrhea, melena, or constipation.

GU: Denies hx of urinary infections, problems urinating, dysuria, hematuria or a hx of syphilis, gonorrhea, or prostate disease. Reports satisfactory sexual relations.

Heme/Endocrine: Denies hx of anemia, fatigue, or easy bruisability. Denies polyuria, polydipsia, or heat or cold intolerance.

Musculoskeletal: see PMH; denies other joint, bone, or muscle problems.

Neurologic: Denies motor or sensory neurologic problems, difficulties in walking or balance, seizures, headaches, TIA, or CVA.

Psychiatric: see PMH.

Skin: Denies rashes, lesions, or other skin problems.

Physical Exam

General Appearance: A cachectic male appearing older than his stated age, lying comfortably in bed, in no acute distress.

Vital Signs: Temp 100.8°F, BP 110/74 and pulse 90/regular while supine

Mary Smith, MS II

MI = myocardial infarction
PVD = peripheral vascular disease
TIA = transient ischemic attack
CVA = cerebrovascular accident

PROGRESS NOTES

Please date and sign each entry

1/3/04 (continued)

BP 105/70 and pulse 96/regular while standing
Respirations 24 and shallow
Skin: A 2 x 1.5 cm. brown, raised, crusted, rough patch on left upper
back, non-tender, non-warm, with irregular borders.
Head: Bi-temporal wasting, normocephalic, atraumatic.
Eyes: Conjunctiva pink, sclera anicteric, pupils 3mm equally round
and reactive to light and accommodation (PERRLA), fundi
demonstrate flat discs, normal vessels, without hemorrhages
or exudates
Ears: External auditory canals (EAC) normal, tympanic membranes
intact, hearing grossly intact.
Nose: Mucosa pink, no discharge or polyps
Mouth: Moist membranes, partial upper dentures, otherwise dentition
normal for age, no oral lesions
Throat: Non-injected, no tonsillar hypertrophy or exudates
Neck: Supple, full range of motion (FROM), trachea midline,
no thyromegaly, carotids 2/2 without bruits, no JVD or
hepatojugular reflux, no abnormal pulses or bruits
Nodes: No cervical, submandibular, supraclavicular, axillary,
or inguinal lymphadenopathy
Breasts: normal male, no masses, discharge, or tenderness

Mary Smith, MS II
→

JVD = jugular venous distention

PROGRESS NOTES

Please date and sign each entry

1/3/04 (continued)

Lungs: I: barrel chest, unable to take a deep breath due to guarding
    P: No tenderness; tactile fremitus increased right base.
    P: Hyperresonance bilaterally, dull to percussion at right base
    A: Crackles, bronchial breathing and egophony at right base,
      otherwise breath sounds diminished throughout.
Heart: I: no apical heave or parasternal (RV) lift
    P: PMI in 4th intercostal space in the mid-clavicular line;
      no palpable heave, lift or thrill
    A: normal S_1, S_2; no splitting or loud P_2; I/VI low-pitched
      early systolic murmur best heard at the lower left
      sternal border; no rubs or gallops
Abdomen: I: abdomen flat, no scars, striae or dilated veins
    A: Bowel sounds normal; no bruits (aorta, iliofemoral, renal)
    P: Soft, non-tender; no guarding or rebound; liver palpable
      4cm below the right mid-clavicular line; spleen not
      palpable; no masses
    P: Liver span 10cm by percussion in right midclavicular line
Back: No spinal or CVA tenderness
Genitalia: normal male, circumcised. Testes descended B/L, no masses,
    no skin lesions
Rectal: Good sphincter tone, no masses or tenderness, prostate smooth,
    It enlarged, no masses, stool Guiac negative.
Extremities: No clubbing, cyanosis or edema; no tenderness, joints have
    FROM; no subcutaneous nodules, no abnormalities of big toe, no tophi
                  Mary Smith, MSII

I = inspection, P = palpatron, P = percussion, A = auscultation
RV = right ventricular
PMI = point of maximal intensity/impulse
CVA = costovertebral angle

PROGRESS NOTES

Please date and sign each entry

1/3/04   (continued)

Pulses:	Brachial	Radial	Femoral	Popliteal	Posterior Tibialis	Dorsalis Pedis
R	+2	+2	+2	+2	+2	+2
L	+2	+2	+2	+2	+2	+2

no bruits

Neuro: Mental Status: awake, alert, fully responsive, oriented to person, place, and time. normal affect.

Cranial Nerves:	
I	not tested
II	visual acuity (corrected 20/20), full visual fields
III, IV, VI	extraocular muscles intact
V	normal sensation on face, jaw-clench
VII	no weakness
VIII	hearing intact
IX, X	gag reflex present bilaterally
XI	symmetric trapezius, sternocleidomastoid
XII	tongue midline

Motor: RUE 5/5, RLE 5/5, LUE 5/5, LLE 5/5

Sensory: Intact to pinprick, light touch, position and vibration

Cerebellar: No dysdiadochokinesis, gait normal, Romberg's sign absent

Reflexes: Biceps 2+, Triceps 2+, Patellar 2+, Achilles 2+, Plantar downward, no snout or glabellar reflexes

Mary Smith, MSII
⟶

RUE = right upper extremity
RLE = right lower extremity
LUE = left upper extremity
LLE = left lower extremity

PROGRESS NOTES

Please date and sign each entry

1/3/04 (Continued)

Laboratory: Hematocrit 27, MCV 79, White blood count 12.8 with 79 polys, 4 bands, 13 lymphs, and 4 monos.
Electrolytes, liver function tests and urinalysis all normal.
Chest X-ray: flattening of the diaphragm and hyperlucency throughout. A 1x2cm. mass in right hilum with dense right lower lobe alveolar consolidation and blunting of right costophrenic angle.
EKG: NSR, rate 90, low voltage diffusely, no ST or T wave changes, normal axis, good R wave progression

Summary
67 year old White male smoker, shipyard worker, with history indicative of COPD and chronic productive cough, gout, and depression presents with 6 month hx. of 25 lb. wt loss, 2 months of hemoptysis, and increased sputum production and night sweats, and 3 days of pleuritic pain in the right chest. The physical exam is remarkable for a pulse of 96, temp of 100.8°F, barrel chest with guarding, clinical signs of consolidation at right base. There is a single skin lesion on the left upper back. Labs show a microcytic anemia, elevated white count with a normal differential, CXR reveals an infiltrate in the right lower lobe and pleural effusion and right hilar mass. The current problems can be summarized as follows:

Mary Smith, MSIII

NSR = normal sinus rhythm

PROGRESS NOTES

Please date and sign each entry

1/3/04   (continued)

Problem List:
1. Acute pulmonary process
2. Right hilar mass
3. Chronic cough
4. Weight loss
5. Anemia
6. Skin lesion

Assessment

1. Acute pulmonary process

Pneumonia is the most likely explanation for the acute process. This is supported by acute onset of change in sputum, hemoptysis, night sweats, fever, pleuritic chest pain, signs of consolidation, CXR showing lobar infiltrate and pleural effusion, and leukocytosis. This probably represents community-acquired pneumonia, most likely due to pneumococcus, but could be due to H. influenzae, S. aureus, B. catarrhalis, L. pneumophila. An alternative diagnosis causing pleuritic chest pain, hemoptysis and fever is pulmonary embolism with infarction. Against this diagnosis is the patient's change in sputum production, and the pulmonary consolidation that is not wedge shaped. Another alternative diagnosis is a chronic pulmonary infection, such as tuberculosis, which can cause fever, weight loss, increased sputum, hemoptysis, and infiltrate. Against tuberculosis is the acute time frame, and the location of the infiltrate. The acute time frame is against other chronic pulmonary infections. Thus, for the acute process, I favor community-acquired pneumonia (95% chance), or tuberculosis (5% chance).

Mary Smith, MSII

→

PROGRESS NOTES

Please date and sign each entry

1/3/04   (continued)

Plan: Diagnostic: sputum for Gram and AFB stains, and cultures; blood cultures; PPD skin test; therapeutic trial of antibiotics; consider V/Q (ventilation-perfusion) scan or spiral CT scan if no response to antimicrobial agents within 24 hours

Therapeutic: IV hydration; empiric broad spectrum antibiotics
a) vancomycin because of concern for resistant pneumo-cocci, while awaiting stain and culture results.
b) erythromycin for atypical organisms
c) duration of course and nature of antibiotics will await evaluation of response to therapy and results of diagnostic tests

2. Right hilar mass
The right lung mass could be a tumor or a hilar node from a chronic infection such as tuberculosis. Given the intensive exposure to tobacco and asbestos and the history consistent with chronic bronchitis it is possible that there is a bronchogenic carcinoma that partially obstructs a bronchus impairing clearance of secretions causing pneumonia. In favor of a neoplasm is the weight loss, anemia, and exposure history. There are no findings against this. Thus, for the lung mass I favor bronchogenic carcinoma (70% chance), tuberculosis (10% chance), other granulomatous disease (10% chance), or lung abscess (10% chance).

Mary Smith, MS II

⟶

AFB = acid-fast bacilli
PPD = purified protein derivative
V/Q = ventilation-perfusion
CT = computed tomography
IV = intravenous

PROGRESS NOTES

Please date and sign each entry

1/3/04 (continued)

Plan: Diagnostic: CT scan of the chest; sputum cytologies; may need bronchoscopy for tissue diagnosis
Therapeutic: Will be based on the specific etiology.

3. Chronic cough

Chronic cough, in an 118-pack year smoker with purulent sputum that clears with antibiotics suggests chronic bronchitis. The barrel chest, hyperresonance, and flattened diaphragm also suggest COPD (emphysema). This patient likely has a mixed picture (typical of COPD with both bronchitis and emphysema). All other possibilities are remote. The cause of the right hilar mass may be contributing to this process of late (hemoptysis for 2 months).

Plan: Diagnostic: PFT's to confirm diagnosis, assess extent of disease and predict response to inhaled dilators; ABG when acute illness resolves to assess prognosis and potential therapeutic response to continuing oxygen therapy.
Therapeutic: Will depend on results of diagnostic tests.

4. Weight Loss

Weight loss, with cachexia and wasting, is indicative of a chronic process. Consider neoplasm or infection. With right

Mary Smith, MS II

CT = computed tomography
PFTs = pulmonary function tests

PROGRESS NOTES

Please date and sign each entry

1/3/04 (continued)

hilar mass, strong history of exposures, consider bronchogenic carcinoma (80% chance); other neoplasms much less likely based on normal exam (10% chance). Also consider tuberculosis (10% chance), but no past history, apices are normal, and TB usually does not present as a mass.

Plan: Diagnostic: Cytologies; bronchoscopy; sputum for AFB
Therapeutic: Pending

5. Anemia
etc., for all issues on problem list.

6. Skin Lesion
etc., for all issues on problem list.

Diagnoses
1. Right Lower Lobe Pneumonia, possibly secondary to 2 or 3.
2. COPD.
3. Probable occult lung neoplasm with weight loss, anemia.
4. Skin lesion, probable seborrheic keratosis.
5. History of gout, on medication.
6. History of depression.
7. Allergy to tetracycline.

Mary Smith, MS II

AFB = acid-fast bacilli

PROGRESS NOTES

Please date and sign each entry

1/3/04   (Continued)

<u>Proposed Pathogenesis:</u>

Chronic tobacco use   Asbestos exposure

Chronic cough ← COPD → Bronchogenic CA ← → Weight loss
Barrel chest   (right hilar mass)   → Anemia
Flat diaphragm
↓Breath sounds

Endobronchial lesion

Partial obstruction

→ Inability to clear
Micro-aspiration of → micro-aspiration
oral flora

Acute pyogenic pneumonia → Cough → Hemoptysis
                              Fever
                              Leukocytosis

Consolidation

Shunt

Tachypnea

Mary Smith, MS II

CA = cancer

PROGRESS NOTES

Please date and sign each entry

2/14/04   MS III Admission Note
8:46 A.M.   Source: pt. (who seems reliable) and old chart.
                CC: "Weakness" and cough X several days.
HPI: This is the 2nd admission for this 55 y/o African-American
woman who was in her USOH until three days PTA when she noted
fatigue. The following morning this "tired feeling" persisted and she
confined herself to her home "to rest." (she works as a seamstress). She
slept well that night but awoke with nasal stuffiness and an
occasional cough productive of clear, mucoid sputum. The pt. then
experienced nausea accompanied by 3-4 episodes of vomiting undigested
food and several mild chills without overt shaking. The pt. says she
felt "feverish" at this time but did not take her temperature. She
also recalls a R temporal HA and sub/periorbital "aching."
        Last night, the pt.'s general malaise increased and she
also noted weakness, dizziness and a change of sputum color from
clear to brown. At this time, she denies any dyspnea, sore
throat, pleuritic chest pain or hemoptysis. She was brought to
the hospital early this morning at her son's insistence. She
denies a Hx of viral syndrome, myalgias or illness occurring
concurrently in a family member. There's no Hx of chronic sputum
production, sinusitis, bronchitis, pneumonia, TB exposure or
respiratory illness, except for an occasional UTI. There is no Hx
of rheumatic fever or heart ⓜ. There is no Hx of travel outside
the U.S. The pt. does admit to a smoking Hx of < 2 pack-
years (quit 11 yrs. ago).
                                                    →
                                    John Smith, MS III

cc = chief complaint
USOH = usual state of health
PTA = prior to admission
HA = headache
Hx = history
TB = tuberculosis
UTI = urinary tract infection
ⓜ = murmur

PROGRESS NOTES

Please date and sign each entry

(continued)

PMHx: Type 1 Diabetes Mellitus (diagnosed at age 28), HTN (diagnosed at age 48, said to be well controlled with the same medication for seven years: Capoten), Hyperlipidemia (diagnosed at age 50, now on Lipitor), R.A. (clinically stable on ASA prn for symptomatic relief) Pt. recalls a "kidney infection" ≈ 20 years ago but few details are available.

Allergies: Sulfa drugs → diffuse rash

PSHx: TAH/BSO in 1990 (at MGH), Dental work in 1997 (at BWH)

Meds: Insulin AM: 26 U NPH and 10 U Reg SQ
                PM: 20 U NPH
        Lipitor 40 mg p.o. QD, Capoten 25 mg. p.o. TID, ASA 81 mg p.o. QD

Social Hx: Widow of 6 years, works as a seamstress full-time, lives with her son (age 26). No hx of toxic exposures at work. Denies EtOH use, denies illicit drug use, tobacco use. < 2 pack-years (quit 11 yrs. ago), G₁P₀₀₁, Menopause in 1990 after TAH 2° to fibroids.

Family Hx:

No family hx of Diabetes Mellitus, CA, TB, HTN or Sickle Cell Disease

ROS: ⊕ fatigue, ⊕ malaise, no weight change, no night sweats, no hx of trauma, no LOC, no fainting, ⊕ wears glasses for presbyopia (last eye exam 3 wks ago), hearing "pretty good," no breast pain or nipple discharge (last mammogram in 2002), ⊕ "leg swelling at the end of the day," no SOB, no CP or palpitations, ⊕ vomiting (see HPI), no heartburn, no early satiety, no numbness of extremities, ⊕ nocturia →

                                John Smith, MS II

RA = rheumatoid arthritis
TAH/BSO = total abdominal hysterectomy/bilateral salpingo-oophorectomy
MGH = Massachusetts General Hospital
BWH = Brigham and Women's Hospital
EtOH = alcohol
MVA = motor vehicle accident
A&W = alive and well
CA = cancer
LOC = loss of conciousness
SOB = shortness of breath
CP = chest pain

PROGRESS NOTES

Please date and sign each entry

(continued)

ROS: no dysuria, last pap smear 3 months ago (negative, reportedly) by gynecologist, ⊕ morning stiffness "all joints," no cold or heat intolerance, no reported memory deficits, no tremors.

Physical Exam:

V.S. T: 102.8°F P: 94, regular R: 24 BP: 122/72 (L) arm ⊆
Wt: 132 lbs. Ht: 5'6" BMI: 21   110/70 (L) arm 0↑

Alert and Oriented ×3, in NAD, cooperative, pleasant, appears younger than her stated age, O₂ saturation: 89% (room air)

SKIN: Warm, dry, no bruises or rashes, nails WNL

HEENT: NC/AT, hair thin and oily, PERRLA, conjunctiva WNL, EOMI, (L) fundus clear c̄ cup: Disc ratio of 2:3 s̄ hemorrhages or exudates, (R) fundus not visualized well, TM's clear c̄ ⊕ ant. cone of light B/L, nares patent c̄ septum midline and pink nasal mucosa, ⊕ dental plate – upper teeth, lower molars, no tonsillar hypertrophy or exudates. Vision (Rosenbaum): 20/20 OS (c̄ glasses), 20/40 OD (c̄ glasses)

NECK: supple, trachea midline, thyroid not palpably enlarged, no JVD, no carotid bruits, 1 cm. (L) ant. cervical adenopathy (non-tender)

BACK: no kyphoscoliosis grossly, no CVA tenderness

LUNGS: ↓ respiratory excursion (R) side, ⊕ end-inspiratory crackles at (R) axilla, no tactile fremitus, egophony or whispered pectoriloquy

BREASTS: pendulous, no masses, tenderness or nipple discharge

CV: nl S₁, S₂, ⊕ soft S₄, ⊕ grade II/VI SEM at LSB and 3rd ICS s̄ radiation to axilla or neck, PMI not displaced, distal pulses +1 to +2 bilaterally throughout.

ABDOMEN: soft, non-tender, not distended, no palpable masses
                                                    →

                                    John Smith, MS III

NC/AT = normocephalic/atraumatic
PERRLA = pupils equally round and reactive to light and accomodation
WNL = within normal limits
EOMI = extra-ocular muscles intact
JVD = jugular venous distention
CVA = costophrenic angle
LSB = left sternal border
ICS = intercostal space
PMI = point of maximal intensity/impulse

PROGRESS NOTES

Please date and sign each entry

(continued)

ABDOMEN: ⊕ normoactive BS × 4 quadrants, no guarding or rebound, mildly obese, liver span: 10-11cm. by percussion

~10-15 cm scar (hysterectomy)

GENITALIA: external: ∃ discharge or lesions
pelvic: deferred to private gynecologist; not indicated at this time. (last pap smear neg. 3 months ago)

RECTAL: good sphincter tone, stool light brown and Guaiac neg.

MS: ROM of all 4 extremities WNL, feet slightly decreased in temp. to touch, ⊕ DIP joint, hypertrophy ∃ tenderness, no subcutaneous nodules, muscle strength 44/15 all 4 limbs, no C/C/E

NEURO: CN II-XII grossly intact, pt is alert (serial 7's intact), ↓ pinprick sensation in feet b/l (position and vibratory sense are WNL), Babinski neg. b/l, Romberg's test negative, DTRs:

LABS/DATA

2/14/04, 7:55 A.M.

PT: 11.3   PTT: 25.3

11.8 < 12.1 / 35.7 > 325K

79P, 6Ba, 7L, 1M, 1E, 1B   ESR: 24

142 | 102 | 12 < 187

3.7 | 29 | 1.0

UricAcid: 6.8

Ca^{++}: 9.6, PO_4^{-}: 3.8, Total Chol: 210, TG: N/A

U/A: 6.0, 1.020, 3-5 wbc/HPF, ⊕ glucose

ABG (on 2L/min NC O_2): 7.47/33/98/28/94%   →

John Smith, MS III

BS = bowel sounds
ROM = range of motion
WNL = within normal limits
DIP = distal interphalangeal
C/C/E = cyanosis, clubbing, edema
CN = cranial nerves
DTR = deep tendon reflexes

wbc > HgB / Hct > platelets

Na⁺ | Cl⁻ | BUN
K⁺ | HCO₃ | Cr > Glucose

PROGRESS NOTES

Please date and sign each entry

(continued)

LABS/DATA: EKG: NSR, 98 bpm, non-specific ST-T∆'s, nl axis (-20°),
.14/.08/.90, ?LVH ($V_1 + V_5 = 36$ mm), small Q in III
CXR: ⊕ RLL (superior segment) infiltrate, no effusions,
borderline cardiomegaly.
Sputum and Urine C&S: pending, Blood C&S: pending
(preliminary report on sputum: numerous Gram ⊕ diplococci
Impression/Plan: This 55 y/o African-American ♀ presents with
fever, productive cough and progressive malaise of 3 days duration.
① RLL Pneumonia, probably bacterial — (Post-obstructive process
possible, but no hx. of weight loss or other chronic symptoms;
P.E. and TB not likely, given the hx.) — with Respiratory Alkalosis
   — Start IV Rocephin 1 gm QD and IV Azithromycin
      1 gm now (followed by 500 mg IV QD)
   — F/U blood cultures and adjust antibiotic regimen as needed
   — Maintain O₂ at 2 L/min via NC and follow closely
   — Admit to Medical Ward to Dr. Martin's Service
      (Case discussed at length with Dr. Martin, who concurs)
② Opacity ® eye — R/O Cataracts (While ® fundus was not
visualized and pt. c̄ specific or marked visual acuity deficit,
and last eye exam reportedly 3 weeks ago, perhaps early
cataracts?)
   — Will request in-house ophthalmology consult
③ Type 1 Diabetes Mellitus (Will assess degree of glycemic
control while hospitalized as infection may ↑ insulin requirement.)
   — Continue current insulin regimen and follow FS glucose
      QAC and QHS c̄ Regular Insulin Coverage Scale/pRN →
                                    John Smith, MS III

LVH = left ventricular hypertrophy
RLL = right lower lobe
C&S = culture and sensitivity
PE = pulmonary embolism
TB = tuberculosis
NC = nasal cannula
FS = finger stick

PROGRESS NOTES

Please date and sign each entry

(continued)

— Will order HgBA1C to assess overall pre-admission glycemic control

— Will order 1800 cal/day ADA diet

— F/U Urine C+S results

④ Hyperlipidemia — Elevated total cholesterol on admission

— Will obtain fasting lipid profile in AM

— Continue Lipitor 40 mg p.o. QD for now

⑤ HTN — Clinically stable.

— Continue Capoten 25 mg. p.o. Q8 hrs

⑥ Rheumatoid Arthritis — reported to be responsive to ASA prn but pt. reports morning stiffness in "all joints"

— Consider Rheumatology consult if discomfort in joints persists or worsens

— Continue ASA full-dose prn for pain

⑦ Preventive Medicine

— In light of multiple cardiac risk factors (post-menopausal, HTN, DM, hyperlipidemia, ⊕ family history of ASHD), will continue ASA 81 mg po QD along with other treatments as indicated

— Once stable, will need mammogram this year (last mammogram in 2002) and baseline 2-D Echo to assess ⓜ

— In light of multiple co-morbidities, pt. should get annual flu shot and pneumococcal vaccine

— Will request podiatry consult (pt. is diabetic and has not seen a podiatrist in six years)

Case discussed ē Attending Physician at 8:29 A.M.

John Smith, MS III

ADA = American Diabetes Association
F/U = follow-up
ⓜ = murmur

PROGRESS NOTES

Please date and sign each entry

2/15/04   MS III Note

9:12 A.M. S: Patient reports feeling "a little better" and denies cough. She denies pleuritic chest pain or SOB but says she still feels "very tired."

O: VS T$_{max}$: 99.2°F P: 85 regular R: 20 BP: 120/70 &
alert, oriented ×3, in NAD, appears a bit sleepy
HEENT: throat has mild posterior oropharyngeal erythema, no tonsillar hypertrophy or exudates
NECK: 1 cm. (L) anterior cervical adenopathy remains smooth, non-tender, easily moveable
LUNGS: improved respiratory excursion on (R), crackles at (R) axilla persist
COR: nl S$_1$S$_2$, RRR, (+) SEM II/VI unchanged
ABD: soft, non-tender, (+) normoactive BS × 4 quadrants
EXT: no C/C/E
NEURO: no sensory or motor deficits grossly
LABS/DATA: 12.1 \ 11.9 / 221K   HgBA1C: pending
                 / 34.8
                            6BP, 0 Ba, 18B, 9L, 5M
Urine C&S: no growth × 24 hrs.
Blood C&S: no growth × 24 hrs.   Fasting lipid profile: pending
FS Glucose readings: before lunch: 146, before dinner: 154, last night: 139 (no additional insulin given for coverage)
ABG (Room Air): 7.42/38/78/26/87% at 10:00 p.m.
ABG (on 2L/min O$_2$ via NC): 7.43/33/95/26/94% at 10:30 p.m.

A: 55 year old African-American ♀ c̄ RLL Pneumonia, clinically improving but still hypoxic, on Day #2 of IV Abx.

John Smith, MS III

NAD = no acute distress
RRR = regular rate and rhythm
SEM = systolic ejection murmur
C/C/E = cyanosis, clubbing, edema

```
        HgB
wbc  <       >  platelets
        Hct
```

C&S = culture and sensitivity
S = finger stick
RLL = right lower lobe
IV = intravenous
Abx = antibiotics

PROGRESS NOTES

Please date and sign each entry

2/15/04 (continued)

P: 1) Continue IV Rocephin and IV Azithromax.
2) Continue O₂ via NC at 2L/min.
3) F/U Blood C+S.
4) F/U Fasting Lipid Profile and HgBA1C level
5) Ophthalmology and Podiatry consults pending.
6) Continue current diet and Insulin regimen with coverage scale
7) Continue Lipitos, ASA and Capoten (BP is clinically stable.)

Case discussed with Intern, Resident and Attending (Dr. Martin).

John Smith, MS III

IV = intravenous
N = nasal cannula
F/U = follow up
C&S = culture and sensitivity
BP = blood pressure

C. **Stance.** The good write-up is not simply an organized rehashing of the information collected in the process of the work-up. It is a structured narrative in which the writer walks the delicate line between objective recording and subjective interpreting; it **takes a stance and persuades as well as informs.** The good write-up organizes the details of the case into a coherent whole that explicitly reflects the writer's impression of which issues are central and which are more peripheral. It should contain all the relevant data necessary for the reader to form an independent opinion concerning the case, but it should arrange the data in a way that lets the reader understand what has led the student to draw the conclusions that are offered. A common pitfall in student write-ups is an attempt to be overly "evenhanded"; to record objectively every bit of information obtained in the work-up, and to avoid deliberately taking any stance until the assessment portion of the write-up. While this evenhandedness may seem admirable, it often results in a sort of laundry list of patient complaints and lab data that leaves the reader with little sense of the actual crucial issues. Although the student may be expected to produce a long differential diagnosis list in the assessment section, the entire write-up should be geared toward differentiating between the two or three most likely possibilities.

II. Progress notes

A. **Purpose.** Once the initial admission write-up is completed, the student or house officer is expected to write a brief progress note every day. As the name implies, these notes summarize what progress has been made in the case since the previous note. The central issues of the progress note address the following questions:

1. What are the patient's **current symptoms and complaints**? Are there **any changes?**

2. Is there any **change in the physical exam**?

3. Are there any **new lab data**?

4. Is there any **change in the formulation of the case** or in the relationship of the patient's various medical problems to one another?

5. What are the **current diagnostic and therapeutic plans** for the patient?

B. **Format.** As with the initial admission write-up, there are three main formats for progress notes: the **comprehensive format**, which is a detailed review of the pertinent positive and negative findings; the **traditional format**, which is simply a set of paragraphs summarizing the progress; and the **problem-oriented format**, in which entries for each medical problem are divided into the four SOAP sections mentioned above:

1. **Subjective data:** the patient's impressions of current symptoms.

2. **Objective data:** the clinical exam and laboratory data.

3. **Assessment:** the writer's impression of the data and their relation to the case.

4. **Plan:** both diagnostic and therapeutic.

No matter whether the initial write-up follows the traditional or the problem-oriented format, many clinicians believe that all progress notes should be written in some variant of the SOAP note format, because it makes chart review much easier.

C. **Off-service notes.** The off-service note is a specialized version of the progress note. Above all, it should be **brief**, usually one page or less in length, and it should contain:

1. A short **summary of the patient's case**, usually one paragraph.

2. A short **summary of the hospital course**, again usually one paragraph.

3. A **problem list** that details ongoing, active problems and any outstanding diagnostic tests or work-up.

4. A list of **current medications and dosages**.

Remember that the purpose of the off-service note is to allow the physician who is coming on-service to orient himself to the patient's case in an expeditious way.

III. Sample write-up and progress notes

A. Note that the first write-up, while primarily organized in the traditional format (with multiple paragraphs and passages), contains elements of the problem-oriented system. The chief complaint and the present illness essentially become problem no. 1 on the patient's problem list, while the past medical history comprises the rest of the patient's active medical problems. The second part of this chapter is keyed to the sample write-up and contains specific practical points about the format and content of each section. As is usually the case with medical notes, many abbreviations and acronyms are used. The Abbreviations and Acronyms List on the inside cover includes most of these standard terms and we have listed a few additional ones as foornotes.

B. While the first sample write-up represents a better than average first-year or second-year write-up, it would be considered inappropriately wordy and compulsively thorough by third or fourth year standards. In particular, note that the review of systems (ROS) is written out in its entirety. While most second-year students are required to describe the complete ROS, the third-year student is generally permitted to record a shorter list of pertinent positives and negatives while the fourth-year student may simply record the essential ones and note that the "remainder of the ROS was negative in detail." Also note that the Assessment and Plan section is too brief and could be fleshed out.

C. In a complicated case, with many consultants writing notes, it is not unusual to see multiple styles being used on the same case, and a student should become comfortable with all of them. Note that whether or not a formal SOAP note is written, all notes organize information in the same order—subjective, objective, assessment, and plan—and so the acronym is useful regardless of the style used.

IV. Introductory information and chief complaint

A. All chart notes should be written on **hospital progress-note paper** that has been marked or stamped with the patient's name and number on each page you utilize. You may find it useful to prepare a supply of this stamped paper when you are first assigned a patient, so that you can carry it around on your clipboard and work on notes when you are away from the chart. Of course, **all entries must be dated, timed, and signed;** the signature should appear on the bottom right-hand corner of each page, with an arrow indicating that the note is continued on the next page, if multiple pages are utilized.

B. It is customary to **title each note with the level of seniority of the writer** (e.g., "Medical Student Admission Note" or "Heme Attending Note"). Consultants who review the chart can thus identify critical entries.

C. Record your source if you derive any of the information in your note from a source other than the patient or the old chart. Although a reliability caveat may be appropriate here (e.g., "patient appeared confused and vague"), it should never be humorous or flippant.

D. The introductory sentence and chief complaint (given with its duration) should provide a **10-second sketch of the patient** and the patient's reason for seeking medical help. A word or two about the patient's past medical history may be appropriate here as well (e.g., "a 55 y/o black seamstress with a long history of hypertension"). You will often use this introductory sentence to refer to the patient in discussions with those not familiar with the case. Include the patient's sex and ethnicity if relevant and, whenever possible, record the patient's chief complaint in the patient's own words (e.g., "a 43 y/o man without any prior medical history presents with a 'stabbing feeling in my chest'").

V. History of the present illness

A. Chronologic organization is the key to a well-written history of the present illness (HPI). Tell the patient's history as a story. Begin with a sentence describing the onset of the constellation of symptoms that you perceive as the present illness and move in a strictly chronological manner to the present. If the present illness is simply the latest episode in a long-standing medical problem, begin with a sentence about how long the patient has suffered from the disease (e.g., "The patient has a 20-year history of asthma usually involving 1 or 2 attacks each spring."). Then organize the salient features of the case, always noting the dates on which the features appeared. For a long-standing problem, this will require a careful chart review, with dates of hospitalizations, surgical procedures, therapies, and definitive diagnostic tests all highlighted. The goal here is to give the reader a feeling for the tempo of the disease process. Avoid giving a chronology using days of the week: noting that the "patient was well until Friday morning" may be useful information to clinicians reviewing the chart or listening to your presentation on Monday afternoon, but it is too vague for those reading your notes weeks, or months, later.

B. All pertinent positives and **some pertinent negatives** from the ROS of the organ system(s) involved in the present illness belong in the HPI. Often it is not clear whether a certain pertinent negative is really important enough to note in the HPI. In these cases a good rule of thumb is to ask yourself whether the information in question helps exclude a possible diagnosis that has entered your mind while considering the patient's symptoms. If it does, then the information belongs in the HPI. Remember to only report the evidence. **Do not interpret the information presented in an HPI.** The actual discussion of the diagnosis must wait until the assessment portion of the write-up. However, consideration of the differential diagnosis will help guide you through asking the "best" questions and writing the history. The HPI should include a complete review of the system(s) (e.g., cardiac, pulmonary, etc.) relevant to the chief complaint.

VI. Past medical history

A. All **active** and **significant inactive medical problems** should be listed in the past medical history (PMHx). Problems should be included if they have led to medical attention or hospitalization. This section can be anywhere from a few sentences to a few pages in length, depending on the severity and the significance of the problems. For each problem, the significant issues that you should concentrate on include:

1. The **date on which the problem was diagnosed**.

2. The **results of definitive tests** that will indicate to the reader the severity of the problem (e.g., "cardiac cath in 2001 showed a 38% ejection fraction").

3. The dates of any **surgeries or hospitalizations** for the problem. If the patient was hospitalized, try to include the hospital's name and location.

4. **Current treatment regimens.**

5. An assessment of the **problem's significance at present**, and its potential for interacting with the present illness.

B. **Other parts of the medical history** included in the PMHx include:

1. **Current medications.** The medication list should document all significant, pharmacologically active substances used by the patient. These include all prescription and over-the-counter medicines, herbal supplements, vitamins, skin creams, laxatives, and sleeping medications. Ask women of child-bearing age whether they are taking oral contraceptives and ask all patients whether they take aspirin regularly; patients sometimes don't think to include these two medications when asked to recall a medication list. List each of these substances with the dosage and route of administration. It is customary to use the Latin acronyms for dosage frequency, for example, "bid" (*bis in die*) for "2 times/day." (See Abbreviations and Acronyms, inside covers.)

2. **Allergies** and the nature of the allergic reaction.

3. A list of **past hospitalizations and surgical procedures** (even if mentioned elsewhere).

4. A list of significant **childhood illnesses**.

5. **Habits.** History of tobacco, ethanol, and recreational drug use should be obtained, as well as diet and exercise information. The smoking history should be listed in pack-years. Drinking history may be quantitated in familiar units (six-packs, quarts).

6. A list of **exposures** to radiation, toxins, poisons, chemicals, and so on. Patient should be questioned about possible occupational exposures.

VII. Family history

A. The family history (FHx) is usually presented in a standard **pedigree format**, especially if the patient comes from a large family. For example:

$\widehat{30}$ = female, 30 years old

MI $\boxed{42}$ = male, died at age 42 of myocardial infarction

→ $\widehat{55}$ = patient, female, 55 years old

For most cases, you will want to list the patient, the patient's siblings, and the patient's parents and children.

B. Any family history of **diabetes mellitus, cancer, cardiovascular problems**, or other disease with significant genetic penetration should also be listed in the FHx. A family history of the disease (or symptoms) that the patient has presented with should always be sought.

VIII. Social history.

The social history (SHx) should be very brief unless a lengthy description would be of crucial importance to the case. The goal is to give the reader an idea of the patient as a person. For most patients, this section of the write-up will involve a few words about the patient's **living situation and work.** Names and telephone numbers of close family members can also be listed here. Recall from Chap. 1 the instances in which this section would assume a larger role, such as cases of occupational exposure or pulmonary disease. Ask about a patient's sexual orientation and the number of sexual partners he or she currently has, if any.

IX. Review of systems.

The ROS should be **listed by organ system**. The ROS is an opportunity to pick up past problems that the patient might not otherwise have the opportunity to tell you about. Once again, the length of this list will depend on the complexity of the case and the level of training of the writer. Experienced clinicians may simply write "ROS negative." When first beginning your clinical training you should list, at a minimum, all the ROS positives and enough of the pertinent negatives to show the reader that you did a complete ROS and that all the important facets of the case are listed. List the ROS telegraphically. For example: "GI: no complaints of nausea, vomiting, diarrhea, constipation, abd. pain." Body systems discussed in the HPI need not be repeated in the ROS; you may simply write, "See HPI."

Significant positive history should be moved into the HPI, PMHx, or PSHx, as appropriate: if, while conducting the ROS, you find information germane to the HPI, when you are writing or narrating the history, include it in the HPI. The ability to appropriately shift information around like this is a learned skill that takes some practice.

X. Physical examination

A. Introductory information and vital signs. Always begin with a statement describing the overall appearance of the patient, which is your first impression when you enter the room and begin to examine the patient. The vital signs (including orthostatic changes in blood pressure and pulse, if any) should be listed before the rest of the exam. For most patients with cardiovascular or renal problems, and for annual physicals in the outpatient setting, the admission weight should be listed with the vital signs. Many physicians include the recording of oxygen saturation by pulse oximetry (the "pulse ox"), particularly in patients in actual or impending respiratory difficulty, as a **fifth vital sign.**

B. **Organ system examination.** Starting with a description of the integument and then proceeding in a generally head-to-toe direction (leaving the neurologic exam results for last), transcribe the results of your physical exam. Just as in the ROS, the first and second year student should include all significant positive and negative findings, while the more advanced third and fourth year student can concentrate on the major positive findings, listing only the most fundamental pertinent negatives. For the lung, heart, and abdomen examinations in a comprehensive write-up, it is particularly useful to describe the results of: **I**nspection, **P**alpation, **P**ercussion, and **A**uscultation. This may also be used for other parts of the physical such as the neck exam. Remember that percussion is not usually a part of the heart exam and that auscultation of the abdomen should precede palpation and percussion.

C. One key to a good physical exam write-up is **specificity**. Always quantitate and localize (e.g., "a 6 × 6-cm round erythematous patch on the left buttock") and avoid using subjective terms such as small or mild. Draw **diagrams** whenever they are helpful. Specifically, the dermatologic exam, breast exam, abdominal exam, and neurologic exam are often illustrated with diagrams and stick figures to indicate the exact location of the findings.

XI. Laboratory data (see also Chaps. 9–15).

A. **Hematologic studies** are usually listed together in shorthand form, as follows:

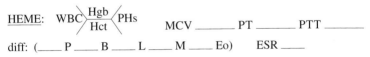

HEME: WBC⟩$\frac{Hgb}{Hct}$⟨PHs   MCV _____ PT _____ PTT _____

diff: (____ P ____ B ____ L ____ M ____ Eo)   ESR ____

Any special hematologic tests or comments on the blood smear, which should be examined whenever the differential is abnormal or suggestive, are recorded below these results.

B. **Serum chemistry** data can be divided into two groups:

1. Seven "core" tests, which make up the basic metabolic panel, are conveniently recorded in a lattice format:

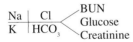

$$\frac{Na \;|\; Cl}{K \;\;|\; HCO_3} \Big\langle \begin{matrix} BUN \\ Glucose \\ Creatinine \end{matrix}$$

2. The remainder of the serum chemistry results are recorded underneath and beside this lattice. Often these other tests are best grouped by organ system (e.g., the liver function tests). You should **circle lab values that are abnormal or significant** for the diagnosis in question.

C. **Urinalysis (U/A)** data are recorded in tabular form: color and appearance; specific gravity; pH and dipstick results; sediment analysis; quantitation (number of cells or structures per high-power field). The time and conditions of collection (e.g., catheter or clean-voided specimen) and the total urine volume in a specified time period may also be recorded here. If you do a dipstick urinalysis and the lab does another, include both sets of data, noting the source of each.

D. **Electrocardiographic data** should be recorded in the following sequence:
1. Rate and rhythm.
2. Axis.
3. P-R, QRS, and Q-T intervals.
4. Comments concerning the following areas:
   a. Q waves, S-T segment, and T-wave morphology.
   b. R wave progression.
   c. QRS morphology and conduction blocks.
   d. Evidence for drug effects.
   e. Other significant findings.
5. Overall impression, **including degree of change from the last recorded electrocardiogram (ECG).**

E. **Chest x-ray** results are recorded either verbally or by means of a labeled diagram. Always include a statement concerning the degree of change from the last chest film.

F. In a similarly telegraphic fashion, record the remainder of the lab data, including:
1. **Arterial blood gas results** (record the FIO_2 together with the results and the time the sample was drawn).
2. **Microbiologic data** (include antibiotic sensitivities if known).
3. **Pathology reports.**
4. **Other radiologic tests.**
5. **Other special diagnostic tests.**

XII. **Assessment and plan.** Up until this point in the write-up, the **analytic** portion of the work-up has been collected and organized. Now the history, physical exam, and lab data are considered together in the **synthetic** portion of the work-up, in which each problem is systematically assessed and a management plan for each is formulated. This section of the write-up may be considered in four parts: (1) a **summary** is written; (2) a complete **problem list** is generated; (3) an **assessment** is made of each problem on the list; and (4) a **plan**—for further diagnosis and for therapy—is formulated.

A. **Summary.** Write a **brief, two- to three-line** summary after the last piece of lab data is recorded and before the assessment and plan are made for each problem. Summarizing serves to refocus both your own and the reader's attention on the case at hand, emphasizing the central concern(s) of the HPI. See the sample write-ups for examples.

B. **Problem list.** You will be familiar with the concept of a problem list from earlier medical studies, but several specific points are useful to remember here:
1. A problem list is the **collected set of findings** that you believe need to be addressed as part of a patient's overall case. **Problems are derived from four general areas: the history, the physical exam, laboratory findings, and a synthesis of any or all of these three.** Thus findings such as chest pain, a supraclavicular node, and a low serum sodium

value might all be possible entries in a case of pneumonia, a diagnosis arrived at by synthesizing data from the history, physical exam, and laboratory. As you gain experience, it will become clear that certain entries previously considered distinct from one another in fact may be subsumed under one new heading on your problem list. What is important at the outset is identifying all abnormalities or problems by methodically examining the data available. The problem list should serve as an **overall outline** for thinking about the case; ideally it will consist of the fewest number of entries that together explain all your findings.

2. The construction of a problem list is not simply an academic exercise; it is the **initial step in management** of the patient. Therefore, if there is a problem that you have no intention of addressing (e.g., poor dentition), it probably does not belong on your problem list.

3. The problem that is central to the present illness usually occupies the number 1 spot on the problem list. Related and distinct problems from the history, physical exam, and laboratory data are then **ranked** in order of the importance you ascribe to them.

C. **Assessment.** Now that the problem list exists, you need to address each problem in turn, considering its significance and reflecting on diagnostic possibilities if the etiology is unclear. The analysis of each problem is at least partially put to paper in the form of the assessment. As is illustrated in the sample write-ups, each problem is discussed in turn, and from this "thinking on paper" arises the logical sequence of further diagnostic steps and therapeutic interventions, which are listed after each problem as the **plan.** The assessment is usually written in the form of one paragraph for each problem.

1. Begin by stating the **diagnoses** that seem to be the most probable explanation for the problem in question (unless, of course, your heading is a diagnosis, such as "pneumonia").

2. Methodically mention the compelling **history, physical exam, and laboratory findings** that are related to the problem in question and that help support the conclusion you are drawing about the significance of a given problem.

3. Mention **other diagnostic possibilities** that you have entertained, and, again using data from the history, physical exam, and laboratory, state why they are unlikely or not yet excluded.

4. By this point the **further diagnostic studies** necessary to arrive at a decisive diagnosis will be fairly clear. These studies form the first part of your plan list.

5. Last, consider **conditions related to the problem** in question that may be important to explore. This part of the assessment requires experience and a firm knowledge of pathophysiology and clinical presentations of disease. For example, if a patient's pneumococcal pneumonia was his third such event in the past 18 months, it might be worthwhile to rule out the possibility of an underlying multiple myeloma (which predisposes to recurrent pneumonia, especially with encapsulated bacteria) by ordering a serum immunoelectrophoresis.

D. The **plan** logically proceeds from the reasoning presented in the paragraph following each problem on the problem list; it is simply a checklist of things to be done. The first entries are further **diagnostic** steps, as mentioned above (p. 199). Following these are the **therapeutic interventions** on which you and your team have decided. To summarize and elaborate on the areas that the assessment and plan address, we have listed below topics to consider when formulating these sections:

1. **Definitive diagnoses.** For problems that are unsolved, try to narrow the diagnostic possibilities and decide what needs to be done to arrive at a final diagnosis. Consider the need for subspecialty consultations here.

2. **Correction or compensation of pathophysiology.** This subject is the cornerstone of medical management. Thinking about pathophysiology, try to understand what perturbation has caused the problem in question and what might be done to compensate for or correct that causative factor.

3. **Therapeutic measures.** In addition to correction or compensation, consider the following areas with respect to therapy:

    a. Pain relief.

    b. Specific medications useful for the problem in question.

    c. Ancillary help (e.g., physical or occupational therapist, nutritionist).

    d. Prevention of complications (e.g., bedsore/decubiti prophylaxis for those who must be on their back constantly).

    e. Long-term care (e.g., potential need for outpatient assistance, nursing home, visiting nurse). As is evident from the sample write-ups, each problem is addressed in turn, and a list of further steps is created.

E. Conclusion. As you come to the end of the assessment and plan, having addressed each problem, two measures are useful to help conclude your write-up. First, conclude with a brief impression of the case, as explained on p. 196. Second, and perhaps more important, define for yourself the **endpoint** for your patient's present hospitalization. Although you may revise the endpoint deliberately, if it is not considered from the day of admission, you will find that the reasons for the patient's hospitalization seem to shift and change emphasis, making the process of concluding the hospitalization very frustrating.

XIII. Concluding information. In a complicated case, it is sometimes useful to conclude the write-up with a few sentences that present your **overall impression,** in which the case priorities and the long-term goals and sequence of therapies that you suggest are briefly mentioned. This is a chance to integrate the patient's medical problems into a unified picture of the patient as a person rather than simply as a set of organ systems.

XIV. You may be asked to create a diagram of **proposed pathogenesis** that ties together as many as possible of the patient's main symptoms, physical findings, and labs with your understanding of the disease processes involved and their pathogenesis. See the sample write-up on page 182. This information can also be incorporated in a short **discussion** of the case and the patient's presentation.

XV. Progress notes

A. Keep your progress notes **brief** and **telegraphic.** Scrupulously avoid any critical comments of other physicians, consultants, or colleagues; the progress note is not the place to take out your personal or professional grievances. Concentrate on any new data that you have, and any change in clinical symptoms or signs. Even if the patient's chart has a separate lab result section in which the lab tests are routinely recorded, you should still **summarize new results in your progress notes.** If a test has been done but the results are not available, note that the test is "pending." No matter what format is used, a good progress note should enable the reader to skim the day's data in a minute or two and answer the following questions:

1. Is there any **new diagnostic information**?
2. Is the patient getting **better or worse**?
3. Are the **chosen therapies** working?
4. What **further diagnostic and therapeutic steps** are in progress or planned?

B. **Flowcharts** are extremely useful, especially for patients with multiple interrelated medical problems. For instance, a patient with severe renal failure might benefit from a flowchart that allows quick day-by-day comparisons of those clinical parameters affected by renal failure. Such a flow chart might be set up as follows:

Date:	7/1	7/2	7/3	7/4
Electrolytes	138 | 94 ⟍ 56 / 90 / 5.6 | 25 ⟍ 3.8			
CBC	⟍ 10.2 / 12.1 ⟩—⟨ 242 / 32.5 ⟍ 35^P 10^B 47^L 5^M 3^{Eo}			
ABGs	8:29 A.M. $PO_2 = 86$ 40% FiO2 $PCO_2 = 28$ pH = 7.31			

Although this sort of chart does not take the place of daily notes, it can be an **invaluable aid** to consultants who see the patient only every few days, as well as to you and your resident or intern, when you wish to summarize the case.

Medical Case Presentations

> **P**erhaps the most difficult thing for medical students and house staff to learn and a lesson the experienced physician frequently relearns, often with discomfort but rarely with surprise, is that for everything we do, based upon sound rationales, for or to acutely ill patients, *there are often equally persuasive competing rationales as to why we should **not** choose a certain treatment or intervention.* Recognizing and dealing with those opposing issues constitutes a most challenging basis for developing clinical judgment. That developmental process begins with awareness of the issues and plans to detect and evaluate adverse effects at the earliest reasonable moment.
>
> *Roland H. Ingram, Jr., M.D.*
>
> *Dr. Ingram is the Martha West Looney Professor of Medicine at Emory University School of Medicine, Atlanta, Georgia, and Chief of Medicine at the Crawford Long Hospital of Emory University.*

In this chapter, Section I outlines the two types of presentations: the **brief presentation** on work rounds and the more **formal presentation** delivered to the attending physician. Section IV provides a description of the teaching points emphasized during attending rounds and some of the general areas that need to be addressed when presenting cases. In fact, presenting a case is an art, and as such it can be described only partially and learned only with practice.

I. Introductory points of medical case presentations. You will need to be familiar with two types of presentations:

   A. Short, 1–2 minute **"bullet" presentations**.

   B. More complete, 5–6 minute **formal presentations.**

   The logical flow of the presentation emerges from a good **work-up (history and physical exam) and write-up (admission or transfer note).** The write-up is the template from which you prepare the presentation you will give to the team later that day or the next morning. Formal presentations should not exceed **5–6 minutes,** even for the most complicated cases.

II. Preparing the data for presentation

   A. Note card. A useful adjunct to every write-up, the note card allows the most important parts of the work-up to be summarized, organized, and recorded in a portable, accessible manner. Prepare the note card at the end of the work-up, when the case is still fresh in your mind, and use your write-up as a guide. Your note cards are vital to your success on the wards, for they function as your portable chart rack and memory prompt. This is true especially at the beginning of your clinical experience, when note cards may be used **to present,** unless you are specifically required to present without notes. Many students today use personal digital assistants (PDAs) for this purpose.

B. **Information to note.** At first, it is useful to have a number of facts on the note card. Later, when presenting from memory is less difficult, it is still useful to carry the following information on a note card. (Information that is especially important is marked with an asterisk.)

   1. **Patient information.*** Use addressograph plate to stamp the top of your card.

   2. **Introductory sentence.*** Record necessary information from your write-up.

   3. **Chief complaint** (CC) and its duration.*

   4. **History of present illness (HPI)**

      a. Record salient points, using **single words** that jog your memory and allow you to tell the patient's story as you summarized it in your write-up.

      b. State pertinent negatives.

      c. State risk factors, positive family history.

   5. **Past medical history.** Record only **active problems.**

   6. **Allergies.*** Record all, and explain type of reaction if drug allergy.

   7. **Medications.*** Note **all,** with dosages. Include ethanol and tobacco use.

   8. **Review of systems.** Note **only** significant positives (usually you will have covered these in your HPI).

   9. **Physical exam findings**

      a. Introductory descriptive sentence.

      b. Vital signs.

      c. Pertinent positive findings only.

   10. **Laboratory tests.*** State all **pertinent positive findings.**

   11. **Problem list.*** Recorded from the assessment and plan section of the write-up.

C. The above information should fit on a 3-by-5-inch index card, unless the case is very complicated or you have large handwriting. For those with poor handwriting a PDA is especially useful and worth the investment.

III. Presenting

A. The **bullet presentation** is a *quick,* 1–2 minute summary, most often delivered on work rounds in the morning. It is to be considered a **brief, orienting introduction** to those members of the team who do not know the patient at all. Think of the bullet presentation as a **summary of the note card** you have prepared: **it is the distillation of your first distillation.** A presentation should include:

1. **Introductory sentence.***
2. **CC** and its duration.*
3. **HPI.** Often condensed in a bullet. Include it if your resident wants it; do not drone on. Summarize the HPI in a few sentences.
4. **Medications.***
5. **Physical exam findings.***
   a. Give the patient's **general condition** (good, fair, stable, guarded, critical).
   b. State **"vital signs** stable," or report those that are not.
   c. State definitive **positive findings**.
6. **Pertinent positive laboratory tests.***
7. **Summary.** If the case is complicated, give a one- or two-sentence summary.

   Be brief: if there are laboratory tests your team members want to know about, they will ask.

B. **General principles** concerning the bullet presentation:

1. The presentation is a skeleton or framework that allows others to think about the person they are about to meet.
2. Someone undoubtedly will ask whether anything important is missing from the bullet. So long as the basic information noted above is given you have done your job.
3. Speak decisively and distinctly.
4. Mention **active** and **potential** problems: this is the time that team members who cover the patients at night hear about them.

C. **Sample bullet**

I'll present Mrs. Jones's case formally during attending rounds, but to give all of you who haven't met her a brief introduction: she's a 55-year-old African-American woman with a history of well-controlled diabetes, hypertension, hyperlipidemia, and rheumatoid arthritis. She entered complaining of weakness, cough, and a feverish feeling of 2–3 days' duration.

On physical exam, she's in good condition now with stable vital signs, a temp of 103°F last night, a few crackles in her right axilla, but nothing else on her last chest exam. The remainder of her physical exam was unremarkable.

Pertinent labs included a CBC with 12,000 WBCs without a left shift, gram-negative rods on an unspun urine (but no UTI symptoms), and a right lower lobe infiltrate on her chest film. In addition, her sputum contained polys and gram-positive diplococci. We think she has pneumococcal pneumonia, and she has begun to defervesce on a gram of ceftriaxone IV every 24 hours.

D. The **formal presentation** is essentially a presentation of the note card outlined on page 204.

1. **Patient information.** If the case is complicated, you may want to interject the phrase "with multiple medical problems."

2. **Introductory sentence**

3. **CC** and its duration. In a presentation, unlike a write-up, **avoid using the patient's words.** Instead, give a description that allows the listeners to focus quickly on the problem at hand.

4. **HPI.** Present a **succinct** version of the HPI. Give pertinent positive findings from the appropriate ROS section(s). Note pertinent risk factors and family history.

5. **PMH.** Mention **prior admissions.** Flesh out other active medical problems.

6. **Allergies.** Note any drug reactions.

7. **Medications.** State **all present medicines,** with dosages.

8. **Positive ROS findings.** State only pertinent positives other than those mentioned during the HPI.

9. **Physical exam findings**

   a. **Introductory sentence,** describing general appearance and condition.

   b. **Vital signs** are stated for every patient.

   c. **Pertinent positive findings.** Some attending physicians may want you to describe the entire physical exam (PE), system by system, even if normal, but this is unnecessary unless specifically requested.

10. **Laboratory tests**

    a. **Pertinent positives** from these categories, in **"CUBS"** order:
       C Complete blood count
       U Urinalysis
       B Blood chemistries
       S Specials, if done (ECG, CXR, ABGs, CT scan, MRI, and so on)

    b. **Pertinent negatives** if you believe they are significant.

11. **Summary.** Give a brief, **two-sentence summary** and then **pause.** The discussion of the case is initiated here, so make your summary useful and make it clear from your voice and expression that you are done. The attending physician will ask you what you and the team did for the patient therapeutically, and will begin discussing specific questions concerning the case.

IV. Areas often discussed during the presentation to the attending. Rounds with an attending physician ("the visit") are often initiated by the case presentation of the previous night's admission and continue, time permitting, with discussions about the case. The purpose of visit rounds preparation is *not* to be able to anticipate and answer every question you will be asked. Spend time reflecting on the case, read what you can, and, first and foremost, understand the pathophysiology. Following are some of the frequently discussed areas; although there is rarely time to learn about all of these for each case, choose those subjects you believe are the most pertinent to the case in question.

   A. **Pathophysiologic mechanisms**

   B. **Historical findings and symptoms** associated with the disease(s) in question.

C. **Physical findings** associated with the disease(s) in question.

D. **Differential diagnosis:** other diseases that might present in a similar manner and important differentiating features among those possibilities.

E. **Complications** associated with the disease(s) under consideration.

F. Mechanism of action and side effects of any **medications** the patient is taking or was placed on during this admission.

V. Caveats of presenting

A. **Speed of presentation.** Do not dawdle, but do not roar through the presentation so quickly that you cannot be understood. Try to relax, and speak as though explaining a subject to friends.

B. **Tone.** Do not read your presentation. This is the most common cause of a monotonic delivery. Tell your listeners a dynamic, interesting story.

C. **Pauses and interruptions.** Roll with the punches here; if a discussion ensues while you are presenting, note where you left off, listen to and perhaps participate in the digression, and be ready to resume, **repeating** the sentence you last spoke as you begin again. The attending or resident will usually ask you to continue.

D. **Enunciation.** Speak precisely. Do not say, for example, "one hundred six" for a temperature of "one hundred point six."

E. **Brevity.** The bullet presentation is meant to be brief, but even the formal presentation should be short enough to maintain the interest of your listeners. Up to 5–6 minutes is a reasonable amount of time to expect people to listen; after that you will begin to lose your audience.

F. **Condensation.** When it is necessary to describe in detail one or two problems, it becomes necessary, as well, simply to mention other issues that you may have wished to elaborate on. Condensing the presentation is preferable to making it too long. Describe problems in further detail only in response to your audience's queries.

G. **Omissions.** You should describe only positive and negative findings pertinent to the differential diagnoses you are entertaining. In other words, omit details that are not relevant to the "argument" you are constructing.

H. **Physical exam findings.** It is natural at all stages of clinical experience, especially at the beginning, to have equivocal physical findings arise. Point out your findings, and if others have disagreed or differed, simply state, "Another observer thought . . . "

I. **Concluding.** At the end of the history, physical exam, and laboratory data presentations, summarize the case in one to two sentences for your listeners, focusing on the problem that is most relevant. For example, "In summary, Mrs. Jones is a 55-year-old African-American woman with a history of diabetes, hypertension, hyperlipidemia, and rheumatoid arthritis who presented last night with a probable pneumococcal pneumonia."

J. **Hospital course.** If the patient has been in the hospital for any length of time, most attending physicians will discuss certain features of the case before they ask about the patient's hospital course. It is reasonable to ask the attending at the end of your presentation whether he or she would like to hear what the patient's hospital course has been. For patients with multiple **active** problems, describe the hospital course in a problem-oriented manner; for example, "First, with respect to the patient's pneumonia. . . . Second, with respect to her elevated blood glucose on admission . . . ," and so on.

K. **Refutations by the bedside.** You will sometimes present by the bedside, and you will almost always see the patient after you present. Patients often refute the stories being told about them, or correct them in major or minor ways. This is not a personal attack; it happens frequently to everyone caring for patients, and it may provide a valuable new clue. Since you are at an advantage, having heard the patient's story previously, try to decipher what the patient has corrected. How was he or she misunderstood originally? Then consider any implications the refutation has for the way in which you have considered the case. Above all, **do not panic, and do not argue with the patient.** Accept this correction respectfully and perhaps take the opportunity to ask a few related questions.

COLOR PLATES

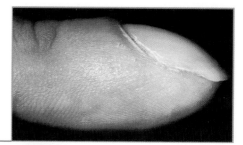

Digital clubbing

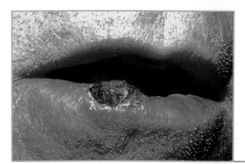

Squamous cell carcinoma (lip)

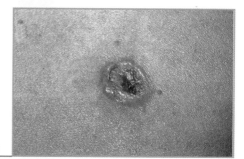

Basal cell carcinoma

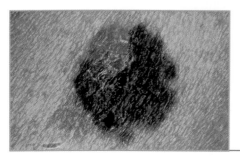

Malignant melanoma

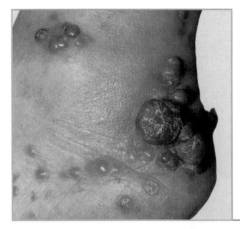

Kaposi sarcoma

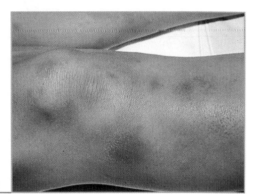

Erythema nodosum

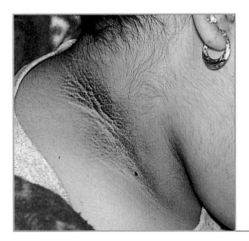

Acanthosis nigricans

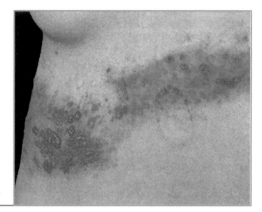

Herpes zoster

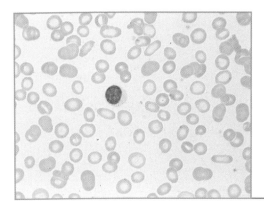

Microcytic, hypochromic anemia

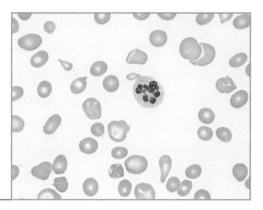

Pernicious anemia

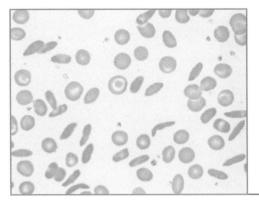

Sickle cell anemia

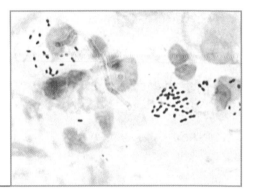

Gram stain *(Streptococcus pneumoniae)*

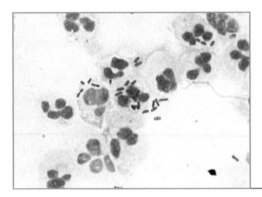

Gram stain *(E. coli)*

PART III

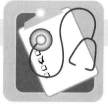

Disease Pathophysiology Review

The diagnosis is nearly always contained in the patients' words and physical findings. The physician must translate their words and the data obtained with the eyes, ears, and hands into a language that describes disorders of organ functions. Remember: the hand of disease can be quicker than the eye of the physician.

Kenneth H. Falchuk, M.D.

A graduate of Harvard Medical School, Dr. Falchuk is board certified in Internal Medicine and Associate Professor of Medicine at Harvard Medical School. He is Director of the Education Council at the Brigham and Women's Hospital, Boston.

The two hardest and yet most important parts of your introduction to clinical medicine are (1) learning how to do a directed history and physical and (2) developing an assessment and a plan. To do either of these well, you need to be able to apply the pathophysiology you learned during the first two years of medical school to the problems of real patients. While you most likely learned a large amount of material in those preclinical years, the information may not be in a form immediately useful to you on the wards.

This part of the book reviews some important facets of disease pathophysiology, going through each of the most common diseases you will encounter on the wards, by organ system. For each disease, it generally describes:

1. A **definition** of the disease, and any important subtypes as well.
2. The **clinical manifestations**—that is, what you should ask for in the history and especially look for on the physical exam. Also included are common lab tests that are used in making the diagnosis.
3. **Differential diagnosis**—other diseases that can present like the disease being described, or how to differentiate between important subtypes of the given illness.
4. **Pathophysiology**—a concise review.

These descriptions should help you in several ways. You can use them as a review of pertinent clinical facts about the major diseases you will see on the wards and in physicians' offices, or you can refer to them during a work-up, to remind yourself what to ask for and look for in a more directed work-up. In addition, you can use them to review basic facts about each disease before writing your analysis and plan, as well as to help you organize your thoughts before presenting your patient at rounds.

The descriptions of diseases here are certainly not a substitute for the more comprehensive discussions found in textbooks, such as *Harrison's* or *Cecil's* (see **Appendix F**). The best way to learn and remember pathophysiology during your clinical training years is to read about each disease you encounter on the wards in textbooks such as these. We do feel, however, that these disease summaries will be helpful for you as you start your clinical career on the wards.

CHAPTER 18

Pulmonary Diseases

> **M**any patients with lung disease have important occupational and environmental factors in their histories. It is important to obtain a detailed and chronological work history and environmental exposure record going back to school days, including summer jobs, hobbies, and pastimes. Latency and chronicity are the hallmarks of many occupationally related disorders of the respiratory system. In thinking of causes of dyspnea, it is necessary not only to think of cardiac and respiratory system disease, but also anemia, primary muscle disease, as well as simple inactivity.
>
> *-Homayoun Kazemi, M.D., FACP*

> *After graduating from Lafayette College, Pennsylvania and Columbia University College of Physicians and Surgeons, Dr. Kazemi completed an internship at Bassett Hospital, Cooperstown, New York, followed by an internal medicine residency at Massachusetts General Hospital, Boston, followed by a cardiopulmonary lab fellowship at Bassett Hospital. A professor of medicine at Harvard Medical School, Dr. Kazemi spent 31 years as the Chief of the Pulmonary Unit at Massachusetts General Hospital, where he is now Chief Emeritus of the Pulmonary and Critical Care Unit.*

 ASTHMA

I. **Definition.** Syndrome of reversible airway hyperreactivity and inflammation in response to a number of known stimuli **(allergic asthma)** or nonidentifiable stimuli **(nonallergic asthma)**.

II. **Clinical manifestations**

   A. **History**

   1. Progressively worsening dyspnea, cough, tachypnea, chest tightness, and wheezing over a period of hours to days.

   2. Elicit **provocative factors**, which may include presence of an upper respiratory illness; exposure to animal dander, pollen, aspirin, or nonsteroidal anti-inflammatory drugs; beta-blockers; exercise; and cold weather.

   B. **Physical exam**

   1. Patient is generally sitting forward, is diaphoretic, and may be unable to speak due to severe dyspnea.

2. Signs of respiratory distress: **grunting** sound during inspiration, **flaring** of nostrils during inspiration, **retractions**, use of accessory respiratory muscles during inspiration.

3. Tachycardia and tachypnea.

4. Pulsus paradoxus, inspiratory decline in systolic blood pressure > 10 mm Hg; reflects large intrapleural pressure swings.

5. Lungs: inspiratory-expiratory rhonchi, hyperinflated chest, prolonged expiratory phase, diffuse wheezing, cyanosis in severe cases.

6. Signs of impending respiratory crisis:

   a. The absence of wheezing, or decreased wheezing, may indicate worsening obstruction.

   b. Paradoxical abdominal movement on inspiration (detected by palpation over the upper part of the abdomen in a semirecumbent position) indicates diaphragmatic fatigue.

7. Mental status changes: generally secondary to hypoxia and hypercapnea, and constitute an indication for emergent intubation.

C. **Diagnostic tests**

1. **Complete blood count** (CBC). Eosinophilia; ↑ WBC with "left shift" may indicate coexistence of bacterial infection, though you may also see leukocytosis if the patient is on inhaled or systemic corticosteroids; most associated pneumonias are viral.

2. **Sputum.** Eosinophilia; bronchial casts; aspergillosis; ± Curschmann's spirals (distal airway casts composed of respiratory epithelial cells); ± Charcot-Leyden crystals.

3. **Chest x-ray** (CXR). Hyperinflation (flattening of diaphragm and increased volume in the retrosternal airspace); look for evidence of pneumonia. Pneumothorax or pneumomediastinum may occur.

4. **Arterial blood gases** (ABGs). Can be used in staging severity of asthmatic attack.

   a. Mild: decreased PO_2 and PCO_2, increased pH.

   b. Moderate: decreased PO_2, normal PCO_2, normal pH.

   c. Severe: markedly decreased PO_2, increased PCO_2, decreased pH.

5. **Pulmonary function tests** (PFTs), FEV_1 ↓ ↓; FVC ↓; RV ↑; TLC ↑ acutely; subtle similar abnormalities may persist chronically.

III. **Differential diagnosis.** Findings that differentiate the two asthmatic populations, **allergic asthma** and **nonallergic asthma**, are compared in Table 18–1.

IV. **Pathophysiology.** The causes of asthma are twofold, consisting of **acute bronchospasm** and **chronic inflammation**. The bronchial musculature of both the large and small airways is hyperreactive to various stimuli. Bronchospasm is manifested by the intermittent attacks of wheezing, dyspnea, and cough. The chronic inflammatory component results in the formation of an adherent exudate that plugs up the airways and submucosal edema. Bronchiolar smooth muscle contractions, bronchial wall edema, and thickened secretions all lead to diminished airway diameter.

Bronchiolar hyperactivity is caused by two distinct mechanisms: the **local**

TABLE 18–1. Diagnosis of asthma

	Allergic	Nonallergic
Inciting agent	Pollen, animal dander	Upper respiratory infections, emotional factors, nonspecific irritants
Age	70% of asthmatics < 30 yr	70% of asthmatics > 30 yr
Historical points	Spring-fall hay fever, ± infantile eczema, FHx allergies	H/O ↑ in winter, chronic cough, H/O respiratory infections, subset with aspirin intolerance, and nasal polyps
Physical exam	Urticaria, eczema, chest exam findings (see II.C)	Rhinitis, nasal polyps, chest exam findings (see II.C)
Laboratory	↑ circulating IgE, skin tests positive, RAST positivity	Normal IgE levels, skin tests negative

RAST= radioallergosorbent test

pathway and the **reflex pathway**. The local pathway, an example of type I immune hypersensitivity, is mediated by IgE immunoglobulins bound to the surface of mast cells. When an allergen binds the IgE molecule, the mast cell degranulates, releasing histamine, prostaglandins, eosinophilic chemotactic factor and leukotrienes, which cause bronchiolar smooth muscle constriction and increased vascular permeability. The reflex pathway is triggered by submucous irritant receptors. Bronchiolar constriction in this pathway is the result of stimuli carried by the parasympathetic nervous system (vagus nerve).

CHRONIC OBSTRUCTIVE PULMONARY DISEASE (COPD)

I. **Definition.** COPD is chronic airflow obstruction secondary to chronic bronchitis, emphysema, or both.

   A. **Chronic bronchitis** is formally defined as a clinical syndrome characterized by excessive tracheobronchial mucus secretion so as to produce cough with sputum production on most days for at least 3 months of the year, during 2 or more consecutive years. "**Blue bloaters**" is the term used to describe patients with chronic bronchitis, derived from the fact that patients with chronic bronchitis often have a bluish tinge (cyanosis) to their skin (secondary to chronic hypoxemia) and frequently have peripheral edema (secondary to cor pulmonale).

   B. **Emphysema** is a pathological diagnosis characterized histologically by distention of the air spaces distal to the terminal bronchiole with destruction of alveolar walls. "**Pink puffers**" is the term used to describe patients with emphysema, derived from the fact that patients with emphysema often are cachectic and have a pink skin color (adequate O_2 saturation) and "puff" when they breathe. They assume a tripod position, purse their lips, and use accessory muscles to breathe.

II. Clinical manifestations and differential diagnosis

COPD is rarely pure; more often it is a mixture of chronic bronchitis and emphysematous disease. Tables 18–2 through 18–4 provide differentiating features of these two types of COPD.

III. Pathophysiology

A. Cigarette smoking plays a central role in the etiology of both emphysema and chronic bronchitis by promoting the breakdown of elastin in the lung. In the normal lung there is a delicate balance between the elastase released by polymorphonuclear leukocytes (PMNs) in the lung and alpha-1 protease inhibitor (A1PI), which inhibits the elastase. Cigarette smoke disturbs this balance by increasing the concentration of PMNs and alveolar macrophages in the lung, thus increasing the reservoir of elastase, and by oxidizing the A1PI, rendering the elastin protector impotent. The net result is that cigarette smoking promotes the breakdown of elastin in the lung. This loss of elastin compromises the internal structure of the respiratory bronchioles, causing them to obstruct upon exhalation.

B. Chronic bronchitis is characterized by hypertrophy and hyperplasia of submucosal mucus-producing glands in larger airways, and small airway changes such as goblet-cell hyperplasia, inflammatory reaction, and retained bronchial secretions.

TABLE 18–2. History and physical exam findings in COPD

Finding	Type A: emphysema (pink puffer)	Type B: chronic bronchitis (blue bloater)
Dyspnea	Insidious onset; often becomes severe	Mild to severe, insidious
Cough	May occur	Often present
Sputum	Scant, mucoid	Copious, purulent
Symptoms at rest	Usual	Milder
Weight change	Often marked loss	Slight loss to moderate gain
Bronchial infections	Less frequent	More frequent
Respiratory insufficiency episodes	At terminal course	Common and repeated
Age at diagnosis	± 60 yr	± 50 yr
Integument	No cyanosis or clubbing	Cyanosis; rarely, clubbing
Pulmonary exam	Hyperresonance, end-expiratory wheezing, lower intercostal space retractions, accessory muscle usage	No hyperresonance, often rhonchi with coarse breath sounds, no lower intercostal retractions, less accessory muscle usage

TABLE 18–3. Diagnostic test findings in COPD

Finding	Type A: emphysema (pink puffer)	Type B: chronic bronchitis (blue bloater)
Total lung capacity	Increased	Normal or slightly increased or decreased
Vital capacity	Decreased	Decreased
Residual volume	Greatly increased	Moderately increased
Elastic recoil	Markedly decreased	Normal
Inspiratory airway resistance	Normal to slightly increased	Markedly increased
Compliance (static)	Increased	Near normal
Compliance (dynamic)	Normal to slightly decreased	Markedly decreased
Diffusing capacity	Decreased	Normal to slightly decreased
Hematocrit	35–45%	40–55% (lower value may indicate superimposed infection with anemia)
PCO_2	35–40 mm Hg	50–65 mm Hg
PO_2	65–75 mm Hg	45–60 mm Hg
Cardiac output	Often decreased	Usually normal
Chest x-ray	Hyperlucent, hyperinflated lung with flat diaphragms; small heart, decreased vascular markings, and bullae may be evident	Large heart; increased bronchovascular shadows in lower field; evidence of old inflammatory disease

  C. Emphysema is subdivided into two main types: **panacinar** and **centrilobular.** The panacinar form, the hereditary form, is due to A1PI deficiency, and is characterized by uniform destruction of the acinus. These patients develop emphysema at a much younger age (30–40), and many do not have a history of smoking. Alpha-1 protease inhibitor was previously known as alpha-1-antitrypsin. The centrilobular form results from smoking, and tends to leave alveoli at the margin of the acinus unaffected; it generally involves alveolar ducts and respiratory bronchioles in the center of the lobule. Clinically, emphysema is best diagnosed by pulmonary function tests (which correlate well with the pathologic changes that define the disease).

PULMONARY TUBERCULOSIS

  I. Definition. An acute and chronic, necrotizing, transmissible infection of the lungs caused by *Mycobacterium tuberculosis.*

TABLE 18–4. **Complications of COPD**

Complication	Type A: emphysema (pink puffer)	Type B: chronic bronchitis (blue bloater)
Pulmonary hypertension at rest	None to mild	Moderate to severe
Pulmonary hypertension with exercise	Moderate	Worsens
Cor pulmonale	Rare (terminal event)	Common
Infectious exacerbations	Less frequent	More frequent

II. Clinical manifestations

A. History. Initial constitutional symptoms: dry, nonproductive cough, night sweats, fever, anorexia, fatigue, dyspnea, hemoptysis, and pleuritic pain.

B. Physical exam. Will be normal in many cases. Initial sign may be crackles near lung apices. As tuberculosis progresses, there may be asymmetric respiratory excursion ± tracheal deviation, dullness to percussion, ↑ tactile fremitus over the involved areas, and crackles.

C. Diagnostic tests

1. **Purified protein derivative (PPD).** A positive reaction is determined by examining the maximum diameter of induration by palpation 48–72 hours after it is placed on the forearm. Induration of 5 mm or more is now considered positive if the patient has been in contact with infectious patients, a chest roentgenograph is consistent with old healed TB, or the patient is HIV positive or at high risk for HIV disease. Induration of 10 mm or more is positive in high prevalence or high risk populations. Induration of 15 mm or more is positive in everyone else. Up to 25 percent of newly diagnosed tuberculosis patients have a negative tuberculin skin test, particularly patients with renal failure, elderly patients, patients on steroid or immunosuppressive therapy, HIV-positive individuals, and patients with severe protein deficiency, concomitant live virus vaccination or infection, lymphoma, or sarcoidosis. Patients who have received **BCG vaccine** are usually PPD positive.

2. **Sputum.** Acid-fast bacilli stain positive in pulmonary tuberculosis, although it is often difficult to find the organism microscopically. Mycobacterial cultures take a minimum of four weeks to grow, and although the cultures make the definitive diagnosis, they are not useful in the acute setting.

3. **CBC.** Normochromic, normocytic anemia common (may be severe); WBC normal usually.

4. **Urinanalysis** (U/A). Hematuria and pyuria may indicate renal involvement (**sterile pyuria** classically associated with tuberculosis). Albuminuria (secondary to amyloidosis) may be seen in prolonged infections.

5. **Chemistry:** ↓ Na^+ (SIADH), ↓ Albumin (severe cases)

6. **CXR.** Crucial to diagnosis.

> a. **Primary tuberculosis.** Patchy infiltrates in lower lung fields and hilar adenopathy.
>
> b. **Postprimary tuberculosis.** Patchy upper-lobe infiltrates (apical and posterior segments involved), cavitation, fibronodular infiltrates, fibrosis, and unilateral infiltrates are common.

III. Differential diagnosis. Tuberculosis needs to be differentiated from the following:

A. **Acute bacterial pneumonia.** Sputum exam and response to antibiotics may be helpful in distinguishing from TB.

B. **Neoplasm.** High incidence of tuberculous changes in upper lobes of older men may make the diagnosis of neoplasm difficult; sputum cytology, bronchoscopy with brushings may help distinguish.

C. **Sarcoidosis.** Negative PPD test; lymph node biopsy through mediastinoscopy or bronchoscopy with transbronchial biopsies may be necessary to distinguish.

D. **Fungal disorder (especially histoplasmosis).** Histoplasmosis and tuberculosis may coexist; skin tests for fungus and cultures help make the diagnosis.

E. **Cavitary lung abscess.** Involves superior segments of lower lobes (most often due to aspiration); positive air-fluid level (rare in tuberculosis); no associated patchy infiltrate adjacent to cavity on CXR (common in tuberculosis). Sputum may be fetid.

IV. Pathophysiology

A. TB infection almost always is by **inhalation of aerosolized bacilli** ("droplet nuclei") from coughing, sneezing, or speech. Tubercle bacilli multiply slowly (maximum of 1–2 cell divisions/day) and require high O_2 concentration, which is why primary tuberculosis occurs in the lower lobes.

B. **Disease stages**

1. **Primary tuberculosis.** Bacterial multiplication with asymptomatic spread to regional hilar nodes; leads to lymphohematogenous spread. Seeds widely, especially to the lung apices, kidneys, vertebral column, long bones, brain, lymph nodes (organs with high oxygen concentrations). Reticuloendothelial system involved in clearance of bacilli.

2. **Postprimary tuberculosis.** Onset weeks to years after infection; a specific population of T lymphocytes determines pathologic response and is responsible for tuberculin reaction and cellular immunity. Quiescent tuberculosis results from immunologically contained infection.

PULMONARY EMBOLISM

I. Definition. Impaction of thrombotic embolism in the pulmonary vascular bed, with subsequent partial or complete obstruction of the blood supply to the lung parenchyma.

II. Clinical manifestations

A. **History.** Sudden onset of dyspnea, generally associated with tachypnea, and often associated with chest pain that may be pleuritic in nature.

Hemoptysis, cough, syncope, fever and diaphoresis may occur as well. In many patients, anxiety or a feeling of impending doom may be present.

B. Physical examination

1. **Pulmonary.** Tachypnea, localized crackles and/or wheezes. Pleural friction rub.

2. **Cardiovascular.** There may be evidence of deep venous thrombophlebitis in the legs. However, most cases of DVT are silent. Patients usually present with tachycardia, increased P2 component of S2 (representing acute cor pulmonale), murmur of tricuspid insufficiency, right ventricular heave, S4 (and/or S3), distended neck veins, cyanosis, hypotension. There may also be evidence of hepatojugular reflux and hepatomegaly.

C. Diagnostic tests

1. **ECG.** Generally shows nonspecific abnormalities or may be normal. Sinus tachycardia is most common abnormality. Changes in S-T segment and T wave inversion common. $S_1Q_3T_3$ pattern and *right axis deviation* usually indicate acute right-sided compromise. Acute-onset atrial fibrillation also noted. ECG most useful for ruling out cardiac causes of patient's signs and symptoms.

2. **Chest X-Ray.** Generally associated with normal findings or nonspecific abnormalities. Most useful to rule out conditions that mimic pulmonary embolism (pneumothorax, pneumonia, congestive heart failure). Lung parenchymal abnormalities common and include consolidation and atelectasis. Pleural-based infiltrates (wedge-shaped) and effusions occur. Abrupt cutoff of a vessel shadow and oligemia distal to the embolus may occur (Westermark's sign),

3. **Arterial Blood Gases.** Hypoxemia common, A-a gradient widened. Hyperventilation commonly observed, even in patients with baseline hypercarbia. Alkalemia often noted.

4. **Ventilation/Perfusion Lung Scanning.** Often performed as initial diagnostic strategy to confirm pulmonary embolism. Normal V/Q scan essentially rules out a pulmonary embolism. V/Q scans are reported as high, indeterminate (intermediate) and low probabilities. Readings involve determining whether ventilation and perfusion defects ar matched or unmatched. Unmatched defects are more suggestive of embolization. In patients with a high clinical suspicion and a high probability scan, pulmonary embolism is almost definite. However, the majority of patients eventually diagnosed with pulmonary emboli have other that high probability scans. Therefore, other approaches must be used as well.

5. **Pulmonary angiography.** Considered the *gold standard* for the diagnosis of pulmonary embolism. Often performed in patients with low or indeterminate V/Q scans and high suspicion of pulmonary embolism. Useful in patients with past history of prior unconfirmed pulmonary embolism or patients at high risk for anticoagulation. In many institutions, often performed only if embolism in question.

6. **CT Scanning with angiography.** Widely used in the initial evaluation of suspected PE, this is a less invasive approach to diagnosis than for-

mal pulmonary angiography. 90% sensitivity for emboli in segmental or larger arteries. Valuable for excluding other entities that may cause similar symptoms.

7. **D-dimer testing.** D-dimer is formed when cross-linked fibrin in thrombi is broken down by plasmin. Elevated levels can be used to detect DVT and PE. Abnormal test is non-specific and cannot be used to diagnose pulmonary embolism or DVT. However, negative predictive value is greater than 98%.

8. **Venous ultrasonography.** Noninvasive method of choice for diagnosing deep vein thrombosis. The presence of DVT in a patient with suspected pulmonary embolism is sufficient for institution of therapy.

III. **Differential diagnosis.** The signs and symptoms associated with a pulmonary embolism are generally nonspecific. A degree of suspicion is needed to at least consider the possibility that the diagnosis exists. The diagnosis itself is not hard to make. It is just that there are many other diagnoses that can present with similar signs and symptoms. The diagnosis can rarely be made on clinical grounds alone. Entities to be considered include: myocardial infarction, anxiety, pneumothorax, pneumonia, pericarditis, and congestive heat failure. Pulmonary infarction is unusual because of the dual blood supply to the lungs (bronchial circulation and pulmonary circulation).

IV. **Pathophysiology**

A. The vast majority of pulmonary emboli are due to venous thrombi originating in the lower extremities. Pelvic vein thrombosis and prostatic vein thrombosis may also occur. Less than ten percent of emboli will cause an infarction.

B. **Predisposing factors** include **prolonged immobilization, trauma** or **surgery** to the lower extremities or pelvis. Also, the presence of a **hypercoagulable state** is recognized as a predisposing factor. These include Factor V Leiden mutation, antithrombin III deficiency, Protein S deficiency, Protein C deficiency, G20210A mutatuion in Prothrombin gene, lupus anticoagulant, polycythemia vera, and deficiency of plasminogen activators. Patients with malignancy, CHF, morbid obesity, and prior venous thromboembolic disease are at risk. Pregnancy and the use of estrogens also increase the risk for venous thromboembolic disease.

ᕽ PNEUMONIA

I. **Definition.** An acute infection of lung parenchyma. There are several types of pneumonia: **lobar pneumonia** (infection confined to a single lobe), **segmental or lobular pneumonia** (infection confined to a segment of a lobe), **bronchopneumonia** (infection involves alveoli and contiguous bronchi), **interstitial pneumonia** (infection involves interstitial tissue). These distinctions are based on x-ray observations.

II. **Clinical manifestations and differential diagnosis.** Less than 40% of patients with community-acquired pneumonia will actually have an etiology found. The most common bacterial, viral, mycoplasma, and fungal pneumonias:

A. Bacterial pneumonias

1. *Streptococcus pneumoniae* (pneumococcus)

   a. **History.** The **most common cause of bacterial pneumonia**, and the most common cause of pneumonia in adults when an etiology is found. Frequently seen in patients with COPD and alcoholism. **Community acquired,** usually with a history of preceding viral upper respiratory infection.

   Sudden onset with single shaking chill, which is followed by fever, pleuritic chest pain, cough, dyspnea, and purulent sputum production that is "rust" colored or blood-tinged; fever $> 102°F$.

   b. **Physical exam.** Patient appears seriously ill. Typical pulmonary signs of lobar pneumonia include those consistent with a consolidation: increased tactile fremitus, percussion dullness, egophony, and whispered pectoriloquy. With pleural effusions or empyema there may be percussion dullness, diminished breath sounds, or a pleural rub. The most frequent observation is simply crackles on auscultation.

   c. **Diagnostic tests**

      (1) **CXR.** The **most frequent cause of lobar pneumonia** is pneumococcus; the most frequent x-ray pattern among all patients with pneumococcal pneumonia is a bronchopneumonia pattern; therefore, pneumococcal pneumonia can appear as a dense consolidation confined to a single lobe with typical air bronchograms or a bronchopneumonia pattern.

      (2) **Microbiology.** Gram stain analysis usually shows gram-positive diplococci in short chains (see Color Plates). Sputum cultures often fail to grow organism. Positive blood cultures in 20 to 25 percent of patients allow definitive diagnosis.

2. *Haemophilius influenzae*

   a. **History.** More common in older patients. Predominantly men affected. COPD present in over 50%, alcoholism in 33%. Abrupt onset of symptoms with patients severely ill within 48 hours. Fever, cough with purulent sputum, pleuritic chest pain and dyspnea common.

   b. **Physical Examination.** Patient acutely ill with high fever. Tachpnea present. Crackles and findings of consolidation often present, predominantly in lower lobes. Pleural effusions in up to 25%.

   c. **Diagnostic Tests.**

      (1) **Chest X-Ray.** Usually shows bronchopneumonia. Cavitation uncommon. Pleural effusions occur, empyema unusual.

      (2) **Microbiology.** Gram's stain of sputum show small Gram-negative coccobacilli. Often seen within cytoplasm of neutrophils. Blood cultures positive in 20%.

3. *Klebsiella pneumoniae*

   a. **History.** Rarely causes pneumonia in previously well adult hosts. Inflicts infants and the aged; is acquired in nursing home or hospital; host is often immunocompromised.

Sudden onset of symptoms with fever $> 102°F$, chills, cough, and thick, bloody ("tenacious") sputum.

b. Physical exam. Characterized by upper-lobe involvement, tissue necrosis with abscess formation.

c. Diagnostic tests

(1) **CXR.** Variable; usually dense upper lobe infiltrate with upper-lobe central cavitation and abscess formation.

(2) **Microbiology.** Gram stain analysis of sputum shows large numbers of gram-negative bacilli. Positive cultures from blood, pleural fluid, or sputum obtained before treatment are considered diagnostic.

4. *Staphylococcus aureus*

a. History. Similar to *Klebsiella*; inflicts infants and the elderly; is acquired in nursing home or hospital; host is often immunocompromised. Intravenous drug abusers are prone to staphylococcal tricuspid valve endocarditis with embolic pneumonia. Patients with influenza pneumonia are predisposed to staphylococcal superinfection.

Onset of symptoms similar to pneumococcal pneumonia.

b. Physical exam. Similar to that noted for pneumococcal pneumonia. *Staphylococcus* differs in its tendency to cause recurrent shaking chills, tissue necrosis with abscess formation (rare with pneumococcal pneumonia), and pneumatoceles (most common in infants and children); empyema is common. Infected skin site (portal of entry) often identifiable in IV drug abusers.

c. Diagnostic tests

(1) **CXR.** Variable; most common pattern is a bronchopneumonia with or without abscess formation or pleural effusion. Bronchopneumonic pattern (often bilateral) seen; cavitation and abscesses common. Lobar consolidation is infrequent.

(2) **Microbiology.** Gram stain analysis shows gram-positive clusters like "grapes." Diagnosis is made by positive cultures from sputum or empyema fluid.

B. Mycoplasma pneumonias (*Mycoplasma pneumoniae*)

1. History. Most common cause of pneumonia in 5- to 35-year-old age group. Community acquired.

Nonspecific constitutional symptoms (malaise and sore throat) are of insidious onset with fever $> 101°F$, nonproductive hacking cough with scant mucoid sputum. Cough is dominant symptom; mild or absent cough makes the diagnosis suspect.

2. Physical exam. Findings may be minimal (crackles, cough, but little else). Unimpressive relative to patients' complaints and x-ray findings.

3. Diagnostic tests.

a. CXR. Interstitial pneumonia, usually unilateral; usually seen in lower lobes, $\pm$ small pleural effusions; radiologic findings often far more severe than clinical manifestations.

    b. Serology. Positive complement fixation tests in 75 to 80 percent of patients.

C. Viral pneumonias (Influenza A)

    1. History. Ninety percent of deaths due to influenza A occur in elderly population.

    Fever up to 105°F with hacking cough; sputum often blood-tinged.

    2. Physical exam. Pulmonary auscultatory findings may be minimal or absent; respiratory distress often far more severe than radiologic findings.

    3. Diagnostic tests. CXR. Diffuse or generalized interstitial pattern usually seen; lobar consolidation or pleural effusion rarely seen.

D. Fungal pneumonias. Primary fungal pneumonia most commonly caused by *Histoplasma capsulatum* and *Coccidioides immitis.*

    1. *Histoplasma capsulatum*

        a. History. Asymptomatic or mild fever, malaise, dyspnea, minimal or absent sputum with nonproductive cough; chills rare. Indistinguishable from viral upper respiratory infection, it is endemic in south-central United States.

        b. Physical exam. Crackles, oral ulceration.

        c. Diagnostic tests

            (1) CXR. Lower lobes favored, with generalized nodular and linear infiltrates; unilateral or bilateral adenopathy may be present. Chronic cavitary form produces pulmonary lesions indistinguishable, except by culture, from cavitary tuberculosis.

            (2) Microbiology. Culture from sputum or oral ulceration is diagnostic.

    2. *Coccidioides immitis*

        a. History. Endemic in southwestern United States.

        Often asymptomatic or indistinguishable from viral upper respiratory infection, with fever, chills, moderate mucoid sputum production.

        b. Physical exam. Scattered crackles, cervical adenopathy, skin lesions resembling erythema nodosum, pleural effusion with friction rub.

        c. Diagnostic tests

            (1) CXR. Lower lobes favored, with generalized nodular and linear infiltrates; unilateral or bilateral adenopathy may be present.

            (2) Microbiology. Sperules of fungus present in sputum and sputum culture positive for fungus are both diagnostic.

III. Pathophysiology. Vastly different for each microbe. For a detailed account, consult Weinberger SE, *Principles of Pulmonary Medicine*, 4th ed., WB Saunders, January, 2004.

CHAPTER 19

Cardiovascular Diseases: Ischemic Heart Disease, Angina Pectoris and Myocardial Infarction

One of the more challenging tasks for a physician is to make a diagnosis of angina pectoris on the basis of the history. In addition to Levine's sign (in describing the pain the patient clenches his/her fist and places it over the sternum), there are several other less well-known clues: 1) The discomfort of angina pectoris rarely occurs superior to the angle of the jaw or inferior to the umbilicus, 2) If the patient can identify the site of discomfort with his/her index finger it is rarely angina.

Eugene Braunwald, M.D., MACP

Author of more than 1,000 publications, and Editor-in-Chief of Harrison's Principles of Internal Medicine *(15th ed.), Dr. Braunwald graduated from New York University School of Medicine and completed his internal medicine residency at the Johns Hopkins Hospital in Baltimore , Maryland. From 1972 to 1996 he was the Chairman of the Department of Medicine at the Brigham and Women's Hospital, Boston. He is the Distinguished Hersey Professor of Medicine at Harvard Medical School and currently serves as Chief Academic Officer, Partners Health-Care Systems, Boston. He is also the Faculty Dean for Academic Programs, Brigham and Women's Hospital and Massachusettes General Hospital, Boston.*

I. Definitions

A. Angina pectoris. Clinical syndrome characterized by pain or discomfort in chest and adjacent areas that occurs when myocardial oxygen demand exceeds supply. It is by definition **transient** and **reversible.** There are three types of angina: **stable, unstable,** and **Prinzmetal's.**

B. Myocardial infarction (MI) is an **irreversible** ischemic necrosis of the myocardium, resulting from an insufficient oxygen supply to that area of the heart for a prolonged period. There are two types of myocardial infarction: **transmural** (Q-wave) and **subendocardial** (non Q-wave).

II. Clinical manifestations. Diagnosis of angina is best made by history.

A. Angina pectoris

1. **History.** Each of the three types of angina presents with its own unique history.

a. **Stable**

    (1) Usually follows a precipitating event, such as climbing stairs, sexual intercourse, a heavy meal, activity in cold weather.

    (2) Generally same severity as previous attack; relieved by customary dose of nitroglycerin.

b. **Unstable**

    (1) New or recent onset.

    (2) Increasing severity, duration, or frequency of stable angina.

    (3) Occurs at rest or with minimal exertion.

c. **Prinzmetal's**

    (1) Occurs when patient is at rest.

    (2) No previous history of coronary artery disease, typically.

d. An angina history is described in the following dimensions: PQRST.

    (1) **Provocative-palliative factors.** Aggravated by emotion, exercise, cold weather, large meals; occasionally also by recumbency (angina decubitus). Related to exertion or emotion. Common for angina to occur soon after awakening; shaving or washing may precipitate. Arm exercise may provoke more angina than leg exercise. Alleviated by rest, cessation of activity, and often by sublingual nitroglycerin. If emotionally precipitated, relieved by relaxation.

    (2) **Quality.** Often characterized as discomfort, not pain. May be described as pressure, tightness, heaviness, squeezing hand-like, vise-like, burning, choking, smothering, or a sensation similar to intestinal gas or dysphagia. Descriptions such as knife-like, stabbing, or cutting rarely reflect angina.

    (3) **Region.** Most frequently substernal. May also be in neck, lower jaw, arm, or hand areas (especially left arm, ulnar aspect) with or without chest symptoms. Precordial areas alone (e.g., left submammary, over heart) **uncommon.**

    (4) **Severity.** Mild to moderate severity; often patients must stop whatever they are doing. May seem less bothersome after patients exert themselves for a while (warm-up phenomenon). Occurs in crescendo-decrescendo pattern; not of sudden onset or dissipation.

    (5) **Temporal characteristics.** Elicit first onset and frequency. Typical attack 1–3 minutes; almost always shorter than 10 and longer than 1 minute.

    (6) **Associated symptoms.** Dyspnea common; nausea, dizziness, diaphoresis sometimes. Palpitations, loss of consciousness rare (unless angina is related to arrhythmia).

e. **Past medical history.** Check for hypertension, tobacco use, diabetes mellitus, hyperlipidemia, obesity, estrogen use.

f. **Family history.** Check for coronary artery disease, MI, angina, premature death in first-degree relatives.

    2. Physical exam. Often no physical signs are found during an attack of angina.

        a. Dyspnea and diaphoresis.

        b. New-onset S_4 frequently occurs because of decreased compliance of the ischemic ventricle.

        c. Arrhythmia may be present, which may or may not be the cause of the angina.

        d. Presence of a heart murmur may indicate valvular cause of angina; mitral valve prolapse, aortic stenosis, mitral stenosis, or idiopathic hypertrophic subaortic stenosis (also known as hypertrophic obstructive cardiomyopathy).

    3. Diagnostic tests

        a. Nitroglycerin test. The unequivocal relief of chest pain or discomfort by the administration of nitroglycerin is strongly suggestive of angina pectoris, but not diagnostic.

        b. ECG. During episode of chest discomfort, may show transient ischemic changes such as T wave inversion or S-T segment depression or elevation.

B. Myocardial infarction. Diagnosis depends on meeting two of three criteria. (1) typical pain, (2) ECG changes, and (3) serum enzyme changes.

    1. History

        a. Chest pain or discomfort is the most common symptom. Preexisting and often worsening angina by history. The pain or discomfort is similar to angina pectoris in its quality, location, and intensity, but it is **not** transient, is not relieved by sublingual nitroglycerin, and lasts 30 minutes or longer. The pain is usually not induced by exertion, nor does it remit with rest. Approximately 15–20 percent of infarcts are painless; painless infarcts more common in diabetics and the aged.

        b. Often accompanied by nausea, vomiting (classically if **MI** is **inferior**), giddiness, anxiety.

        c. Key items of interest in the past medical history and family history are the same as in angina.

    2. Physical exam

        a. Patient will appear diaphoretic and pale, resulting in cold, clammy skin.

        b. Often heart rate accelerates and the blood pressure declines, sometimes to shock levels when there is extensive myocardial damage. A quadruple rhythm (summation gallop) is sometimes heard (S_4-S_1-S_2-S_3). Apical systolic murmur caused by mitral regurgitation secondary to papillary muscle dysfunction may be present.

        c. Arrhythmia may be present.

        d. Crackles may appear in lung bases (pulmonary edema), indicative of congestive heart failure.

        e. Pericardial friction rub may be heard.

        f. Mild fever may be present.

3. **Diagnostic tests**
   a. **ECG.** Changes appear soon after pain begins. **Sequence of evolution**: T wave inversion, S-T segment depression, S-T segment elevation, development of Q waves. Q waves usually develop over 12 to 36 hours. A subendocardial myocardial infarct (a non-Q wave infarct) is limited to the inner third to half of the myocardial wall. A transmural myocardial infarct (a Q wave infarct) encompasses the entire thickness of the ventricular wall.
   b. **Serum enzyme changes** (Fig. 19-1). Creatinine phosphokinese (CPK) isoenzyme specific to cardiac muscle (**CPK-MB**) is released when damage occurs to the myocardium. This marker is thus a more specific indication of myocardial damage than the unfractionated CPK value. Amount of CPK-MB released correlates to size of the infarct. **Cardiac troponin** is able to detect lesser degrees of myocardial necrosis and if the MI was suspected to have occurred 2–10 days prior to presentation. In 2003, plasma **myeloperoxidase** was found to independently predict the early risk of myocardial infarction in patients presenting with chest pain and the Food and Drug Administration approved the **Albumin Cobalt Binding** (ACB) test to detect early cardiac ischemia.

III. Differential diagnosis

A. **Angina.** The two types of **thoracic pain** most difficult to differentiate from angina are musculoskeletal and gastrointestinal pain.

   1. **Musculoskeletal.** Costochondritis pain is often sharp in quality and usually persists for 1 or more hours; often worse at the end of day and

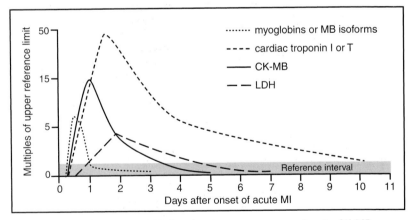

Fig. 19-1. Effect of myocardial infarction on serum enzyme levels. CK-MB = creatinine phosphokinase-MB fraction, LDH = lactate dehydrogenase. (Adapted with permission from Wu, AHB. Introduction to coronary artery disease (CAD) and biochemical markers. In: Wu, AHB, ed. *Cardiac Markers.* Totowa: Humana Press, 1998: p. 12).

relieved by positional changes or heat; localized (point) tenderness may be present on physical exam.

2. **Gastrointestinal.** Pain due to peptic ulcer disease, esophageal reflux, esophageal spasm, cholecystitis, cholelithiasis, and pancreatitis. GI pain is not related to exertion, but may be related to anxiety; often related to meals; may last up to several hours; often relieved by bowel movement, antacid, and or positional change. GI pain (e.g., esophageal spasm) may be relieved by nitroglycerin or calcium channel blockers and may even be accompanied by ECG changes. Also, GI pain may precipitate anginal pain, or patient may have both GI disease and angina.

3. **Pulmonary.** Pain due to pulmonary embolism, pleurisy, pneumothorax, pneumonia with pleuritis, pulmonary hypertension.

4. **Cardiovascular.** Pain due to myocardial infarction, pericarditis, dissecting aortic aneurysm.

5. **Infectious.** Pain from herpes zoster.

6. **Psychological.** Anxiety-induced pain.

B. **Myocardial infarction.** Same differential diagnosis as angina.

Tables 19-1 and 19-2 differentiate among the many cardiac and noncardiac causes of chest pain.

IV. **Pathophysiology.** Angina pectoris and myocardial infarction are part of a continuum of responses resulting from myocardial oxygen demand exceeding oxygen supply.

A. **Myocardial oxygen supply** is a function of the ventricular diastolic perfusion pressure, the rate of coronary blood flow, and the oxygen-carrying capacity of the blood. Myocardial oxygen demand is a function of heart rate, ventricular wall tension, and the intrinsic contractility of the myocardium. Wall tension is proportional to left ventricular systolic blood pressure and left ventricular volume, and inversely proportional to left ventricular wall thickness. Exertion, the major cause of myocardial ischemia, increases all three determinants of myocardial oxygen demand. Due to coronary artery disease, this increase in oxygen demand cannot be met with an increase in oxygen supply, an imbalance occurs, and myocardial ischemia results.

B. In addition to coronary artery disease, other conditions may result in an imbalance between myocardial oxygen supply and demand and result in ischemia. Decreased myocardial oxygen supply can result from decreased aortic perfusion pressure, due to hypotension or aortic **regurgitation**, or a decrease in the blood's oxygen-carrying capacity, due to **anemia or hypoxemia.** An increase in myocardial oxygen demand that can result in ischemia occurs in **aortic stenosis.**

C. In general, **stable** and **unstable** angina are caused by a fixed coronary artery obstruction secondary to atherosclerosis, where **Prinzmetal**'s angina is caused by coronary artery spasm, with or without superimposed coronary artery disease. **Myocardial infarction** is most often the result of coronary artery disease (85 percent of cases). It may also result from coronary artery spasm, due to cocaine use, congenital abnormalities of coro-

TABLE 19-1. Cardiovascular causes of chest pain

Condition	Location	Quality	Duration	Aggravating or relieving factors	Associated symptoms or signs
Angina pectoris	Retrosternal region; radiates to or occasionally isolated to neck, jaw, epigastrium, shoulder or arms—left common	Pressure, burning, squeezing, heaviness, indigestion	<10 min	Aggravated by exercise, cold weather, or emotional stress, or occurs after meals; relieved by rest or nitroglycerin; atypical (Prinzmetal's) angina may be unrelated to activity and caused by coronary artery spasm	S$_4$, paradoxical split S$_2$, or murmur of papillary muscle dysfunction during pain
Rest or crescendo angina	Same as angina	Same as angina	>10 min	Same as angina, with gradually decreasing tolerance for exertion	Same as angina
Myocardial infarction	Substernal, and may radiate like angina	Heaviness, pressure, burning, constriction	Sudden onset, 30 min or longer but variable; usually goes away in hours	Unrelieved	Shortness of breath, sweating, weakness, nausea, vomiting, severe anxiety
Pericarditis	Usually begins over sternum or toward cardiac apex and may radiate to neck and down left upper extremity; often more localized than the pain of myocardial ischemia	Sharp, stabbing, knife-like	Lasts many hours to days	Aggravated by deep breathing, rotating chest, or supine position; relieved by sitting up and leaning forward	Pericardial friction rub, cardiac tamponade, pulsus paradoxus
Dissecting aortic aneurysm	Anterior chest; radiates to thoracic area of back; may be abdominal; pain may move as dissection progresses	Excruciating, tearing, knife-like	Sudden onset, lasts for hours	Unrelated to anything	Lower blood pressure in one arm, absent pulses, paralysis, murmur of aortic insufficiency, pulsus paradoxus, MI

Reproduced with permission from T. E. Andreoli et al.

TABLE 19-2. Noncardiac causes of chest pain

Condition	Location	Quality	Duration	Aggravating or relieving factors	Associated symptoms or signs
Pulmonary embolism (chest pain often not present)	Substernal or over region of pulmonary infarction	Pleuritic (with pulmonary infarction) or angina-like	Sudden onset; minutes to < hour	May be aggravated by breathing	Dyspnea, tachypnea, tachycardia, hypotension; signs of acute right heart failure and pulmonary hypertension with large emboli; crackles, pleural rub, hemoptysis with pulmonary infarction; clinically present in minority of cases
Pulmonary hypertension	Substernal	Pressure; oppressive		Aggravated by effort	Pain usually associated with dyspnea; signs of pulmonary hypertension
Pneumonia with pleurisy	Localized over area of consolidation	Pleuritic, well localized		Painful breathing	Dyspnea, cough, fever, dull to percussion, bronchial breath sounds, crackles, occasional pleural rub

(continued)

TABLE 19-2. Noncardiac causes of chest pain (*Continued*)

Condition	Location	Quality	Duration	Aggravating or relieving factors	Associated symptoms or signs
Spontaneous pneumothorax	Unilateral	Sharp, well localized	Sudden onset, lasts many hours	Painful breathing	Dyspnea; hyperresonance and decreased breath and voice sounds over involved lung
Musculoskeletal disorders	Variable	Aching	Short or long duration	Aggravated by movement; history of muscle exertion	Tender to pressure or movement
Herpes zoster	Dermatomal in distribution		Prolonged	None	Rash appears in area of discomfort
Gastrointestinal disorders (e.g., esophageal reflux, peptic ulcer, cholecystitis)	Lower substernal area, epigastric; right or left upper quadrant	Burning, colic-like, aching		Precipitated by recumbency or meals	Nausea, regurgitation, food intolerance, melena, hematemesis, jaundice
Anxiety states	Often localized to a point	Sharp burning, commonly location of pain moves from place to place	Varies; usually very brief	Situational anger—very brief	Sighing, respirations, often chest wall tenderness

Reproduced with permission from T. E. Andreoli et al.

nary circulation, periarteritis and other coronary artery inflammatory diseases, or coronary embolism.

CONGESTIVE HEART FAILURE

I. Definition. A clinical syndrome that results from the inability of the heart to achieve cardiac output capable of supplying sufficient oxygen to the metabolizing tissues. Congestive heart failure (CHF) may be further divided into **right ventricular failure, left ventricular failure**, and **biventricular failure.** There is also a distinction between **systolic** heart failure (LV ejection fraction <40%) and **diastolic** heart failure (normal LV ejection fraction).

II. Clinical manifestations, listed in order of decreasing specificity for each type of heart failure.

  A. Right ventricular failure

   1. **Jugular venous distention**
   2. Hepatomegaly
   3. Increased prothrombin time
   4. **Peripheral edema**
   5. Increased aspartate aminotransferase (AST)
   6. Increased bilirubin
   7. **Pleural effusion**
   8. Decreased albumin
   9. Abdominal discomfort
   10. Anorexia
   11. Proteinuria

  B. Left ventricular failure

   1. Chest x-ray with redistribution of perfusion or interstitial edema
   2. **Third heart sound (S_3)**
   3. Cardiomegaly
   4. Pulmonary crackles
   5. Paroxysmal nocturnal dyspnea (PND), orthopnea
   6. Dyspnea on exertion

III. Differential diagnosis

  A. Right ventricular failure

   1. Pulmonary embolus
   2. Tricuspid stenosis
   3. Tricuspid regurgitation
   4. Right atrial tumor
   5. Cardiac tamponade
   6. Constrictive pericarditis
   7. Pulmonic insufficiency

    8. Right ventricular infarction

    9. Intrinsic lung disease

   10. Epstein's anomaly

   11. High cardiac output states: anemia, systemic fistulae, beriberi, Paget's disease, carcinoid, thyrotoxicosis

  B. Left or biventricular failure

    1. Aortic stenosis

    2. Aortic insufficiency

    3. Mitral stenosis

    4. Mitral regurgitation

    5. Most cardiomyopathies

    6. Restrictive cardiomyopathy

    7. Myocardial infarction

    8. Myxoma

    9. Hypertensive heart disease

   10. Myocarditis

   11. Supraventricular arrhythmias

   12. Left ventricular aneurysm

   13. Cardiac shunts

   14. High cardiac output states

IV. Pathophysiology. The etiologies of CHF can be divided into six general categories that have distinct pathophysiologic mechanisms. For each general category, its pathophysiology, most common etiologies, and clinical manifestations are listed. Note that cardiomyopathies, valvular heart disease, systemic hypertension, and pericardial disease are the subjects of further discussion in this chapter.

  A. Cardiomyopathies

    1. Pathophysiology. ↓ Myocardial contractile function (most cardiomyopathies), or ↓ diastolic filling secondary to ↓ ventricular compliance (e.g., infiltrative processes); results in left or biventricular failure.

    2. Most common etiologies. Hypertrophic obstructive cardiomyopathy, dilated cardiomyopathy, restrictive cardiomyopathy.

    3. Clinical manifestations. Dilated versus hypertrophic cardiomyopathies on physical exam. Evidence of systemic disease (e.g., sarcoid, hemochromatosis, connective tissue disease, amyloidosis).

    4. Diagnostic tests. Echocardiography, radionuclide ventriculography (RVG), cardiac catheterization, myocardial biopsy. A serum BNP (B-type natriuretic peptide) level below 100 pg/mL has strong negative predictive value for CHF in the assessment of patients with dyspnea.

  B. Valvular heart disease

    1. Pathophysiology. ↑ Cardiac work load (secondary to ↑ volume or pressure work) results in left or biventricular failure.

2. **Most common etiologies.** Aortic stenosis, aortic insufficiency, mitral regurgitation, mitral stenosis.

3. **Clinical manifestations**

    a. Presence of significant murmur(s) on physical exam.

    b. Specific cardiovascular exam findings.

    c. Echocardiography and cardiac catheterization.

C. **Systemic hypertension (HTN)**

1. **Pathophysiology.** ↑ Cardiac work load (secondary to ↑ afterload) results in left or biventricular failure.

2. **Most common etiologies.** Essential HTN.

3. **Clinical manifestations.** ↑ Blood pressure and systemic signs of HTN disease (e.g., fundoscopic, renal changes).

D. **Pericardial disease**

1. **Pathophysiology.** ↓ Diastolic ventricular filling (causes a fixed restriction in cardiac output); results in right ventricular failure.

2. **Most common etiologies.** Viral, traumatic, radiation-induced, tuberculosis- or uremia-associated constrictive disease.

3. **Clinical manifestations.** Constrictive pericarditis: signs of right heart failure (RHF)—edema, ascites, ↑ venous pressure, hepatomegaly; signs of small, quiet heart.

4. **Diagnostic tests**

    a. Echocardiography, cardiac catheterization, characteristic pressure tracings.

    b. CXR may show triangle-shaped heart and calcium in pericardium.

E. **Pulmonary arterial hypertension**

1. **Pathophysiology.** ↑ Cardiac work load secondary to ↑ pulmonary (right-sided) resistance; results in right ventricular failure.

2. **Most common etiologies.** Primary pulmonary hypertension, pulmonary embolism (acute or chronic), left heart disease (↑ pulmonary venous pressure), parenchymal lung disease (e.g., COPD).

3. **Clinical manifestations.** Signs of right ventricular (RV) overload and ↑ pulmonary pressures, parasternal lift, prominent jugular venous pressure (JVP) *a* wave and *v* wave if tricuspid regurgitation (TR), ↑ intensity P_2; murmurs of pulmonic insufficiency (PI) or TR, peripheral signs of RHF (hepatomegaly, edema, pulsatile liver if TR present).

4. **Diagnostic tests.** Echocardiography, RVG; right-sided and pulmonary artery catheterization.

F. **High output states**

1. **Pathophysiology.** ↑ Workload (secondary to ↑ metabolic demands).

2. **Most common etiologies.** Thyrotoxicosis, anemia, arteriovenous (AV) fistula.

3. **Clinical manifestations.** Search for systemic disease, such as:

    a. **Thyrotoxicosis:** hyperactive heart, wide pulse pressure, atrial fibrillation.

    b. Anemia: rapid pulse, hyperactive heart, signs of peripheral vasodilatation.

    c. AV fistula: history of prior surgery, presence of continuous bruit in abnormal location.

V. Exacerbations of CHF. Patients with well-controlled chronic CHF can experience sudden exacerbations due to some slight change in the baseline compensated state of the patient. This generally occurs secondary to:

  A. ↓ Myocardial function

    1. Poor medication compliance: ↓ digoxin

    2. Alcohol

    3. New-onset arrhythmia

    4. Myocardial ischemia, myocardial infarction, or both

  B. ↑ Cardiac work load

    1. ↑ Salt intake

    2. Poor medication compliance: ↓ Lasix results in fluid overload.

    3. ↑ Activity

    4. Infection, fever

    5. Pulmonary embolism

    6. Anemia

    7. Pregnancy

    8. Thyrotoxicosis

    9. Acute or chronic renal failure

 CARDIOMYOPATHIES

I. Definition. Disease in which the clinical presentation is due to dysfunction of the myocardium, as a result of a process that primarily affects the myocardial tissue. Classically, myocardial changes due to systemic or pulmonary hypertension, ischemic heart disease, and valvular disease are **excluded** from this group of myocardial disorders. There are three types of cardiomyopathy: **dilated cardiomyopathy, hypertrophic cardiomyopathy,** and **restrictive cardiomyopathy.**

  A. Dilated cardiomyopathy is characterized by ventricular dilatation with decreased systolic contractile function.

  B. Hypertrophic cardiomyopathy is characterized by thickened hypercontractile ventricles.

  C. Restrictive cardiomyopathy is characterized by an abnormally stiff myocardium with impaired ventricular relaxation and filling but preserved contractile function.

II. Clinical manifestations. Table 19-3 compares the clinical manifestations of the three types of cardiomyopathy.

TABLE 19-3. Clinical manifestations of cardiomyopathies

	Dilated cardiomyopathy	Hypertrophic cardiomyopathy	Restrictive cardiomyopathy
History	History of viral illness, recent pregnancy, alcoholism, collagen vascular disorder, exposure to toxins, recent mediastinal radiation; nutritional history, drug history, dyspnea on exertion, orthopnea, paroxysmal nocturnal dyspnea, peripheral edema, symptoms of pulmonary and systemic venous congestion (biventricular CHF), palpitations	Family history of sudden death due to heart disease, angina (decreased in the recumbent position), dyspnea, syncope (usually seen with exercise), palpitations	Dyspnea on exertion, orthopnea, fatigue or weakness (due to low cardiac output)
Physical exam	Pulmonary crackles, hepatomegaly, peripheral edema, sinus tachycardia, pulsus alternans, diffuse PMI, S_3, S_4, MR murmur, prominent v wave with JVP and jugular venous distention	Left ventricular heave, bisferiens carotid pulse ("spike and dome" morphology), paradoxical splitting of S_2 if left ventricular obstruction is present, bifid-trifid apical impulse, systolic ejection murmur at left sternal border or apex that increases with Valsalva's maneuver and decreases with squatting, S_4	Edema, ascites, hepatomegaly, distended neck veins
Diagnostic tests	Atrial arrhythmias (AE, premature atrial contractions), ventricular arrhythmias (premature ventricular contractions), left ventricular hypertrophy with nonspecific S-T–wave changes, right or left BBB (or both)	Left ventricular hypertrophy with strain pattern, abnormal Q waves may be seen in anterolateral and inferior leads, Wolff-Parkinson-White syndrome	Atrial and ventricular arrhythmias, nonspecific S-T wave changes
Chest x-ray	Cardiomegaly (may be massive), interstitial pulmonary edema	Normal, or signs of left ventricular hypertrophy	Moderate cardiomegaly, evidence of CHF (pulmonary vascular congestion and pleural effusions)
ECG	Large, poorly contractile LV	Asymmetric ventricular hypertrophy (general left ventricular hypertrophy with even greater septal hypertrophy)	Normal-size, poorly relaxing and filling LV (due to high diastolic pressures)

III. Differential diagnosis

- **A. Dilated cardiomyopathy: congestive or hypodynamic**
    1. **Idiopathic**
    2. **Inflammatory**
        a. Infectious: postviral myocarditis (Coxsackie B or echovirus).
        b. Noninfectious: collagen vascular disease (systemic lupus erythematosis [SLE], rheumatoid arthritis, polyarteritis), peripartum, sarcoidosis.
    3. **Toxin-induced.** Alcohol, chemotherapeutic agents (doxorubicin and Adriamycin), drugs (cocaine, heroin, organic solvents—"glue sniffer's heart").
    4. **Metabolic.** Hypothyroidism and chronic hypocalcemia or hypophosphatemia.
- **B. Hypertrophic (obstructive) cardiomyopathy.** Familial (autosomal dominant trait).
- **C. Restrictive cardiomyopathy**
    1. **Myocardial fibrosis, scarring, or infiltration**
        a. Infiltrative disorders: amyloidosis, sarcoidosis
        b. Noninfiltrative: idiopathic, scleroderma
        c. Storage diseases: glycogen storage disease, hemochromatosis
    2. **Endomyocardial fibrosis, scarring, or infiltration**
        a. Endomyocardial fibrosis
        b. Hypereosinophilic syndrome
        c. Metastatic tumors
        d. Radiation therapy
    3. Restrictive cardiomyopathy **shares almost identical symptoms, physical signs, and hemodynamic profiles with constrictive pericarditis.** It is imperative to distinguish between these two entities, because constrictive pericarditis is curable whereas restrictive cardiomyopathy is not. Diagnosis is made by a computed tomography (CT) scan or magnetic resonance imaging (MRI) of the mediastinum. Constrictive pericarditis has a thickened pericardium, while restrictive cardiomyopathy does not.

IV. Pathophysiology

- **A. Dilated (congestive) cardiomyopathy.** The hallmark is biventricular dilatation with decreased contractile function.
    1. When ventricular stroke volume falls because of impaired myocyte contractility, two compensatory mechanisms activate.
        a. There is an increase in heart rate, mediated by sympathetic tone.
        b. Because of the decreased stroke volume, the ventricular diastolic volume increases and further stretches the myofibrils to increase their stroke work (Starling's principle).
    2. These compensations may render the patient asymptomatic during the early stages of ventricular dysfunction, but progressive myocyte

degeneration and volume overload occur, and clinical symptoms of heart failure soon follow. As cardiac output falls, a decline in renal blood flow activates the renin-angiotensin system, resulting in an **increase in peripheral vascular resistance and intravascular volume**. These compensatory effects are detrimental for two reasons.

  a. The increased resistance makes it more difficult for the left ventricle to eject blood.

  b. The rise in intravascular volume burdens the dilated ventricles further.

 3. As the ventricles enlarge over time, the mitral and tricuspid valves fail to coapt adequately in systole, and **valvular regurgitation** ensues. Such regurgitation has two detrimental effects.

  a. Volume and pressure loads are placed on the atria, causing them to dilate and often leading to atrial fibrillation.

  b. Regurgitation of blood into the left atrium further decreases stroke volume and thereby cardiac output into the systemic circulation.

B. Hypertrophic cardiomyopathy. There is marked hypertrophy of the myocardium and a disproportionately greater thickening of the interventricular septum than that of the free wall of the ventricle: asymmetric septal hypertrophy (ASH). During midsystole the apposition of the anterior mitral leaflet against the hypertrophied septum can cause a narrowing of the subaortic area and result in left ventricular outflow obstruction. Because of this, the disease has been termed idiopathic hypertrophic subaortic stenosis (IHSS) or hypertrophic obstructive cardiomyopathy (HOCM).

C. Restrictive cardiomyopathies are less common than dilated cardiomyopathy and hypertrophic cardiomyopathy. They are characterized by abnormally rigid ventricles that impair diastolic filling but retain normal size and normal systolic function. Reduced ventricular compliance, due to fibrosis or infiltration, results in abnormally high diastolic pressure, which has two consequences: elevated systemic and pulmonary venous pressures, with signs of right- and left-sided vascular congestion, and reduced ventricular cavity size with decreased stroke volume and cardiac output.

MITRAL VALVE DISEASE

 I. Definition. Alterations in the integrity or normal functioning of the mitral valve or its associated structures that lead to alterations in normal cardiovascular physiology. The two most common pathologies of the mitral valve are **mitral stenosis** and **mitral regurgitation.**

 II. Clinical manifestations. Table 19-4 compares some common features of mitral stenosis and mitral regurgitation. Unless otherwise stated, mitral regurgitation refers to the **chronic** lesion.

 III. Differential diagnosis and pathophysiology

  A. Mitral stenosis results from rheumatic heart disease (RHD). Fifty percent of those with mitral stenosis will have a history of rheumatic fever.

TABLE 19-4. Common features of mitral stenosis and mitral regurgitation

	Mitral stenosis	Mitral regurgitation
History	Dyspnea on exertion, pulmonary edema, hemoptysis, fatigue, reactive pulmonary hypertension, right heart failure	In *chronic* mitral regurgitation, fatigue, dyspnea on exertion appear gradually; if *acute,* sudden onset of CHF symptoms
Heart sounds	Loud S_1; opening snap	Diminished S_1; S_3 due to volume
Murmurs	Localized near apex; onset at opening snap (middiastolic) of a low-pitched decrescendo murmur; presystolic accentuation of murmur if normal sinus rhythm present	Loudest over PMI; holosystolic; blowing; radiates to axilla
Chest x-ray	Straight left heart border; large LA, RV; mitral valve calcification; Kerley's B lines; prominent upper lung field vasculature	LV and LA enlarged; minimal pulmonary congestion if chronic
ECG	Broad, notched P waves; axis normal or right axis deviation (RAD); AF common	Left atrial dilatation; tall P waves sometimes notched; AF common

B. Mitral regurgitation can result from RHD, mitral valve prolapse, or ruptured chordae tendinae or papillary muscle dysfunction post-MI.

AORTIC VALVE DISEASE

I. **Definition.** Alterations in the integrity or normal functioning of the aortic valve or aortic infravalvular or supravalvular structures that lead to alterations in the normal physiology of the cardiovascular system. The two most common pathologies of the aortic valve are **aortic stenosis** and **aortic regurgitation.**

II. **Clinical manifestations**

    A. History

        1. Aortic stenosis. CHF, angina, and syncope are the three main symptoms; presence of **any one** indicates need for surgical therapy.

        2. Aortic regurgitation. CHF or angina late in course; may be asymptomatic or have subtle decreases in exercise tolerance over long period of time.

    B. Physical exam and diagnostic tests. Findings in aortic stenosis and aortic regurgitation are compared in Table 19-5.

III. **Differential diagnosis and pathophysiology**

    A. Aortic stenosis results from congenital lesions, such as bicuspid aortic valve, rheumatic heart disease, and calcific aortic stenosis.

TABLE 19-5. Physical exam and diagnostic test findings in aortic stenosis and aortic regurgitation

	Aortic stenosis	Aortic regurgitation
Heart sounds	A_2 normal or decreased in calcific AS (may be increased in congenital AS); S_4	A_2 normal or decreased; S_4
Murmurs	Diamond-shaped systolic ejection murmur at right second intercostal space parasternally or at apex	Decrescendo diastolic murmur begins after A_2 and ends before S_1; located at left sternal border in third to fourth intercostal space
Pulse wave	Carotid pulse with gradual up-stroke and prolonged down-stroke (pulsus tardus and parvus)	Dictrotic pulse (pulsus bisferiens), bounding pulse (water-hammer pulse), Duroziez's sign
Chest x-ray	± Left ventricular hypertrophy, prominent ascending aorta, calcified valve	Dilated LV
ECG	Left ventricular hypertrophy	Left ventricular hypertrophy, left axis deviation (LAD)

   B. Aortic regurgitation results from rheumatic heart disease, endocarditis, valvular congenital structural defects, dissecting aneurysms, syphilis, inflammatory diseases, and subvalvular structural disease.

SYSTEMIC HYPERTENSION

I. Definitions. The definition of HTN is arbitrary but is at present based on studies defining the relationship between systolic and diastolic pressures and cardiovascular morbidity and mortality rates.

   A. Using the **blood pressure (BP) levels** obtained from these studies, hypertensive patients may be diagnosed as men and women at any age with a BP > 140/90. It is worth pointing out that a clear impact on cardiovascular mortality by blood pressure control has been demonstrated in patients with either systolic or diastolic HTN, or both. In May of 2003, "prehypertension" (those at increased risk for progression to hypertension) was defined as a BP in the 120-139/80-89 mm Hg range.

   B. Hypertensive crisis. While malignant HTN is a term that is no longer officially used, significantly elevated pressures (usually in the > 210/120 range) with or without evidence of end-organ damage (e.g., papilledema) are considered **hypertensive emergencies** and **urgencies** respectively.

   C. Remember that 95 percent of HTN is **essential** (idiopathic). The term "idiopathic" is preferable to "essential," the latter a holdover from the days when it was considered essential for the blood pressure to increase as one ages; we now realize there is nothing essential about hypertension—all forms of hypertension increase morbidity and mortality.

  D. Hypertension affects approximately 50 million Americans and about 1 billion people worldwide. Recent data from the Framingham Heart Study suggest that individuals who are normotensive at age 55 have a 90 percent lifetime risk for developing hypertension.

II. Clinical manifestations. Findings associated with hypertension vary; the degree of symptomatology and physical exam evidence of HTN is roughly correlated with the degree of blood pressure elevation.

  A. History

   1. Essential hypertension is asymptomatic until complications develop.

   2. With **increasing pressures**, cardiovascular dysfunction may become apparent as orthopnea, dyspnea, anginal symptoms, and even frank pulmonary edema. Ocular fatigue, decreased visual acuity, visual blurring, and occipital headaches may all be present.

   3. With **high pressures**, severe headaches may develop, with associated visual impairment, drowsiness, and even encephalopathic changes. Transient paresthesias and cerebrovascular accidents tend to occur with higher pressures.

  B. Physical exam. Classical findings are described for the cardiovascular, visual (retinal), and neurologic systems.

   1. Cardiovascular findings are due to left ventricular hypertrophy, which results from increased afterload. Possible findings include a left ventricular heave, sustained apex beat, and fourth heart sound (S_4). As the hypertrophy worsens, murmurs of aortic insufficiency (AI), mitral regurgitation (MR), or both, as well as signs of left ventricular failure (e.g., S_3, pulsus alternans) may occur.

   2. Retinal changes follow a progression based on the severity and duration of the elevation in blood pressure.

     a. Earlier retinal changes consist of vascular changes: constriction of retinal arterioles and arteriovenous nicking.

     b. With **higher blood pressures**, in addition to vascular changes, there are flame-shaped hemorrhages and exudates.

     c. Papilledema, the most severe retinal change, defines what used to be known as malignant hypertension.

   3. Neurologic changes include transient weakness or numbness, paresthesias, and an increasing incidence of cerebrovascular accidents: cerebral thrombotic or hemorrhagic events.

   4. Hypertensive encephalopathy occurs with very high blood pressures and is characterized by transient, focal central nervous system deficits, severe headache, visual disturbances, and even convulsions, stupor, and coma.

  C. Diagnostic tests

   1. Urinalysis may reveal proteinuria; hematuria can occur, usually with higher pressures.

2. **Chemistries** may show evidence of renal disease, with increased BUN and creatinine values.

3. **ECG** may show increased voltage consistent with left ventricular hypertrophy, as well as "strain" patterns of T wave flattening or inversion, especially in lateral leads (V4-V6).

4. **CXR** may show cardiomegaly, with left ventricular prominence. Dilatation or tortuosity of the ascending aorta may be a prominent feature as well.

III. Differential diagnosis. Table 19-6 lists the causes of secondary hypertension and their major clinical manifestations.

IV. Pathophysiology. The cause of idiopathic HTN is unknown, and complications are due to tissue changes that result from prolonged exposure to a hypertensive vascular system. Table 19-7 lists the multisystem complications of hypertension.

PERICARDIAL DISEASE

I. Definition. Cardiovascular dysfunction due to acute or chronic changes involving the pericardium, either from a primary disease process or as a manifestation of systemic illness. There are two types of pericarditis: **acute** and **chronic.**

II. Clinical manifestations. Table 19-8 lists pertinent findings on history, physical exam, and diagnostic tests that differentiate acute and chronic pericarditis.

III. Differential diagnosis

    A. Acute pericarditis

        1. Idiopathic (possibly postviral)

        2. Infectious: viral (e.g., Coxsackie B), bacterial, tuberculous, fungal, amebic, protozoan

        3. Collagen-vascular disease (SLE, rheumatoid arthritis, scleroderma)

        4. Postmediastinal radiation

        5. Uremia

        6. Post-MI

        7. Postpericardiotomy

        8. Rheumatic fever

        9. Trauma

    B. Chronic (constrictive) pericarditis

        1. Idiopathic

        2. Occasionally, history of acute pericarditis

IV. Pathophysiology. The clinical manifestations of acute pericarditis are due to inflammation of the pericardium, while the clinical manifestations of chronic pericarditis are due to constriction of the pericardium around the myocardium. Since the right ventricle experiences lower pressures than the left ventricle, it is primarily affected by the constricted pericardium, and so the symptoms seen in chronic pericarditis are right-sided symptoms. The right ventricle can-

TABLE 19-6. Secondary causes of hypertension

Cause	Symptoms/signs	Associations	Confirmation
Renovascular	Flank bruit, diffuse atherosclerosis	↓ K+, ↑ creatinine	Arteriogram, ↑ renal vein renin level
Renal disease	Edema	Acute/chronic reral disease	↑ Creatinine, ↑ BUN
Paroxsymal Pheochromocytoma	Paxoysmal sweating, palpitations, flushing, headache, weight loss, episodic hypertension, tachycardia, orthostatic hypotension	↑ Urine VMA, metanephrines, catecholamines	CT scan, arteriography
Mineralocorticoid excess	Weakness, muscle cramps	Hypokalemia, alkalosis, ↓ renin	↑ Aldosterone level, CT scan
Aortic coarctation	↑ BP in arm, ↓ BP in legs	Rib notching on CXR	Arteriography

VMA - vanillyl mandelic acid.
Reproduced with permission from T. E. Andreoli et al.

TABLE 19-7. Hypertensive complications

Target organ	Hypertensive	Atherosclerotic
Brain/eye	Intracerebral hemorrhage; lacunar infarcts; encephalopathy; fundal hemorrhages, exudates, papilledema	Thrombotic stroke, TIA
Heart	Congestive failure, ventricular hypertrophy	MI, angina
Kidney	Nephrosclerosis	Renal artery stenosis
Vessels	Aortic dissection	Diffuse atheromata

Reproduced with permission from T. E. Andreoli et al.

not fill to its normal capacity due to the constriction, and as a result there is venous congestion, reduction of preload, and reduction of output.

PERIPHERAL VASCULAR DISEASE

I. **Definition.** Acute or chronic changes in the arterial or venous vasculature that lead to compromise of blood circulation in a given extremity. There are two types of arterial peripheral vascular disease, **acute** and **chronic**, as well as two types of venous peripheral vascular disease, acute and chronic.

II. **Clinical manifestations**

A. **Arterial disease.** The common clinical manifestations of acute and chronic arterial vascular disease are as follows. To diagnose acute arterial disease look for the **five P's: pain, paresthesias, polar, pallor,** and **pulselessness.**

1. **History**

a. **Acute arterial disease.** Sudden onset, pain, paresthesias, numbness. **Risk factors** for mural thrombi include AF, arrhythmias post recent MI, chronic CHF, cardiomyopathy, history of endocarditis.

b. **Chronic arterial disease.** Intermittent claudication; results in muscle ischemia and focal necrosis, causing chronic pain at rest, ± paresthesias. **Risk factors** for arterial compromise include diabetes mellitus, cigarette smoking, hypertension, obesity, hyperlipidemia.

2. **Physical exam**

a. **Acute arterial disease.** Pale extremity, pulselessness, ↓ temperature distal to occlusion.

b. **Chronic arterial disease.** ↓ Or absent peripheral pulse(s), ↓ temperature distal to occlusion, bruit(s) over involved area.

(1) **Feet.** Pallor on elevation; delayed capillary blush on lowering to dependent position; rubor on dependency.

(2) **Trophic skin changes.** ↓ Hair or nail growth, or both.

TABLE 19-8. Differentiating features of acute and chronic pericarditis

	Acute pericarditis	Chronic (constrictive) pericarditis
History	Antecedent upper respiratory infection; dyspnea; sharp, substernal chest pain, often with left supraclavicular radiation; ↑ pain in supine position; ↓ pain when sitting, leaning forward; malaise, constitutional symptoms, myalgias	Exertional dyspnea
Physical exam	Fever, pericardial friction rub ± pericardial effusion, muffled heart sounds, cyanosis, pulsus paradoxus	Jugular venous distention, Kussmaul's sign, edema of the legs, hepatomegaly, ascites, pulsus paradoxus, pleural effusions, cyanosis, prominent JVP *a* wave and rapid *y* wave descent, pericardial knock in early diastole
Lab tests	Mild to moderate leukocytosis, ↑ ESR	↓ Serum albumin, lymphopenia
ECG	S-T segment elevation with decreased QRS voltage and T wave flattening; supraventricular arrhythmias (e.g., PACs) PAT, AF or flutter)	Low voltage in QRS complex, notched P wave, AF, flattened or inverted T waves in leads I and II
Chest x-ray	± Enlarged cardiac silhouette	Small heart, ± calcium in pericardium, irregular or triangle-shaped heart, dilated SVC
ECG	Effusion ± pericardial thickening	Pericardial thickening, small ventricular chamber size, enlarged atrial chamber size

PACs = paroxysmal atrial contraction, PAT = paroxysmal atrial tachycardia.
AF = atrial fibrillation
JVP = jugular venous pulse
SVC = superior vena cava

(3) **Ulcers.** Inferior to malleoli; toes most common site.

3. **Diagnostic tests.** Arterial angiography for both acute and chronic arterial disease.

B. **Venous disease.** The common clinical manifestations of acute and chronic venous disease are compared in Table 19-9.

✥ **TABLE 19-9.** Clinical manifestations of acute and chronic venous disease

	Acute venous disease	Chronic venous disease
History	Thrombophlebitis may be asymptomatic; pain: aching, tenderness over muscles; conditions leading to venous stasis: post-MI, postoperative period, hemiplegia, hypercoagulable states (e.g., polycythemia vera)	Aching pain after standing or sitting, pregnancy, ascites, abdominal tumor, excessive weight or height
Physical exam	Superficial venous distention, swelling, edema, cyanosis, measurable difference in calf circumference	Thickened, discolored (brown) overlying skin, secondary varicosities, pruritus, ulcers anterior and superior to lateral malleoli
Diagnostic tests	Noninvasive: impedance plethysmography, real-time (duplex) ultrasonography, invasive: contrast venography	Noninvasive (same as for acute venous disease) for documentation purposes only

III. **Differential diagnosis.** Symptomatically related syndromes include:

   A. **Raynaud's disease.** Symptom complex of pain and pallor in fingers, toes, or both, following exposure to cold or emotional upset.

   B. **Raynaud's phenomenon.** Symptom complex of Raynaud's disease, found in association with systemic disease (e.g., collagen vascular diseases).

   C. **Leriche's syndrome.** Impotence and bilateral buttock and thigh pain due to aortoiliac atherosclerotic disease.

   D. **Thromboangiitis obliterans.** Vascular disease characterized by occlusion of small to medium arteries below the elbow and knee, which may lead to necrosis of the digits of hands and feet. Most commonly seen in young Jewish males who are heavy smokers. Thrombophlebitis often coexists.

IV. **Pathophysiology**

   A. **Acute arterial disease** is the result of inadequate distal oxygenation secondary to occlusion by embolus (90 percent originates from mural thrombus in heart). **Chronic arterial disease** is the result of inadequate distal oxygenation secondary to arterial lumen stenosis caused by atherosclerotic plaques. **Common sites** for acute arterial disease include narrowed areas and bifurcations: femoral artery (profunda femoris junction), aortoiliac junction. Common sites for chronic arterial disease include superficial femoral and popliteal in vast majority of patients, as well as the aortoiliac junction.

B. **Acute venous disease** results from impaired venous return secondary to **thrombophlebitis** mostly, but also external venous compression and trauma. **Chronic venous disease** results from impaired venous return secondary to thrombotic disruption of venous vessels and valves. **Common sites** for both acute and chronic venous disease include deep and superficial veins of lower extremities.

CHAPTER **20**

Gastrointestinal Diseases

SECTION 1. DISEASES OF THE LIVER, GALLBLADDER, AND BILIARY TRACT

 ### ACUTE VIRAL HEPATITIS

I. **Definition.** Acute infection and inflammation of hepatocytes caused by a viral agent.

II. **History.** Classically, acute viral hepatitis is marked by three stages. The first is a **prodromal stage**, in which patients typically complain of general malaise, nausea, vomiting, anorexia, diarrhea, myalgia, arthralgia, low grade fever, and right upper quadrant (RUQ) abdominal pain. The **icteric stage** follows, in which patients notice yellowing of the skin and sclera, darkening of the urine, and loss of color in the stool. Of note, jaundice is not present in the majority of cases, which is why this is known as anicteric hepatitis. In most cases, symptoms resolve in the **convalescent stage**; in some instances, complications arise including chronic hepatitis or fulminant hepatic failure.

III. **Physical exam.** When present, icterus is first manifested in the sublingual area, followed by the sclera and skin; hepatomegaly is present in over half of the cases of acute viral hepatitis; enlarged liver presses against Glisson's capsule, causing tenderness in the RUQ; splenomegaly, as well as limited lymphadenopathy, can be present in about 20% of patients.

IV. **Lab findings.** An increase in aspartate transaminase (AST) and alanine transaminase (ALT) levels will precede the rise in bilirubin. Jaundice becomes evident when the total bilirubin exceeds 2.5 mg/dl. A prolonged prothrombin time (PT) signifies a decrease in the synthetic function of the liver and portends a worse prognosis. Serological studies confirm the diagnosis of acute viral hepatitis.

V. **Differential diagnosis.** Toxin or medication-induced hepatitis, ischemic hepatitis, cholecystitis, choledocholithiasis, cholangitis, appendicitis.

VI. **Pathophysiology**

   A. **Hepatitis A virus (HAV).** HAV is an RNA virus that causes epidemics as well as sporadic cases of acute hepatitis. Transmission is fecal-oral with common outbreaks resulting from contaminated food or water. The incubation period averages 30 days. Although a vaccine is available, once HAV is contracted, therapy is supportive. There is no chronic form of this disease. Symptoms are generally mild, prognosis is excellent and only 0.1% of cases are complicated by fulminant hepatic failure. IgM anti-HAV signifies acute disease, while IgG anti-HAV signifies remote infection.

   B. **Hepatitis B virus (HBV).** HBV is a DNA virus that causes both acute and chronic hepatitis. HBV has an inner core protein (hepatitis B core antigen, HBcAg) and outer surface coat (hepatitis B surface antigen, HBsAg). Transmission occurs by inoculation of blood or blood products, by sexual contact or from mother to fetus. The incubation period ranges from 6 weeks to 6 months, with an average of 12–14 weeks. About 5% of patients will develop chronic infection. A vaccine is available and is administered to all newborns. Acute hepatitis B is diagnosed by the combination of HBsAg (+) and IgM anti-HBcAg (+). Chronic hepatitis B is diagnosed by the combination of HBsAg (+) and IgG anti-HBcAg (+). A patient who has recovered from hepatitis B infection will be HBsAg (−), anti-HBs (+) and IgG anti-HBcAg (+). A patient who is immunized against hepatitis B will be HBsAg (−), anti-HBs (+), and IgG anti-HBcAg (−). To the extent that HBV is a risk factor for the development of hepatic carcinoma, the HBV vaccine is the only vaccine known today that is anti-neoplastic.

   C. **Hepatitis D virus (HDV).** HDV (also known as the delta agent) is a defective RNA virus that can only cause hepatitis in association with HBV. HDV, like HBV, is transmitted in blood products, via sexual contact or from mother to fetus. If HDV infects at the same time (co-infection) as HBV, the clinical course is similar to that of HBV alone. However, if HDV causes infection in a patient who is already infected with HBV (i.e., superinfection), the clinical course is much more severe. Vaccination against HBV confers immunity against HDV.

   D. **Hepatitis E virus (HEV).** HEV is an RNA virus responsible for waterborne hepatitis that is endemic to India, Burma, Afghanistan, Algeria, and Mexico. Like HAV, transmission is via the fecal-oral route. The incubation period averages 40 days. There is no chronic form of HEV and no vaccine currently available. Symptoms are usually mild; however, there is about a 10–20% incidence of fulminant hepatic failure in pregnant women who become infected with HEV.

CHRONIC VIRAL HEPATITIS

I. Definition. Infection and inflammation of hepatocytes caused by viral agents that does not resolve after six months.

II. History. Since majority of patients are asymptomatic, diagnosis must be suspected after careful review of risk factors, including blood transfusions, sexual practices, intravenous or intranasal drug use, immunizations, occupational exposure, and family history. Those patients who are symptomatic report non-specific complaints including fatigue, anorexia, and abdominal pain. Those with more advanced disease may complain of increased abdominal girth, episodes of bleeding, and marked confusion.

III. Physical exam. Findings range from normal to presence of stigmata of cirrhosis (hypersplenism, encephalopathy, gynecomastia, palmar erythema, testicular atrophy, Dupuytren's contracture, ascites, and varices). Extrahepatic manifestations include arthritis and vasculitis.

IV. Lab findings. Transaminase elevations tend to be modest in chronic viral hepatitis, although fluctuations occur. Alkaline phosphatase levels are usually normal or slightly elevated. The synthetic function of the liver declines in advanced disease, resulting in a prolonged PT and a depressed albumin level. Thrombocytopenia can result from splenic sequestration. As with any chronic illness, anemia of chronic disease may develop. Immune complex deposition in the kidney results in abnormal renal parameters. Cryoglobulinemia is sometimes associated with hepatitis C.

V. Differential diagnosis. Autoimmune hepatitis, hemachromatosis, Wilson's disease, α_1-antitrypsin deficiency, and chronic alcoholic hepatitis.

VI. Pathophysiology

    A. Hepatitis B virus (HBV). See HBV in the Acute Viral Hepatitis section.

    B. Hepatitis C virus (HCV). Incubation with HCV, an RNA virus, averages about 6 weeks and the acute illness is largely unremarkable. Unlike HBV, the risk of sexual contact and vertical transmission of HCV is relatively low. Currently, there exists no vaccine for HCV. Importantly, 85% of HCV infections will progress to chronic disease.

XENOBIOTIC-INDUCED HEPATITIS

I. Definition. Injury and inflammation of hepatocytes caused by xenobiotics (therapeutic agents and environmental toxins).

II. History. A detailed medication and exposure history is paramount in making the diagnosis of xenobiotic-induced hepatitis. The history should include prescription medications as well as over-the-counter drugs and herbal remedies. A history of depression or suicide attempts is significant and may suggest drug overdose. The physician must ascertain what medications were accessible to the patient. Patients commonly report nausea, vomiting, abdominal pain, arthralgias, and rash.

III. Physical exam. Findings depend on what substance has been ingested and may include fever, confusion, jaundice, hepatomegaly, abdominal tenderness, and rash. Encephalopathy and ascites are features of advanced disease.

IV. Lab findings. Hepatocellular injury is marked by significantly elevated transaminase levels. Hepatocellular necrosis is characterized by decreased synthetic function of the liver, including a prolonged PT and a depressed albumin. An acetaminophen level is extremely useful in evaluating the etiology of liver injury, especially when the history is incomplete or unreliable.

V. Differential diagnosis. Acute viral hepatitis, Budd-Chiari syndrome (occlusion of the hepatic vein), alcohol-induced hepatitis.

VI. Pathophysiology. Xenobiotics produce hepatic injury either in a direct or idiosyncratic manner. Toxins exerting a direct effect include acetaminophen, carbon tetrachloride, and the mushroom toxin *Amanita phalloides,* in which the hepatitis is dose-dependent and the latent period between exposure and liver injury short. Idiosyncratic hepatic injury (i.e., due to isoniazid, halothane, phenytoin, and trimethoprim-sulfamethoxazole) is unpredictable, dose-independent, and may occur a significant period of time after exposure.

ALCOHOLIC LIVER DISEASE

I. Definition. Alcohol-induced injury of hepatocytes that may lead to **alcoholic fatty liver** (in which the cytoplasms of the hepatocytes are filled with fat vacuoles), **alcoholic hepatitis** (in which polymorphonuclear cells destroy hepatocytes), or **alcoholic cirrhosis** (in which hepatocytes are replaced with collagen).

II. History. A history of episodic drunkenness or chronic alcohol intake. It is useful to objectively quantify the amount of alcohol ingested over a specific time period and to remember that alcohol may potentiate the effects of other medications. Anorexia, nausea, vomiting, weight loss, and abdominal pain are common presenting symptoms.

III. Physical exam. Findings are absent or very minimal. May see fever, tender hepatosplenomegaly, jaundice, or signs consistent with fulminant hepatic failure (encephalopathy, massive hemorrhage, and ascites). The clinical manifestations are usually not apparent until very late in the course. It is not uncommon for a cirrhotic to present initially with rupture of esophageal varices, for example.

IV. Lab findings. Patients with alcoholic fatty liver disease usually have minimal elevation in AST. In more advanced disease, anemia and thrombocytopenia are common. The AST level is usually elevated, but rarely above 300. An AST/ALT ratio greater than 2 is strongly suggestive of alcoholic hepatitis, especially when the AST and ALT are each above 100. Serum bilirubin is elevated in 60–90% of patients. Serum alkaline phosphatase is typically elevated, but rarely over three times normal. Serum albumin can be depressed, PT is elevated, and the gamma globulin level is elevated in 50–75% of patients.

V. Differential diagnosis. Cholecystitis, cholelithiasis, xenobiotic-induced hepatitis, and viral hepatitis.

VI. Pathophysiology. Alcohol is the most common cause of cirrhosis in the United States. Although onset can occur within one year of heavy consumption, 80% of patients with alcoholic hepatitis have been drinking five or more years before symptoms appear. Prolonged duration and heavy consumption correspond to an increased risk of developing alcoholic hepatitis and cirrhosis. Many of the adverse effects of alcohol on the liver are thought to be caused by its metabolite acetaldehyde.

 AUTOIMMUNE HEPATITIS

I. Definition. A chronic inflammation of hepatocytes believed to be caused by circulating autoantibodies.

II. History. Autoimmune hepatitis typically has an insidious onset and most often occurs in young women. Many have additional autoimmune disorders including thyroiditis, anemia, and systemic lupus erythematosis. Fatigue, anorexia, arthralgias, and jaundice are common features.

III. Physical exam. Findings can range from normal to stigmata of cirrhosis. Extrahepatic manifestations include arthritis, vasculitis, pleuritis, pericarditis, and sicca syndrome.

IV. Lab findings. Elevated transaminases, hypoalbuminemia, slightly elevated alkaline phosphatase, hypergammaglobulinemia, and positive autoantibodies including ANA, anti-dsDNA, anti-smooth muscle antibody, and ANCA. An anti-mitochondrial antibody can be present in low titers; however, high titers should raise the suspicion for primary biliary cirrhosis (PBC).

V. Differential diagnosis. Chronic viral hepatitis, chronic alcoholic hepatitis, PBC, and xenobiotic-induced hepatitis must be ruled out before the diagnosis of autoimmune hepatitis can be established.

VI. Pathogenesis. Largely unknown. It is believed that an environmental trigger (virus, medication) causes a genetically predisposed individual to start creating antibodies that are inappropriately targeted against host tissue, in this case, the liver.

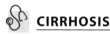 **CIRRHOSIS**

I. Definition. Fibrosis of the liver, the common endpoint of chronic hepatocellular injury of numerous etiologies.

II. History. Onset of symptoms usually insidious and may include weakness, fatigue, muscle cramps, and weight loss. Advanced disease associated with anorexia, nausea, and vomiting. Abdominal pain may be present. Amenorrhea in women and impotence, sterility, and loss of libido in men can occur. Up to one-quarter of cirrhotic patients present with hematemesis as a result of ruptured esophageal varices.

III. Physical exam. Hepatosplenomegaly, skin manifestations (spider nevi, palmer erythema), and superficial dilation of the superficial veins (i.e., caput medusa). Gynecomastia can occur in men. Late findings include ascites, pleural effusions, peripheral edema, and ecchymoses. Encephalopathy can present as asterixis, tremor, delirium, drowsiness, and coma.

IV. Lab findings. Liver function tests are abnormal in early stages but often return to normal as the number of functioning hepatocytes decreases. Macrocytic or microcytic anemia is often noted. Liver biopsy is used to confirm the diagnosis and may help elucidate the etiology of the cirrhosis. Ultrasound can assess liver size and nodularity and detect subclinical ascites. CT scan and MRI can be used to further characterize hepatic nodules. Esophagogastroduodenoscopy (EGD) identifies varices and specific bleeding in the gastrointestinal tract.

V. Differential diagnosis. The most important causes are chronic alcohol use and hepatitis C and B. Other causes include congestive heart failure, primary biliary cirrhosis, sclerosing cholangitis, hemochromatosis, Wilson's disease, and α_1-antitrypsin deficiency.

VI. Pathophysiology

  A. **Alcoholic cirrhosis.** (See the "Alcoholic Liver Disease" section.)

  B. **Infectious cirrhosis.** (See the "Acute Viral Hepatitis" and "Chronic Viral Hepatitis" sections.)

  C. **Cardiac cirrhosis.** Prolonged right-sided congestive heart failure can lead to chronic liver injury and eventually cardiac cirrhosis. Liver injury results from both liver congestion due to elevated venous pressure and hypoperfusion of the liver due to reduced cardiac output. On gross examination, the liver has alternating red (congested) and white (fibrotic) areas, referred to as "nutmeg" liver.

  D. **Primary biliary cirrhosis (PBC)** is a disease of chronic inflammation and fibrous obliteration of intrahepatic biliary ductules that usually presents in middle-aged women. The etiology is unknown, but it is associated with a variety of autoimmune disorders. The earliest detectable lesion is called chronic non-suppurative destructive cholangitis that progresses to micronodular or macronodular cirrhosis over years.

  E. **Primary sclerosing cholangitis (PSC)** is an uncommon disease characterized by diffuse inflammation of the biliary tract leading to fibrosis and strictures of the biliary system. Closely associated with ulcerative colitis, it causes cirrhosis by extrahepatic biliary obstruction with increased biliary intraductal pressure and inflammation.

  F. **Hemochromatosis** is one of the most common genetic disorders in humans and involves the accumulation of abnormal amounts of iron due to inappropriate absorption from the intestine. Cirrhosis results from excess iron deposition in hepatocytes.

  G. **Wilson's disease** is an uncommon inherited disorder of copper metabolism that involves impairment of copper excretion due to a specific transporter. Deposition of copper results in a typically macronodular cirrhotic liver.

  H. **Alpha-1-antitrypsin deficiency.** α_1-antitrypsin is an inhibitor of proteases that are secreted by neutrophils during inflammation. A deficiency in this enzyme facilitates injury (particularly of the liver and lung) and is a rare cause of cirrhosis and emphysema.

  I. **Cryptogenic cirrhosis** is the term used to describe the approximately 10–15% of cases of cirrhosis that do not have an identifiable etiology.

CHOLELITHIASIS

  I. Definition. Formation of calculi in the gallbladder.

  II. History. Most patients with gallstones are asymptomatic. Calculi are usually found incidentally. Risk factors include female gender, obesity, increasing age, and Native American ancestry.

III. **Physical exam.** Usually normal.

IV. **Diagnostic findings.** Ultrasound is the diagnostic test of choice. Stones as small as 2 mm can be easily identified by their characteristic acoustic shadows. Lab findings are typically normal.

V. **Pathophysiology.** About 75% of gallstones in the United States are cholesterol stones. Bile salts and lecithin form micelles that solubilize cholesterol in an aqueous solution. Any disruption of this system can cause cholesterol to precipitate out of solution, forming gallstones. Pigment stones account for about 20% of gallstones, and they contain mostly calcium bilirubinate and unconjugated bilirubin with less than 10% cholesterol.

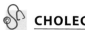 ## CHOLECYSTITIS

I. **Definition.** Inflammation of the gallbladder.

II. **History.** Patients typically report episodes of self-limited pain in the epigastrium or RUQ of the abdomen that can be precipitated by fatty food (symptoms known as **biliary colic**). In acute cases, the pain is constant and becomes progressively worse. Pain (which may radiate to the right infrascapular area) may accompany nausea, vomiting, jaundice, and fever.

III. **Physical exam.** Findings include a low-grade fever, RUQ tenderness (with or without rebound and guarding), and a palpable gallbladder (which is found in 15% of cases). The arrest of inspiration on palpation of RUQ (Murphy's sign) is a classic sign.

IV. **Diagnostic findings.** Leukocytosis, hyperbilirubinemia, elevated alkaline phosphatase, and elevated transaminases are typical. An ultrasound usually reveals gallstones, an enlarged gallbladder, and thickening of the gallbladder wall. A hydroxy iminodiacetic acid (HIDA) scan is the best test to use and it can reveal cystic duct obstruction and, when positive, shows radiolabeled dye in the common bile duct but not the gallbladder. A transhepatic cholangiography or fiberoptic endoscopy may also be used for direct visualization of the biliary tree, especially if other testing is inconclusive.

V. **Differential diagnosis.** Acute pancreatitis, perforated peptic ulcer, appendicitis, perforated carcinoma of the colon, diverticulum at the hepatic flexure, liver abscess, and hepatitis.

VI. **Pathophysiology.** Acute cholecystitis is due to obstruction of the cystic duct by a gallstone in over 90% of cases. Inflammation develops distal to the obstruction. Acalculous cholecystitis accounts for 5 to 10% of cases of cholecystitis, and is especially associated with trauma or burn injury. Complications include gangrene of the gallbladder, cholangitis, and chronic cholecystitis. Bacterial inflammation may play a role in 50-85% of cases.

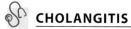 ## CHOLANGITIS

I. **Definition.** Inflammation of the bile ducts.

II. **History.** Very commonly, patients report a history of biliary colic or known gallstones. The classic triad includes **frequent episodes of pain in the RUQ of the abdomen, fever with shaking chills,** and **jaundice** (Charcot's triad).

III. Physical exam. Findings include fever, icterus, RUQ or epigastric tenderness, and hepatomegaly.

IV. Diagnostic findings. Leukocytosis and markedly elevated total bilirubin, direct bilirubin, and alkaline phosphatase are common. An ultrasound or CT scan will often reveal dilated bile ducts. If necessary, endoscopic retrograde cholangiopancreatography (ERCP) or percutaneous transhepatic cholangiography can directly determine the location and cause of the obstruction.

V. Differential diagnosis. Cholecystitis, pancreatitis, pancreatic cancer, gallbladder cancer, and hepatitis.

VI. Pathophysiology. Cholangitis most often occurs after a gallstone becomes stuck in the common bile duct (choledocholithiasis). Increased intraductal pressure causes abdominal pain, and the inability to excrete bile causes jaundice. Stasis allows enteric bacteria, trapped distal to the stone, to flourish. The resulting acute suppurative cholangitis is an endoscopic or surgical emergency. Long-term common duct obstruction can cause liver damage leading eventually to cirrhosis.

PANCREATITIS

I. Definition. Acute or chronic inflammation of the pancreas.

II. History. Usually manifested by nausea, vomiting, and constant abdominal pain in the periumbilical region (radiating to the back) that may continue for hours or days. The pain is often exacerbated by lying supine and ameliorated by sitting up. Weight loss and steatorrhea are commonly found in patients with chronic pancreatitis. Of note, 90% of pancreatic tissue is destroyed before patients present with symptoms of malabsorption.

III. Physical exam. In mild cases, diffuse abdominal tenderness. In advanced disease, common findings include fever, hypotension and tachycardia, diffuse abdominal tenderness, mostly with rebound or guarding. Ecchymoses on the flanks (Grey Turner's sign) or around the umbilicus (Cullen's sign) are consistent with hemorrhagic pancreatitis.

IV. Laboratory. Leukocytosis, elevated serum amylase and lipase, a transient hyperbilirubinemia, and an abnormal calcium level are common. Ranson's criteria can be used to predict prognosis (Table 20-1). CT scan is helpful in determining the extent of damage. In chronic disease, CT scan may show pancreatic calcification, a phlegmon (a solid mass of swollen, inflamed pancreas with or without areas of necrosis), an abscess (resulting from an infected phlegmon) or a pseudocyst (collection of fluid, debris, pancreatic enzymes, and blood) formation. ERCP shows ductal dilatation with an irregular "beaded" appearance.

V. Differential diagnosis. In acute disease: perforated viscus, acute hepatitis, peptic ulcer disease, acute cholecystitis, cholangitis, myocardial infarction, dissecting aortic aneurysm, diabetic ketoacidosis, and a lower lobar pneumonia. In chronic disease: other causes of malabsorption.

VI. Pathophysiology. Approximately 70% of acute cases caused by either alcohol abuse or cholelithiasis. Other causes include hypertriglyceridemia, hypercalcemia, various medications, iatrogenic (post-ERCP), and

TABLE 20-1. Ranson's criteria for acute pancreatitis

	Age	>55
On Admission	White blood cell (WBC) count	>16,000
	Serum lactate dehydrogenase (LDH)	>350 IU/L
	Plasma glucose	>200 mg/dl
	Aspartate transaminase (AST)	>250 IU/L
After 48 hours	Hematocrit (Hct) decrease	>10%
	Blood urea nitrogen (BUN)	>5 mg/dl
	Serum calcium	<8 mg/dl
	Arterial PO_2	<60 mm Hg
	Base deficit	>4 mEq/L
	Third-spacing of fluid	>6 liters

Used to predict mortality in patients with acute pancreatitis. Mortality rate rises with number of positive criteria. (Reproduced with permission from Ranson JH et al. Prognostic signs and the role of operative management in acute pancreatitis, *Surg Gynecol Obstet 139:69, 1974.*)

apolipoprotein CII deficiency. Attacks may be precipitated by impaction of gallstones in the ampulla of Vater, causing release of pancreatic enzymes and tissue necrosis. Edema, hemorrhage, and necrosis are mediated partially by release of trypsin, elastase, phospholipase A, and plasma kinins. Pathologic changes include fat necrosis and formation of pseudocysts and abscesses. Chronic pancreatitis is usually caused by alcoholism.

SECTION 2. DISEASES OF THE GASTROINTESTINAL TRACT

 ## ESOPHAGITIS

I. Definition. Inflammation of the esophageal mucosa.

II. History. Heartburn or retrosternal chest discomfort are usual chief complaints; odynophagia, dysphagia, nausea, emesis, hematemesis, atypical chest pain, fever, and weight loss. Alternatively, patients may be asymptomatic. Risk factors include immunosuppression, alcohol abuse, recurrent emesis, oral medication intake without water, ingestion of caustic agents, or exposure to chemotherapy or radiation.

III. Physical exam. Normal in uncomplicated disease, otherwise signs of hypovolemia (orthostasis, tachycardia, hypotension), anemia (skin and conjunctival pallor, delayed capillary refill), and a positive guaiac test for occult blood are consistent with gastrointestinal blood loss. Abdominal exam may reveal epigastric tenderness. In immunocompromised patients, oral examination may reveal white exudates (suggestive of candidiasis) or vesicles (suggestive of herpes simplex virus infection, HSV).

IV. Diagnostic findings. Lab findings may be normal in uncomplicated cases. Elevated WBC suggests infection. Microcytic anemia (low Hb, low Hct, low MCV) and iron deficiency (low iron, low ferritin, and elevated TIBC) are consistent with GI blood loss. Hypokalemic hypochloremic metabolic alkalosis (low K^+, low Cl^-, and high HCO_3^-) suggests emesis. A nasogastric (NG) lavage is performed if GI blood loss is suspected to assess where the blood loss is originating and whether the bleeding is ongoing. An EGD (esophagogastroduodenoscopy or upper GI endoscopy) with biopsy or brushing, the gold standard, may reveal: creamy white/yellow plaques adherent to mucosa (candida); small vesicles and multiple, small, superficial ulcerations (HSV); large, deep ulcerations with intranuclear inclusions on biopsy (cytomegalovirus); or edematous mucosa, sometimes with ulceration (pill-induced). A barium swallow may demonstrate a granular appearance to the mucosa in a patient with radiation or chemotherapy-induced esophagitis.

V. Differential diagnosis. In the **immunocompetent**: gastroesophageal reflux disease (GERD), Barrett's esophagitis, corrosive esophagitis, chemotherapy or radiation-induced esophagitis, pill-induced esophagitis, and recurrent emesis-induced esophagitis. In the **immunocompromised**: esophagitis caused by candida, HSV, varicella zoster virus, CMV, and bacteria.

VI. Pathophysiology. Exposure of esophageal mucosa to gastric acid, infectious agents, corrosive agents, chemotherapy, or radiation therapy damages the epithelial cell lining, inducing a subsequent inflammatory response. Complications include stricture, obstruction and perforation.

DYSPHAGIA

I. Definition. Difficulty swallowing, or the sensation that food is obstructed in its passage from mouth to stomach.

II. History. The defining feature of dysphagia is a sensation that food becomes "stuck" behind the sternum. Dysphagia that begins with difficulty ingesting both liquids and solids is very suggestive of a motility disorder. Dysphagia that begins with difficulty ingesting solids alone is most consistent with a mechanical obstruction. Postprandial heartburn, exacerbated by reclining and relieved by antacids, suggests peptic stricture. Sensitivity to hot or cold liquids suggests esophageal spasm. Concomitant findings of polyarthralgia and Raynaud's phenomenon suggest scleroderma. Halitosis, nocturnal choking, and protrusion in the neck are consistent with a Zenker's diverticulum. Cough, dyspnea, and hemoptysis suggest aspiration. Late stage symptoms include drooling and weight loss.

III. Physical exam may be normal. Cutaneous calcifications, telangiectasias, sclerodactyly, and abnormal pulmonary or cardiac exams suggest scleroderma. Skin and conjunctival pallor and spooning of the nails (koilonychias) suggest esophageal webs (Plummer-Vinson syndrome). Crackles on respiratory examination may indicate aspiration pneumonia.

IV. Diagnostic findings. Barium esophagography, performed to image the lumen of the esophagus, may show: a "corkscrew" esophagus (seen in diffuse esophageal spasm), a "bird's beak" sign (seen in achalasia), and pockets filled with barium in the hypopharynx (seen in Zenker's diverticulum). EGD allows direct visualization and biopsy of the esophagus. Manometry records the changes in pressure that occur in multiple sites in the lumen of the esophagus and possible findings include non-peristaltic, high amplitude contractions after many or most swallows (seen in diffuse esophageal spasm), high pressure at lower esophageal sphincter (LES) and absence of peristalsis or relaxation upon swallowing (seen in achalasia) and high amplitude contractions, and inability to relax LES (seen in scleroderma). Although not commonly used, esophageal pH monitoring measures the pH of the esophageal lumen. Patients with chronic GERD will typically have low pH readings.

V. Differential diagnosis. Zenker's diverticulum, diffuse esophageal spasm, Schatzki ring, scleroderma, achalasia, esophageal webbing (Plummer-Vinson syndrome), esophageal carcinoma, and stricture.

VI. Pathophysiology. Differs depending on underlying etiology. Complications include aspiration pneumonia, malnutrition, and vitamin deficiencies.

GASTROESOPHAGEAL REFLUX DISEASE (GERD)

I. Definition. Reflux of acidic gastric contents into the esophagus.

II. History. Most often seen in white men. Postprandial substernal burning pain (heartburn), exacerbated upon reclining and relieved by antacids. Metallic or bitter taste. Hematemesis or melena suggests mucosal erosion and a GI bleed. Late symptoms include dysphagia. Cough, hoarseness, and nocturnal wheezing suggest aspiration of gastric contents. Risk factors include alcohol abuse, use of anticholinergic medications, nitrates, calcium channel blockers, and a history of cigarette smoking. Exacerbating factors include stress, ingestion of coffee, chocolate, and peppermint.

III. Physical exam. Normal or subtle, such as an isolated finding of halitosis. Signs of hypovolemia, anemia, and a positive guaiac test for occult blood suggest GI blood loss. Epigastric tenderness. Peritoneal signs (rigid abdomen, diminished bowel sounds, rebound tenderness) suggest perforation. Poor dentition may be the result of long-standing acid reflux. Crackles on lung exam may indicate aspiration pneumonia.

IV. Diagnostic findings. The diagnosis can be made clinically after obtaining a history. If symptoms are alleviated with empiric treatment, no further testing is necessary. Additional tests are warranted when patients do not respond to empiric therapy. EGD demonstrates friability and erosions of the squamocolumnar junction in about 50% of patients with GERD. Because the other 50% of patients with GERD have normal appearing mucosa, biopsy is required for definitive diagnosis. 24-hour esophageal pH monitoring can detect the relationship between symptoms and episodes of reflux. The Bernstein test induces heartburn by infusing acid into the esophagus and then provides relief by infusing saline. Barium esophagography may be useful in identifying a stricture.

V. Differential diagnosis. Other causes of esophagitis, gastritis, peptic ulcer disease, esophageal motility disorders, cholelithiasis, and coronary artery disease.

VI. Pathophysiology. Excessive transient relaxations of the LES, an incompetent LES (secondary to hiatal hernia), and delayed gastric emptying (leading to high gastric pressure) can all lead to reflux of gastric contents. Prolonged exposure of esophageal mucosa to acid, pepsin, and bile salts damages the endothelial layer and induces an inflammatory reaction, which may lead to stricture. In severe cases, this process results in the erosion of the esophageal mucosa and subsequent bleeding. Some patients eventually develop **Barrett's esophagus**, the columnar epithelialization of the mucosa. This transformation increases the patient's risk of developing **esophageal adenocarcinoma**. Suspicion of Barrett's esophagus is an indication to perform an EGD.

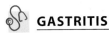 **GASTRITIS**

I. Definition. Acute or chronic inflammation of the gastric mucosa.

II. History. While many patients are asymptomatic, others present with anorexia, nausea, emesis, and gnawing epigastric pain. Pain is often exacerbated by eating and relieved with antacids. Erosion of the gastric mucosa is a cause of upper GI bleeding. Risk factors include use of NSAIDs, steroids, cigarettes, and alcohol. Gastritis occurring in the setting of a serious systemic illness such as trauma, burn, sepsis, liver failure, or renal failure is called stress-induced gastritis. Symptoms including dementia and ataxia suggest vitamin B_{12} deficiency.

III. Physical exam. Normal or signs of hypovolemia, anemia, and a positive guaiac test for occult blood suggest GI blood loss, possibly from severe acute gastritis. Abdominal exam may reveal epigastric tenderness. Peritoneal signs suggest perforation.

IV. Diagnostic findings. NG lavage is performed if gastrointestinal blood loss is suspected. EGD allows for direct visualization of the gastric mucosa, along with the ability to biopsy suspicious lesions. *Helicobacter pylori* testing has shown that colonization occurs in virtually 100% of patients with active chronic gastritis, however, mere colonization does not necessarily predict disease, as most patients with such colonization remain asymptomatic. Serological studies include *H. pylori* IgG or IgA antibodies. The urease breath test involves the parenteral ingestion of radiolabeled carbon; the detection of CO_2 isotopes in the breath suggests the presence of urease-producing *H. pylori*. Laboratory results are often normal. Hypokalemic hypochloremic metabolic alkalosis suggests emesis. Microcytic anemia and iron deficiency suggest gastrointestinal blood loss. Macrocytic anemia (low Hgb, high MCV) and low B_{12} levels suggest pernicious anemia.

V. Differential diagnosis. Esophagitis, GERD, peptic ulcer disease (PUD), gastric cancer, biliary tract disease, food poisoning, viral gastroenteritis, pancreatitis, coronary artery disease.

VI. Pathophysiology. Stress-induced gastritis is thought to result from the combination of an ischemic gastric mucosa that is further injured by the direct toxic effects of acid. Type A chronic gastritis is an autoimmune disease in which autoantibodies are directed against parietal cells. The destruction of parietal cells leads to achlorhydria (inability to make hydrochloric acid) as well as the inability to make intrinsic factor. Ultimately, vitamin B_{12} deficiency develops (pernicious anemia). Type B chronic gastritis is much more common than Type A and is believed to result from *H. pylori* infection. The infection is thought to induce an immune reaction, which results in inflammation of the gastric mucosa. Gastritis increases the risk of developing gastric cancer.

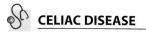

PEPTIC ULCER DISEASE (PUD)

I. Definition. Erosion of the gastric or duodenal mucosa.

II. History. Burning or gnawing epigastric pain may persist for months prior to presentation. Patients suffering from **duodenal ulcers** (which are four times more common than gastric ulcers) report epigastric pain worsened by fasting and relieved thirty minutes after eating (manifested by weight gain). Patients with **gastric ulcers** describe epigastric pain that improves with fasting and is exacerbated within thirty minutes of eating (manifested by weight loss). In both gastric and duodenal ulcers, risk factors include male sex, increasing age, NSAID or steroid use, cigarette smoking, alcohol abuse, and physiological stress. Zollinger-Ellison syndrome (ZES) should be suspected in patients who are refractory to treatment.

III. Physical exam. Epigastric tenderness, which tends to be midline and between the umbilicus and xyphoid process. Peritoneal signs (rigid abdomen, diminished bowel sounds, rebound tenderness) suggest perforation. Signs of hypovolemia are consistent with a large GI blood loss.

IV. Diagnostic findings. PUD is a clinical diagnosis. In the majority of cases, diagnosis is based on history, physical exam, and response to empiric treatment. Barium esophagography is the most common initial method to establish the diagnosis. A typical duodenal ulcer appears as a discrete crater. EGD allows for direct visualization and biopsy of the gastric and duodenal mucosa. Biopsy is important since up to 3% of gastric ulcers are associated with an underlying gastric cancer. *H. pylori* testing has shown that colonization occurs in up to 95% of patients with duodenal ulcers and 70% of patients with gastric ulcers. The secretin stimulation test is indicated in the evaluation of intractable PUD when ZES is suspected. A parenteral delivery of secretin (a gastrin inhibitor) induces a paradoxical rise in gastrin in ZES patients. Laboratory values may be normal in uncomplicated disease. Microcytic anemia and iron deficiency suggest GI blood loss. Leukocytosis suggests ulcer penetration or perforation. Elevated amylase is consistent with posterior ulcer penetration into the pancreas.

V. Differential diagnosis. Gastritis, esophagitis, GERD, CAD, biliary tract disease, pancreatitis, and gastric carcinoma.

VI. Pathophysiology. A decrease in mucosal defense mechanisms or an increase in acid production. NSAIDs disrupt the host mucosa by inhibiting prostaglandin synthesis. *H. pylori* causes breakdown of the protective mucosal lining via its urease activity. Hypersecretion of acid in ZES is thought to overwhelm normal host defense mechanisms.

CELIAC DISEASE

I. Definition. An inflammatory condition of the entire small intestine precipitated by gluten ingestion, leading to malabsorption. Also known as celiac sprue, non-tropical sprue, and gluten-sensitive enteropathy.

II. History. Most often found in white women at any age. Classic symptoms include diarrhea, steatorrhea, bloating, abdominal distention, and weight loss.

Patients may also present with a pruritic rash (dermatitis herpetiformis), fatigue (suggesting anemia), bone pain (reflecting vitamin D deficiency), and neurological symptoms (paresthesias, cerebellar ataxia, dementia, and seizures) suggesting vitamin B_{12} deficiency.

III. **Physical exam.** Signs of dehydration (orthostasis, tachycardia, hypotension, dry mucous membranes, and poor skin turgor) and anemia (skin and conjunctival pallor). Extensive skin bruising secondary to vitamin K deficiency. Abdominal distention, hyperactive bowel sounds or tenderness. Guaiac test for occult blood is usually negative. Cerebellar signs such as a positive Romberg's test, inability to perform finger-nose-finger exam, and abnormal gait.

IV. **Diagnostic findings.** A 24-hour stool collection, while cumbersome to perform, is consistent with malabsorption if more than 6 grams of fat are retrieved, though this is not specific for celiac sprue. Serological tests, including anti-glia-dial, anti-endomysial, and anti-reticulin antibodies are more sensitive. Barium esophagography may reveal dilation of the lumen of the small intestine, loss of mucosal folds and clumping of barium. Biopsy of the small intestine, the gold standard, will show flattened villi, crypt hyperplasia, lymphocyte and plasma cell infiltration of the lamina propria. Repeat biopsy after initiation of gluten-free diet will demonstrate return to normal histology. Lab findings include a prolonged PT and decreased levels of folate, cholesterol, β-carotene, serum albumin, calcium, magnesium, potassium, and vitamins A, B_{12}, D, E, and K.

V. **Differential diagnosis.** Non-tropical sprue, Whipple's disease, lactase deficiency, infectious gastroenteritis, pancreatic insufficiency, inflammatory bowel disease, irritable bowel syndrome, carcinoid syndrome, VIPoma, hyperthyroidism, laxative overdose, and medication induced.

VI. **Pathophysiology.** Glutens are high molecular weight proteins found in wheat, rye, and barley. Ingestion of foods containing gluten by individuals with a genetic predisposition precipitates an inflammatory reaction in the small intestine. The inflammation leads to villous atrophy, which in turn leads to loss of both the absorptive surface area as well as the brush border enzymes. Malabsorption results. A worrisome complication is the development of intestinal lymphoma.

TROPICAL SPRUE

I. **Definition.** A malabsorption disorder of unknown etiology usually affecting the jejunum.

II. **History.** Occurs in natives and long term visitors of the tropics. Classic malabsorptive symptoms, which may develop years after exposure, include diarrhea, steatorrhea, bloating, abdominal distention, and weight loss. Complaints of an enlarged tongue, chapped lips, and symptoms of anemia suggest folate deficiency.

III. **Physical exam.** Signs of dehydration and anemia. Abdominal distention, tenderness, and hyperactive bowel signs are sometimes seen. Stool guaiac exam is negative. Oral cavity examination may reveal cheilosis, glossitis, or stomatitis.

IV. **Diagnostic findings.** Tropical sprue is a clinical diagnosis based on history and characterized by malabsorption and megaloblastic anemia. Malabsorption of more than two nutrients is needed for the diagnosis. A peripheral blood smear will show megaloblastic anemia with hypersegmented neutrophils (because of folate deficiency). Small intestinal biopsy will show a monocytic infiltration and mildly flattened villi (less pronounced than in celiac sprue).

V. Differential diagnosis. Celiac sprue, Whipple's disease, lactase deficiency, infectious gastroenteritis, pancreatic insufficiency, inflammatory bowel disease, irritable bowel syndrome, carcinoid syndrome, VIPoma, hyperthyroidism, laxative overdose, or medications. Common infectious causes of diarrhea in tropical regions must be ruled out, including *Giardia lamblia, Yersinia enterocolitica, Clostridium difficile, Corynebacterium parvum,* and *C. cayetanensis.*

VI. Pathophysiology: While poorly understood, it is postulated that infectious agents may be involved.

 WHIPPLE'S DISEASE

I. Definition. A multisystem illness caused by *Tropheryma whippleii.*

II. History. Most common in middle-aged white men. Insidious onset of fever, diarrhea, steatorrhea, abdominal pain, weight loss, and migratory large joint arthropathy. Increased skin pigmentation with ophthalmologic, cardiac, and neurologic symptoms. Dementia, confusion, and memory deficits are associated with late stage disease.

III. Physical exam. Signs of dehydration (orthostasis, tachycardia, hypotension), dry mucous membranes, and poor skin turgor reflect extensive diarrhea. Skin exam may reveal hyperpigmentation or extensive bruising secondary to vitamin K deficiency. Abdominal exam may reveal distention, hyperactive bowel sounds, or tenderness. Stool guaiac test is negative. Fever and uveitis are sometimes seen. Jugular venous distention, hepatic congestion, pedal edema, and crackles on respiratory exam suggest congestive heart failure. A new cardiac murmur, petechiae, splinter hemorrhages, Osler's nodes, Janeway lesions, and Roth spots suggest endocarditis. Cranial nerve palsies, nystagmus, and ophthalmoplegia. Mental status exam may be abnormal.

IV. Diagnostic findings. Biopsy of small intestine and involved organs will show infiltration of the lamina propria with PAS-positive macrophages containing small bacilli. PCR testing of the peripheral blood can be used to detect *T. whippleii,* which cannot be cultured. Hypokalemic, metabolic acidosis (low K^+ and low HCO_3^-), as well as leukocytosis are common. Lab findings consistent with malabsorption include a prolonged PT and a decrease in folate, cholesterol, β-carotene, serum albumin, calcium, magnesium, potassium, and vitamins A, $B_{12,}$ D, E, and K.

V. Differential diagnosis. Celiac sprue, lactase deficiency, infectious gastroenteritis, pancreatic insufficiency, inflammatory bowel disease, irritable bowel syndrome, carcinoid syndrome, VIPoma, hyperthyroidism, laxative overdose, medications. Also consider sarcoidosis, Reiter's syndrome, familial Mediterranean fever, systemic vasculitis, intestinal lymphoma, and subacute bacterial endocarditis.

VI. Pathophysiology. *T. whippleii* has a low virulence but high infectivity, which explains patients' gradual onset of symptoms and multiorgan involvement.

INFLAMMATORY BOWEL DISEASE (IBD)

I. Definition. Chronic, relapsing, inflammatory disorders of the gastrointestinal tract, namely Crohn's disease (CD) and ulcerative colitis (UC).

II. History. The epidemiology of UC and CD is similar. Both entities are more common in whites and are three to six times more common in the Jewish population. Men and women are affected equally and age of onset is most common in the twenties. Intestinal and extraintestinal symptoms as well as complications vary with each disease. Major symptoms of UC include bloody diarrhea, lower abdominal cramping, and rectal pain. Crohn's disease presents with fever, malaise, weight loss, and diarrhea often without blood. Extraintestinal symptoms: uveitis (more common in CD), pyoderma gangrenosum, and ankylosing spondylitis (more common in UC). Common complications in CD include fistulae formation (enteroenteric, cystic, vaginal), obstruction, perianal fissures, perirectal abscesses, and colon cancer. Complications in UC include perforation, stricture formation, and the development of toxic megacolon and colon cancer.

III. Physical exam. Fever, tachycardia, and orthostatic hypotension indicate severe illness. Skin and conjunctival pallor suggest anemia. Abdominal exam often reveals tenderness. A palpable mass in Crohn's patients represents adherent loops of bowel. Peritoneal signs (rigid abdomen, absent bowel sounds, rebound tenderness) suggest perforation. Rectal exam in Crohn's patients may reveal a fistula or perirectal abscess. Ophthalmologic exam might reveal uveitis or episcleritis. Dermatologic exam may be significant for pyoderma gangrenosum or erythema nodosum. (see COLOR PLATES) Pain on movement and limited range of motion suggests arthritis. Hepatomegaly suggests hepatosteatosis. Jaundice suggests either cholelithiasis or primary sclerosing cholangitis.

IV. Diagnostic findings. The diagnosis should be considered in all patients with bloody diarrhea. Lab findings are usually non-specific. Severe diarrhea from any cause may result in hypokalamia and hypomagnesemia. Markers of inflammation (platelet count, ESR, C-reactive protein) are typically elevated but are non-specific for IBD. The cornerstone of diagnosing IBD (and distinguishing between CD and UC) rests in radiologic imaging studies, endoscopy, and biopsy results. In CD, inflammation involves all layers of the bowel; in UC, inflammation only involves the mucosa. CD shows deep skip lesions, most often of the terminal ileum and sparing the rectum about half the time. UC shows superficial lesions that always start in the rectum and move proximally in a continuous pattern.

V. Differential diagnosis. Diverticulosis, colon cancer, polyps, arteriovenous malformation, hemorrhoids, infectious colitis, ischemic colitis, pseudomembranous colitis, celiac sprue, Whipple's disease, lactase deficiency, pancreatic insufficiency, irritable bowel syndrome, carcinoid syndrome, VIPoma, hyperthyroidism, laxative overdose, medication-induced.

VI. Pathophysiology. Not well understood. The increased incidence of IBD in first-degree relatives suggests a genetic predisposition. Its association with other autoimmune diseases suggests an immunologic origin.

DIVERTICULAR DISEASE

I. **Definition.** A herniation, or outpouching, of the bowel wall. The presence of one or more diverticulum defines the condition known as diverticulosis. The two main complications of diverticuli are infection and bleeding. The inflammation of one or more diverticulum is known as diverticulitis.

II. **History.** Conditions that chronically increase the intraluminal pressure, including chronic constipation and a low fiber diet, are thought to contribute to the development of diverticulae. More common in the elderly, it can present at an earlier age in those with connective tissue disorders. Patients are generally asymptomatic; however, some report left lower quadrant (LLQ) abdominal, colicky pain with alternating bouts of constipation and diarrhea. Patients with diverticulitis commonly report fever, LLQ pain, nausea, vomiting, constipation, and obstipation. Patients with diverticular hemorrhage present with a sudden onset of abdominal cramping and urgency followed by painless bright red blood per rectum (BRBPR).

III. **Physical exam** may be normal in diverticulosis. Patients with diverticulitis are usually febrile and may be hypotensive and tachycardic. Abdominal exam is significant for LLQ tenderness with or without an abdominal mass; peritoneal signs (rigid abdomen, absent bowel sounds, rebound tenderness) suggest perforation. Patients experiencing diverticular hemorrhage usually do not manifest the signs and symptoms present in diverticulitis. Massive bleeding may result in hemodynamic instability. Rectal examination is notable for gross blood.

IV. **Diagnostic studies.** Only necessary in the symptomatic patient. Patients with diverticulitis frequently have a leukocytosis; occult blood loss, present in 25% of patients with diverticulitis, may result in a microcytic anemia. A plain abdominal film is helpful to look for free air, ileus, and obstruction. In addition to diverticuli, an abdominal CT commonly shows bowel wall thickening, inflammation of the pericolic fat, and abscess formation. Note that barium enema is not performed in the acute setting for fear of rupture. In patients with diverticular bleeding, colonoscopy and angiography are useful diagnostically and therapeutically.

V. **Differential diagnosis.** Inflammatory bowel disease, AV malformation, malignancy, colonic polyp, ischemic colitis, infectious diarrhea, aortoenteric fistulas, hemorrhoids and anal fissures.

VI. **Pathophysiology.** Conditions that generate persistently high intraluminal pressures favor the formation of diverticuli. Diverticulitis results when a fecalith obstructs the diverticular lumen and compromises its blood supply, thereby creating a nidus for bacterial growth and infection. Diverticuli tend to develop where the bowel wall is the weakest, which is also the site of penetration of the vasa recta blood supply. When a fecalith deposits within a diverticulum, it induces minor inflammation and occasionally erodes into this blood supply causing hematochezia.

ISCHEMIC BOWEL DISEASE

I. **Definition.** A spectrum of disorders that results in the inadequate oxygenation of intestinal tissue.

II. **History.** There are three major patterns of intestinal ischemia: acute mesenteric ischemia, chronic arterial insufficiency (abdominal angina), and ischemic colitis. Patients with **acute mesenteric ischemia** present with an acute onset of severe abdominal pain. Initially periumbilical and colicky, the pain later becomes diffuse and constant. Vomiting, anorexia, and either diarrhea or constipation may also be present. Risk factors include valvular heart disease, atrial fibrillation, prosthetic valve, use of oral contraception, factor V Leiden deficiency, factor C and S deficiencies, dehydration, and digitalis toxicity. In contrast, patients with **chronic arterial insufficiency** report intermittent dull, epigastric pain starting about half an hour after eating and lasting several hours. Weight loss and "fear of eating" are common features of this illness. Those with coronary artery disease or peripheral vascular disease are most at risk. Patients with **ischemic colitis** tend to be elderly with comorbid conditions. In mild cases, patients describe minimal pain and bleeding occurring over weeks, while those with more severe cases present with severe pain and profuse bleeding.

III. **Physical exam.** Pain is often out of proportion to physical exam findings. Abdominal exam may be normal or may reveal only mild tenderness and distention. Bowel sounds are usually normal. Rectal examination and guaiac testing often reveals occult bleeding. Extreme tenderness, positive peritoneal signs, distention, and absent bowel sounds suggest mesenteric infarction.

IV. **Diagnostic findings.** Typical laboratory findings in acute mesenteric ischemia include a leukocytosis with a polymorphonuclear (PMN) predominance. An increased anion gap metabolic acidosis from elevated lactate levels may also be present. A barium enema can show dilation, poor motility, thickened mucosal folds, a finding referred to as "thumbprinting". Note that a barium enema is contraindicated acutely since it may cause perforation. Arteriography is performed to localize vessel occlusion and is the gold standard in evaluating acute mesenteric ischemia.

V. **Differential diagnosis.** Inflammatory bowel disease, infectious colitis, diverticulitis, appendicitis, PUD, gastritis, and biliary disease.

VI. **Pathophysiology.** Acute mesenteric ischemia is most commonly an occlusive disease resulting from a thrombus or embolus lodged in the celiac or superior mesenteric artery. Non-occlusive acute mesenteric ischemia results from "low output states" including CHF, arrhythmias, and digitalis toxicity. Chronic arterial insufficiency results when underlying atherosclerotic disease in the splanchnic bed prevents an increase in blood flow to the gut. The symptoms develop after eating when the vascular demand to the gut is increased to facilitate digestion. Ischemic colitis is a non-occlusive disease, which results in inadequate oxygenation of the mucosa. The severity of the illness is dictated by the degree and acuity of the hypoperfusion.

IRRITABLE BOWEL SYNDROME (IBS)

I. **Definition.** A clinical diagnosis marked by chronic intermittent abdominal pain and altered bowel habits in the absence of structural abnormalities.

II. **History.** Diagnosed most commonly in young adults, predominantly women. Many have a history of sexual or physical abuse; thus, understanding the psychiatric component of the history is helpful. The **Rome criteria** are used to establish the diagnosis of IBS. The patient must have at least a three month history of abdominal pain that is either a.) relieved by defecation, b.) accompanied by a change in frequency of stool, or c.) accompanied by a change in consistency of stool. In addition, the patient must complain of disturbed defecation at least 25% of the time consisting of two or more of the following: a.) altered frequency, b.) altered consistency, c.) passage of mucus, d.) altered stool passage, or e.) abdominal distention. Finally, constitutional signs including fever and weight loss as well as nocturnal symptoms are incompatible with the diagnosis of IBS.

III. **Physical exam.** Apart from generalized anxiety, physical exam findings are notably absent. Significant abdominal tenderness or distention is unusual. Guaiac examination is negative.

IV. **Diagnostic findings.** Thyroid stimulating hormone (TSH), stool studies, and sigmoidoscopy (or colonoscopy) are normal in IBS and are useful in excluding other diagnoses.

V. **Differential diagnosis.** Thyrotoxicosis, lactose intolerance, laxative abuse, malignancy, inflammatory bowel disease, *C. difficile* infection, any disorder leading to malabsorption, and endometriosis.

VI. **Pathophysiology.** Not well understood. Some patients exhibit "heightened visceral perception" in which mild increases in distention of the intestinal lumen exacerbate abdominal pain and diarrhea.

 UPPER GASTROINTESTINAL BLEEDING (UGIB)

I. **Definition.** Gastrointestinal blood loss that originates proximal to the ligament of Treitz.

II. **History.** Presentation varies tremendously depending on the amount and chronicity of blood loss. Those with slow, small bleeds may be asymptomatic or complain of increasing fatigue and progressive weight loss. Those with faster, larger bleeds may experience syncope or report maroon-colored, sticky, foul-smelling feces (melena) or bright red blood in the vomitus (hematemesis). In cases of massive UGIB, blood moves through the alimentary tract too quickly to be digested; as a result, bright red blood may pass from the rectum (hematochezia). Important elements of the history include prior episodes of gastrointestinal blood loss and medication use, particularly NSAIDs, corticosteroids, and anticoagulants. The patient should also be questioned for alcohol and tobacco abuse, recurrent or forceful retching, cirrhosis, and a family history of ulcerative disease or cancer.

III. Physical exam. The most important initial assessment is a review of the vital signs. Tachycardia suggests a volume loss greater than 10%, orthostatic hypotension indicates a volume loss greater than 20%, and hypovolemic shock corresponds with a volume loss greater than 30% (remember that beta-blockers blunt the tachycardic response to hypovolemia). Skin and conjunctival pallor suggest chronic blood loss. Oral and nasal cavities should be carefully examined so as to rule out non-intestinal causes of blood loss. Gynecomastia, palmar erythema, spider angiomata, testicular atrophy, ascites, jaundice, and hepatosplenomegaly are consistent with cirrhosis, a diagnosis that raises the suspicion of esophageal and gastric varices. Abdominal exam may be significant for diffuse or localizable tenderness with or without peritoneal signs. Periumbilical lymphadenopathy (Sister Mary Joseph node) is seen in gastric cancer. Rectal examination should always be performed (except in a neutropenic patient) to assess the color of the stool and to exclude local pathology including anal fissures, hemorrhoids, and masses.

IV. Diagnostic findings. The HgB concentration is most helpful if a prior value is available. Hypochromic, microcytic erythrocytes are consistent with chronic blood loss. Note that changes in HgB concentration occur up to 12 hours after a bleed; thus a normal HgB concentration should be interpreted with caution in a patient with acute blood loss. An abnormal platelet count or coagulation profile may point to a disorder in hemostasis. Abnormal liver function tests may represent impaired synthetic function of the liver or inflammation of hepatocytes. EGD is the most useful procedure because it affords direct visualization of the mucosa, the ability to biopsy suspicious lesions, as well as the power to intervene therapeutically. If EGD fails to localize the bleed and HgB concentration continues to fall, angiography is indicated.

V. Differential diagnosis. Over 90% of UGIB cases are caused by ruptured esophageal or gastric varices, Mallory-Weiss tears, gastritis, and peptic ulcer disease. Other causes include ingested epistaxis, esophagitis, AV malformation, and cancer.

VI. Pathophysiology. Differs for each disorder.

LOWER GASTROINTESTINAL BLEEDING (LGIB)

I. Definition. Gastrointestinal blood loss that originates distal to the ligament of Treitz.

II. History. An otherwise asymptomatic patient who occasionally finds bright red blood on toilet paper after straining probably suffers from hemorrhoids. Weight loss and chronic fatigue is consistent with malignancy or inflammatory bowel disease. A history of fever, travel, or the consumption of undercooked meat is consistent with infectious diarrhea. Chronic constipation, pain, and fever in the LLQ is consistent with diverticulitis. A prior history of blood loss, family history, a complete medication list and the use of tobacco and alcohol are important features to note.

III. Physical exam. The evaluation begins with supine and standing vital signs. Skin and conjunctival pallor suggest chronic blood loss. Stigmata of cirrhosis in the setting of bright red blood per rectum is suggestive of ruptured internal hemorrhoids. Tiny and multiple telangiectasias on the skin and in the oral cavity are consistent with Osler-Weber-Rendu syndrome, a condition that may also affect the mucosa throughout the entire gastrointestinal tract. An abdominal mass in the context of fatigue, microcytic anemia, and weight loss must prompt an evaluation of malignancy. A rectal examination is essential not only to look for the color of the stool, but also to examine for hemorrhoids, anal fissures or masses.

IV. Diagnostic findings. The laboratory assessment includes HgB concentration, platelet count, white blood cell count, coagulation panel, and liver function tests. Colonoscopy is the most useful procedure in evaluating LGIB because it affords the direct visualization of the mucosa, the ability to biopsy suspicious lesions and the power to intervene therapeutically. If colonoscopy fails to localize the bleed and HgB concentration continues to fall, angiography is indicated. If no source of LGIB is found, the upper gastrointestinal tract should be evaluated.

V. Differential diagnosis. Inflammatory bowel disease, diverticular disease, AV malformation, malignancy, colonic polyp, ischemic colitis, infectious diarrhea, aorto-enteric fistulas, hemorrhoids, and anal fissures.

VI. Pathophysiology. Differs for each disorder.

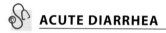 **ACUTE DIARRHEA**

I. Definition. An increase in the frequency, weight, or volume of stool produced by a patient. (A common research definition is stool production greater than 150 grams/day, or greater than 150 ml/day, occurring for less than two weeks.)

II. History. It is essential to determine whether the patient is experiencing increased stool production or simply loose stool or incontinence. If the patient reports increased stool production, other important elements of the history include a complete medication list (especially crucial are *changes* in medication as well as antibiotics use), recent travel to a developing country, change in diet (especially shellfish or improperly prepared meat), sick contacts (especially a child in day care), immune status, occupational history, and prior surgery or gastrointestinal illness. Most patients with acute diarrhea report abdominal cramping and vomiting, symptoms consistent with a non-invasive infection, an ingested toxin, or medication-induced illness. The presence of fever, persistent abdominal pain or vomiting, and blood in the stool are consistent with an enteroinvasive infection or IBD.

III. Physical exam. The general appearance is usually that of an otherwise healthy person. The presence of generalized wasting or temporal muscle atrophy should prompt an evaluation for an underlying chronic illness. Vital signs may be unremarkable in mild disease. Patients may be febrile, orthostatic, and manifest other signs of dehydration, including dry mucous membranes and poor skin turgor. Abdominal exam may be significant for distention, hyperactive bowel sounds, or diffuse tenderness. A rectal examination is essential to determine the presence of blood or mucus.

IV. Diagnostic findings. In the absence of fever, persistent vomiting, severe abdominal pain, bloody stool, or recent travel to a developing country, an immunocompetent patient may be closely observed and rehydrated without further testing. The presence of any of these symptoms (especially in an immunocompromised patient) should prompt further evaluation, namely fecal leukocytes, fecal occult blood, and fecal ova and parasites. Recent use (ranging from three days prior to three months prior) of antibiotics should prompt analysis of *C. difficile* toxin. The absence of fecal leukocytes and fecal blood is consistent with medication-induced illness, or a diarrhea caused by a virus or enterotoxic bacteria. The presence of fecal leukocytes and fecal blood is consistent with both enteroinvasive bacteria or IBD; stool cultures with or without sigmoidoscopy are helpful in distinguishing these entities.

V. Differential diagnosis. Most likely causes include pre-formed toxin (food poisoning), non-invasive bacteria (enterotoxigenic *Escherichia coli, Vibrio cholerae, C. difficile*), invasive bacteria (*Salmonella, Shigella, Campylobacter jejuni,* enteroinvasive *E. coli, Yersinia*), viruses (rotavirus, Norwalk virus), parasites (*Giardia, Entamoeba histolytica*), and medication-induced (especially antibiotics). Less likely causes include IBD and intestinal ischemia.

VI. Pathophysiology. The prototypic organism leading to enterotoxin diarrheal illness is *Vibrio cholerae. Vibrio* produces an enterotoxin, choleragen, which works via the adenylate cyclase pathway to increase secretory activity of the gastrointestinal tract. As a result, copious amounts of "rice water stool" without leukocytes or erythrocytes is produced. Enteroinvasive *E. coli* invades the bowel wall to produce an inflammatory diarrhea containing leukocytes and erythrocytes.

CHRONIC DIARRHEA

I. Definition. An increase in stool frequency, weight, or volume occurring for more than two weeks.

II. History. The etiology of chronic diarrhea is usually non-infectious. It is useful to divide the causes of chronic diarrhea into five categories: inflammatory, osmotic, secretory, motility, and factitious. A history of fever, abdominal pain, and stool containing blood or mucus raises the suspicion of an **inflammatory process**. A history of weight loss and bulky, greasy, especially foul-smelling stool is suggestive of a malabsorptive (i.e. **osmotic**) disorder. A patient who reports very watery diarrhea that persists despite fasting may be suffering from a **secretory disorder**. A diagnosis of scleroderma, advanced diabetes, or hyperthyroidism is compatible with a **motility disorder**. A thorough medication history may help in diagnosing **factitious diarrhea**, usually caused by laxative abuse.

III. Physical exam. The general appearance of the patient may be normal or that of a wasted person. Vital signs may be unremarkable in mild disease. In more severe cases, patients may be febrile, orthostatic, and manifest other signs of dehydration, including dry mucous membranes and poor skin turgor. You must search for other clues in the physical exam, including exophthalmos and hyperreflexia (seen in hyperthyroidism), calcinosis and telangectasias (seen in scleroderma), pyoderma gangrenosum (seen in IBD), dermatitis herpetiformis (seen in celiac sprue), generalized edema (seen in protein-losing enteropathy), and retinopathy, neuropathy, and arterial insufficiency (seen in advanced diabetes).

IV. Diagnostic findings. A systematic approach to diagnosis, driven by the history and physical examination, has the highest yield. The presence of fecal leukocytes with or without occult blood in the context of chronic diarrhea should prompt an investigation for inflammatory bowel disease or cancer. In the absence of fecal leukocytes or occult blood, the next step is to determine the fecal osmotic gap. The fecal osmotic gap is the measured fecal osmolality minus the calculated fecal osmolality $[2 \times (Na^+ + K^+)]$. A fecal osmotic gap greater than 50 mosmol/kg H_2O is considered significant. If the fecal osmotic gap is normal, the next step is to weigh the stool. Normal stool weight is consistent with IBS. An increased stool weight is consistent with secretory causes of diarrhea. If the fecal osmotic gap is increased, the next step is to measure the fecal fat. Normal fecal fat is indicative of laxative abuse or lactase deficiency. Increased fecal fat is consistent with malabsorption syndrome, pancreatic insufficiency, and bacterial overgrowth.

V. Differential diagnosis. Inflammatory: ulcerative colitis, shigellosis, amebiasis, radiation colitis. Osmotic: lactose intolerance, malabsorption syndromes, pancreatic insufficiency. Secretory cholera, VIPoma, carcinoid, ZES, fatty acid-induced diarrhea. Motility: hyperthyroidism, IBS, scleroderma, diabetic gastropathy. Factitious: laxative abuse.

VI. Pathophysiology. Inflammatory diarrhea results in the destruction of the gut mucosa and a subsequent release of blood and WBCs. Osmotic diarrhea results when an osmotically active substance draws fluid into the bowel lumen. In secretory diarrhea, there is an increased secretion of chloride, resulting in large volume watery diarrhea that is not affected by fasting. An increase in gut motility causes diarrhea due to decreased time for absorption, whereas a decrease in gut motility causes diarrhea via bacteria overgrowth.

CHAPTER **21**

Genitourinary Diseases

Most *serious errors made by physicians* are the result of their being unable
or unwilling to consider the possibilities that they are misinformed, unin-
formed, or incorrect. If the patient's history and physical fail to fit neatly into
some diagnostic niche, it may be that the history is incomplete, the physical
incorrect, or the physician unaware of the correct niche. The patient who
refuses to get better despite intensive and expensive therapy may have
been treated for the wrong problem and/or, worse yet, may be toxic from
the medications. Maimonides was correct: "Teach thy tongue to say I do not
know and thou shall progress."

Marshall A. Wolf, M.D., FACP

*A graduate of Harvard College and Harvard Medical School, Dr. Wolf completed his
residency training in Internal Medicine at the Brigham and Women's Hospital, where
he served as Program Director of the Internal Medicine Residency Program and Vice
Chairman of Medical Education. A Professor of Medicine at Harvard Medical School,
he is the recipient of the Second Annual Harvard Medical/Dental School Excellence in
Mentoring Award. He has trained 1,200 doctors over a 28-year period.*

ACUTE RENAL FAILURE

I. **Definition.** Acute suppression of kidney filtration resulting in rapidly
increasing azotemia, with or without oliguria (< 500 ml urine daily).

II. **Clinical manifestations.** The presentation of acute renal failure (ARF) can be
divided into two phases.

    A. Oliguric phase. Associated findings are ↓↓ urine output (< 20 ml/hr)
with rising BUN and/or serum creatinine levels; anorexia, nausea, vomiting; urine sediment consisting of protein, red cells, epithelial cells, brown
granular casts; specific gravity 1.010–1.016; ↓ serum Na^+ (120–130
mEq/L); hyperkalemia; Hct 25–30%.

    B. Diuretic phase. Begins approximately 2 weeks post-onset. Gradual ↓ in
urine formation to 6–8 L/day, indicating nephron recovery. Continuous for
7–10 days.

III. **Differential diagnosis and pathophysiology**

    A. Table 21–1 compares lab values for prerenal versus intrinsic renal
azotemia.

TABLE 21-1. Differential diagnosis of prerenal azotemia versus intrinsic renal azotemia

Determination	Prerenal	Renal
Urine osmolality	>500 mOsm/L	<350 mOsm/L
Urine: plasma creatinine	>20	<10
Urine: plasma urea	>40	<20
Urine Na+	<20 mEq/L	>40 mEq/L

B. Etiologies

1. **Prerenal.** Renal compromise results from diminished renal blood flow: volume depletion; cardiac dysfunction resulting in a diminished cardiac output; diminished intravascular volume due to redistribution of fluid into interstitial spaces, as can occur with hepatic cirrhosis, sepsis, and burns.

2. **Postrenal.** Renal compromise results from obstruction of the urinary system: benign prostatic hypertrophy, prostate cancer, calculi at the level of the prostatic urethra, pelvic or retroperitoneal tumors, and congenital anomalies. Blockage of both ureters is uncommon but can be caused by a widespread retroperitoneal process, such as lymphoma.

3. **Renal.** Renal compromise results from intrinsic renal pathology: glomerular disease, vascular disease, tubulointerstitial disease. By far the most common cause of acute intrinsic renal disease is the category of tubulointerstitial disorders, although in hospitalized patients acute tubular necrosis is the major cause of intrinsic renal failure.

   a. **Glomerular disease.** Poststreptococcal glomerulonephritis, glomerulonephritis associated with endocarditis and abscesses, membranoproliferative glomerulonephritis, rapidly progressive glomerulonephritis (systemic lupus erythematosus, Wegener's granulomatosis, Goodpasture's syndrome, and Henoch-Schönlein purpura).

   b. **Vascular disease.** Renal artery thrombosis or embolism, renal vein thrombosis, scleroderma, malignant hypertension, thrombotic thrombocytopenic purpura (TTP), disseminated intravascular coagulation (DIC) with cortical necrosis.

   c. **Tubulointerstitial disease.** Separated into acute interstitial nephritis and acute tubular necrosis (ATN).

      (1) **Acute interstitial nephritis.** Caused by infiltrative disease (sarcoidosis or lymphoma), systemic infection (syphilis and toxoplasmosis), and drugs (penicillin, diuretics, nonsteroidal anti-inflammatory drugs [NSAIDs]).

      (2) **Acute tubular necrosis.** Caused by ischemia (shock, trauma, hypoxia, or sepsis) nephrotoxins (radiocontrast agents and aminoglycosides), myoglobinuria, and myeloma proteins (Bence Jones).

   C. Damage occurs through direct **nephrotoxicity** (usually involving necrosis of tubular epithelium) and **ischemia** (often secondary to constriction of afferent arterioles).

   D. Although oliguria is common, the volume of urine bears no relation to the degree of functional impairment.

CHRONIC RENAL FAILURE

  I. **Definition.** Chronic insufficiency of renal excretory and regulatory functions leading to **uremia.** Chronic renal failure (CRF) results from a progressive decrease in glomerular filtration and the loss of tubular function.

  II. **Clinical manifestations.** The functional effects of CRF are divided into the following progressively worsening categories: diminished renal reserve, renal insufficiency, and uremia. With **diminished renal reserve,** there is a measurable loss of renal function, but homeostasis is preserved at the expense of hormonal adaptations such as secondary hyperparathyroidism and intrarenal changes in glomerulotubular balance. At the stage of **renal insufficiency**, there is slight retention of nitrogenous compounds (azotemia), reflected in elevated plasma urea and creatinine. With further renal dysfunction, fluid and electrolyte balance is disturbed, azotemia increases, and systemic manifestations of **uremia** occur.

   A. History

     1. Patients with a **diminished renal reserve** are asymptomatic, and renal dysfunction can only be detected by careful testing.

     2. Patients with **renal insufficiency,** despite the elevated BUN and creatinine, suffer only from nocturia, due to the failure of the kidney to concentrate urine during the night.

     3. Patients with **uremia** suffer from weakness, fatigue, and mental status changes, as well as anorexia, nausea, vomiting, early satiety, stomatitis, and an unpleasant taste in the mouth. Patients also suffer from intractable pruritus.

   B. Physical exam and pathophysiology. Following are the physical manifestations of the multisystem **effects** of the **uremic state:**

     1. **Cardiovascular:** hypertension (due to volume overload), dilated cardiomyopathy (due to volume overload), pericarditis.

     2. **Pulmonary:** pulmonary edema and large pulmonary effusions (due to volume overload, increased capillary permeability), and Kussmaul's respirations (due to acidemia).

     3. **Neurologic:** both peripheral and central nervous system derangements are seen. Progressive sensory polyneuropathy and distal motor dysfunction are usually present. Uremia unchecked will eventually result in asterixis and coma (metabolic encephalopathy).

     4. **Hematopoietic:** normochromic normocytic anemia results in pallor (due to progressively decreasing erythropoietin levels), thrombasthenia (decreased platelet aggregation and adhesiveness) presents as purpura.

5. **Gastrointestinal:** increased incidence of duodenitis and angiodysplasia of stomach and proximal intestine results in ulceration and bleeding.

6. **Metabolic disturbances:** hypertriglyceridemia (hepatic dysfunction); increased insulin resistance and glucose intolerance.

7. **Skin:** yellow-brown discoloration and urea from sweat may crystallize on skin as uremic frost.

8. **Musculoskeletal:** bone pain and multiple fractures (due to renal osteodystrophy resulting from secondary hyperparathyroidism).

C. **Diagnostic tests.** Lab findings include azotemia, acidosis ($[HCO_3^-]$ = 15–20 mEq/L), hyperphosphatemia, hyperkalemia, and normochromic normocytic anemia. Urine osmolarity $\sim$ 300–320 mOsm/L.

III. Differential diagnosis. The cause of CRF must be elucidated, because some etiologies are reversible. Etiologies of CRF include advanced and prolonged hypertension, diabetes mellitus, glomerulonephritis, tubulointerstitial disease, polycystic kidney disease, and obstructive uropathy. All result in parenchymal scarring and progressive glomerular failure.

GLOMERULOPATHIES

I. Definition. A group of diverse conditions including, but not limited to, glomerulonephritis, in which the disease predominantly affects glomerular function. Based on their clinical presentation, the glomerulopathies have been divided into five subtypes:

A. **Acute glomerulonephritis (GN).** Acute onset and early resolution.

B. **Rapidly progressive glomerulonephritis (RPGN).** Acute onset and rapid progression.

C. **Idiopathic renal hematuric syndrome.** Persistent, asymptomatic, minimal urinary abnormalities.

D. **Nephrotic syndrome.** Acute onset and gradual resolution.

E. **Chronic glomerulonephritis.** Insidious onset and gradual progression.

II. Clinical manifestations and differential diagnosis vary, depending on the subtype. Acute glomerulonephritis and nephrotic syndrome are discussed in detail later in this chapter as they are by far the most common glomerulopathies.

III. Pathophysiology. Glomerular damage produces changes in glomerular capillary permeability, resulting in various degrees of proteinuria, hematuria, leukocyturia, and urinary casts.

Microthrombosis occurs, commonly accompanied by epithelial "crescents" formed from leaked fibrinogen and precipitated fibrin, and if damage is severe, hemodynamic changes may produce oliguria. Commonly tubular function is deranged by inflammatory changes in the interstitium. Measurable changes consist of reduction in the urinary concentrating capacity, acid excretion, and varying disturbances in nephron solute exchange. Because there is some inherent capacity for glomerular hypertrophy, such defects in tubular function usually occur before the **glomerular filtration rate** (GFR) is much reduced. As glomerular derangement progresses, however, the total filtration surface is significantly reduced, the GFR falls, and azotemia occurs.

 ## ACUTE GLOMERULONEPHRITIS

I. Definition. A group of diseases characterized pathologically by diffuse inflammatory changes in the glomeruli and clinically by the acute onset of **hematuria, RBC casts,** and **proteinuria.**

II. Clinical manifestations of acute glomerulonephritis vary according to the disease entity that causes it. The most common cause of acute glomerulonephritis is **poststreptococcal glomerulonephritis (PSGN).**

    A. History. History of streptococcal pharyngitis 3–4 weeks prior to onset of smoky or frankly bloody urine, oliguria, headaches, and visual disturbances (secondary to hypertension).

    B. Physical exam

        1. Hypertension

        2. Gross (or microscopic) hematuria

        3. Periorbital edema

    C. Diagnostic tests

        1. Urinalysis: proteinuria of 1–3 gm/day, hematuria, active urinary sediment including white blood cell, granular, and red blood cell casts

        2. Positive throat culture for β-hemolytic streptococci

        3. Low C3

        4. Elevated antibodies to streptococcal antigens (antistreptolysin O or antihyaluronidase)

III. Differential diagnosis

    A. Postinfectious glomerulonephritis. PSGN, subacute bacterial endocarditis, infected ventriculoatrial shunts, varicella, hepatitis B, syphilis, and malaria.

    B. Mesangiocapillary glomerulonephritis

    C. Lupus nephritis

    D. IgA nephropathy (Berger's, pronounced "Bur-jhare's", **disease)**

IV. Pathophysiology. The glomerular damage seen in acute glomerulonephritis is due to immune complex deposition and the activation of the complement system that results from this deposition. An endogenous or exogenous antigen stimulates production of a specific antibody, which combines with the antigen in one of two ways: within the kidney, after the antigen has been planted; or in the circulation, to form a circulating immune complex that subsequently becomes deposited. The former mechanism is the more common process. Deposition of the immune complex in the glomerular wall in subepithelial sites activates the complement system. From the complement cascade, chemotactic factor C567 is formed, which causes polymorphonuclear leukocyte localization in the area of the immune complex deposition and the release of lysozyme. Lysozyme injures the foot processes of the podocytes, resulting in "holes" in the glomerular filter. These holes are the means by which red blood cells and protein escape into the tubular portion of the nephron.

NEPHROTIC SYNDROME

I. **Definition.** Nephrotic syndrome (NS) is characterized by proteinuria, hypoalbuminemia, lipemia, and generalized edema.

II. **Clinical manifestations**

A. **History and physical exam.** Patients usually report symptoms associated with new-onset focal edema, "foamy" urine (urine with bubbles on its surface), anorexia, and malaise.

Focal edema is usually the trigger that brings the patient with NS to a physician. Patients seek help for such varied complaints as difficulty breathing (pleural effusion or laryngeal edema), substernal chest pain (pericardial effusion), scrotal swelling, swollen knees (hydroarthrosis), swollen abdomen (ascites), and, in children, abdominal pain from edema of the mesentery.

B. **Diagnostic tests**

1. **Urinalysis: proteinuria > 3 gm/day;** urine sodium low and urine potassium high (due to increased aldosterone secretion as the body attempts to increase intravascular volume); lipiduria.

2. **Serum chemistries:** hypoalbuminemia (< 2.5 gm/dl); BUN and creatinine are elevated in proportion to the degree of renal impairment; increased cholesterol and triglyceride levels.

III. **Differential diagnosis.** The diagnosis of NS is made by clinical features and proteinuria (Fig. 21–1), but determination of the etiology of the nephrotic syndrome depends on renal histology determined by renal biopsy.

A. **Primary renal diseases** account for 90% of cases of nephrotic syndrome in children and 75% in adults.

	Children	Adults
Minimal change disease (MCD)	65%	15%
Focal glomerulosclerosis (FGS)	10%	15%
Membranous glomerulonephritis (MGN)	5%	35%
Membranoproliferative glomerulonephritis (MPGN)	10%	10%
Total	90%	75%

B. **Secondary disease** accounts for 10% of NS in children and 25% of NS in adults. Secondary causes include:

1. **Metabolic:** diabetes mellitus, amyloidosis.

2. **Immunogenic:** systemic lupus erythematosis, Henoch-Schönlein purpura, polyarteritis nodosa, Sjögren's syndrome, sarcoidosis.

3. **Neoplasms:** leukemias, lymphomas, multiple myeloma.

4. **Nephrotoxins:** mercury, gold, penicillamine.

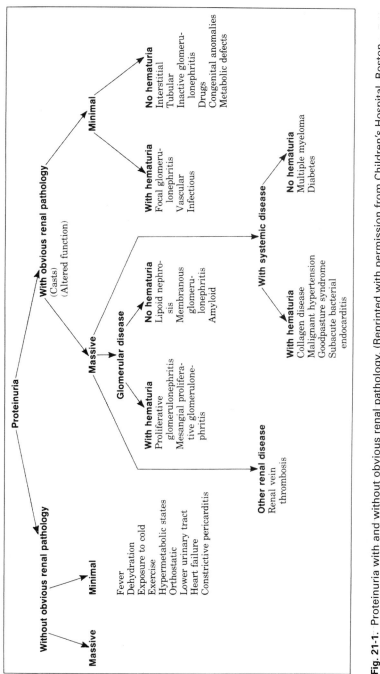

Fig. 21-1. Proteinuria with and without obvious renal pathology. (Reprinted with permission from Children's Hospital, Boston, *Manual of Pediatric Therapeutics*, 5th ed., Boston: Little, Brown, 1994.)

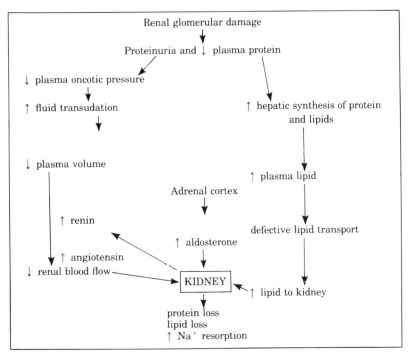

Fig. 21-2. Pathophysiologic sequence in the nephrotic syndrome.

5. **Infections:** PSGN, shunt nephritis, endocarditis, syphilis, hepatitis B, varicella, malaria, schistosomiasis.

6. **Hereditary:** Alport's syndrome, Fabry's disease.

7. **Miscellaneous:** toxemia of pregnancy, malignant hypertension.

IV. Pathophysiology. The sequence of events leading to the nephrotic syndrome is illustrated in Fig. 21–2.

URINARY TRACT INFECTION (UTI)

I. **Definition**. Acute or chronic infection of any portion of the urinary tract.

II. **Clinical manifestations and differential diagnosis**

A. UTI must be distinguished from other causes of dysuria, polyuria, urgency, and lower abdominal or suprapubic pain. These disorders include genital infections, external bladder compression, and prostatitis.

B. **Differentiating features of lower and upper UTI**

1. **History and physical exam**

a. Lower UTI (cystitis): dysuria; dark, foul-smelling urine.

TABLE 21-2. Clinical manifestations of gonorrhea and syphilis

Disease	Time from exposure to onset	Clinical manifestations	Diagnostic tests
Gonorrhea	2–8 days	Dysuria, frequency, discharge; often asymptomatic; men often present with urethritis, women with PID	Discharge smears show gram-negative diplococci; selective medium and high CO_2 necessary to culture organisms
Primary syphilis	10–90 days (average 21)	Painless chancre, often in genital area; nontender adenopathy in draining nodes	Fluid from lesions contains *Treponema pallidum*; must use dark fields or immunofluorescence
Secondary syphilis	6 wk–6 mo	Mucosal lesions; generalized rash consisting of lesions (condylomata latum); generalized nontender adenopathy; fever, hepatitis, arthritis, iritis, meningitis	VDRL and FTA-ABS serologic tests almost always positive
Tertiary syphilis	2–10 yr	Charcot's arthropathy; infiltrative tumors (gummas) in liver, skin, bone; aortic aneurysms with aortic insufficiency; meningovascular involvement; neurologic: degenerative changes, tabes dorsalis, paresthesias, dementia, etc.; Argyll Robertson pupil and Romberg's sign	Often positive CSF serology

VDRL = Venereal Disease Research Laboratories; FTA-ABS = fluorescent treponemal antibody-absorption.

    b. Upper UTI (pyelonephritis): headaches, chills, fever, vomiting, back pain, costovertebral angle (CVA) tenderness.

  2. Diagnostic tests

    a. Lower UTI (cystitis): bacteriuria, pyuria, normal C-reactive protein.

    b. Upper UTI (pyelonephritis): bacteriuria, proteinuria, pyuria, leukocytosis (with left shift). Chronic UTI may result in anemia, uremia, acidosis, hypertension, elevated C-reactive protein.

III. Pathophysiology

A. Usually due to ascending urinary tract infection by fecal-perineal flora. Since female urethra is shorter, UTIs are generally more common in women than men (except for cases of congenital anomalies and prostatism). Instrumentation of urethra increases risk.

B. Most common organism is ***Escherichia coli*** (see COLOR PLATES). Others include *Klebsiella, Proteus*, enterococci.

GONORRHEA AND SYPHILIS

I. Definition. Gonorrhea and syphilis are two sexually transmitted diseases (STDs) that are still common today, though their incidence and prevalence has declined greatly in recent years.

II. Clinical manifestations and differential diagnosis. The clinical features of gonorrhea and syphilis are compared in Table 21-2. Note that syphilis manifests itself in one of three stages (primary, secondary, and tertiary).

III. Pathophysiology

A. Gonorrhea. There are more than 300,000 newly reported cases in the United States each year; caused by ***Neisseria gonorrhoeae***, a gram-negative, kidney-shaped diplococcus usually found intracellularly (especially in polymorphonuclear leukocytes) on Gram stain.

B. Syphilis. There are more than 50,000 cases of syphilis in the United States; caused by ***Treponema pallidum***, a spirochete. *T. pallidum* often invades the central nervous system and aorta, leading to the symptoms of meningovascular neurosyphilis, tabes dorsalis, dissecting aortic aneurysm, aortic insufficiency, and aortic scarring.

CHAPTER **22**

Musculoskeletal Diseases

In this chapter we will discuss some important examples among the four major types of rheumatologic disease:

1. **Monoarticular arthritis:** gout, pseudogout, septic arthritis.

2. **Polyarticular arthritis:** rheumatoid arthritis (RA), osteoarthritis (also known as degenerative joint disease).

3. **Connective tissue disorders:** systemic lupus erythematosus (SLE), scleroderma.

4. **Vasculitides:** temporal arteritis.

 GOUT

I. Definition. A usually monoarticular arthritis caused by deposition of uric acid crystals in joints.

II. Clinical manifestations

   A. History and physical exam. Predominantly affects middle-aged and elderly men and postmenopausal women. Linked with excessive alcohol consumption, salicylate ingestion, diuretic use, and obesity. Clinical manifestations of gout can be divided into three phases.

   1. An acute attack consists of a very painful monoarthritis, usually in the first metatarsophalangeal joint (i.e., the big toe). Recurrences may affect other joints, but usually spare the hips and shoulders.

   2. In the interval phase patients are asymptomatic, but as the disease progresses this period gets shorter and shorter.

   3. About 10–20 years after original onset, some patients enter the chronic phase, in which tophaceous deposits (tophi) are found in various periarticular areas, as well as commonly on the extensor surface of the forearm and pinna of the ear. Later complications can include uric acid nephrolithiasis and tubulointerstitial nephritis.

   B. Lab findings. Gout is characterized by excess circulating uric acid and deposition of uric acid crystals in the joint fluid. A patient with a uric acid level > 10 mg/dl has a 90% chance of suffering from gout, though uric acid levels may not be elevated during an acute attack. Measurement of 24-hr urine uric acid after a 5-day purine-restricted diet can be used to separate uric acid overproducers from undersecretors. See needle-shaped, negatively birefringent crystals under polarized microscopy.

III. Differential diagnosis. Definitive diagnosis, made by the presence of uric acid crystals in joint fluid, is important because anti-inflammatory agents used to treat gout can mask signs of joint sepsis. Pseudogout, the result of deposition of calcium pyrophosphate, is indistinguishable clinically from gout, except for its predilection for larger joints, such as the knee, septic arthritis, psoriatic arthritis, rheumatoid arthritis, and pseudogout.

IV. Pathophysiology. Causes of increased uric acid include genetic defects in purine metabolism, increased cellular turnover (psoriasis, myeloproliferative diseases), and decreased excretion of uric acid (as in patients with interstitial nephritis, or those taking various drugs, like certain diuretics).

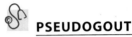

PSEUDOGOUT

I. Definition. A usually monoarticular arthritis caused by calcium pyrophosphate deposition in joints. Also known as chondrocalcinosis.

II. Clinical manifestations

    A. History and physical exam. Seen most frequently in the elderly and in those with hyperparathyroidism, hypothyroidism, and hemochromatosis. Painful attacks can last up to 2 weeks and are accompanied by fever. Pseudogout usually attacks larger joints, like the knee, and not uncommonly affects more than one joint at a time.

    B. Diagnostic tests

        1. X-ray shows linear, punctate calcifications in the knee, hip, intervertebral disks, and other joints.

        2. Definitive diagnosis is made by identifying calcium pyrophosphate crystals in synovial fluid, which appear rhomboid-shaped and weakly positively birefringent.

III. Differential diagnosis. See "Gout," sec. III.

SEPTIC ARTHRITIS

I. Definition. Inflammation of one or more joints due to infection in the joint space.

II. Clinical manifestations

    A. History. Patients with preexisting arthritis are especially prone to septic joints, as are those with diabetes, a history of joint injury, immunosuppression, and chronic alcohol and IV drug abuse. Onset is rapid, and patients can range from showing no signs of systemic illness to appearing quite sick.

    B. Physical exam. Involved joints are warm, red, swollen, and tender, with intense pain, especially on motion. Eighty to ninety percent of cases are monoarticular.

    C. Diagnostic tests. Definitive diagnosis is made by Gram stain and culture of synovial fluid.

III. Differential diagnosis. Septic arthritis can be differentiated from other causes of monoarthritis when signs of infection occur both locally (redness, warmth, swelling, intense pain on movement) and systemically (fever, enlarged nodes). Gout, pseudogout, Lyme's arthritis, reactive arthritis, seronegative spondyloarthropathy.

IV. Pathophysiology

A. In young sexually active patients, the most common cause is *Neisseria gonnorrheae*. In other populations, *Staphylococcus aureus* is the most frequently encountered pathogen. Gram-negative organisms are seen especially in patients with underlying diabetes, cancer, or other serious diseases.

B. Mechanism of infection is primarily through the hematogenous spread of microorganism.

RHEUMATOID ARTHRITIS

I. Definition. A chronic systemic disease characterized by inflammation of synovial membranes with resultant cartilage and joint destruction.

II. Clinical manifestations

A. History. Onset is usually insidious and may begin with small joints. Prodrome symptoms include fever, malaise, weight loss, morning stiffness that persists, and lymphadenopathy. Joint symptoms are usually symmetric, and include pain, swelling, stiffness, and muscular weakness. In the fingers, proximal interphalangeal (PIP) and metacarpophalangeal (MCP) joints are usually involved, distal interphalangeal (DIP) usually spared.

B. Physical exam. Swelling, warmth, and tenderness of involved joints. As disease progresses, joint deformities develop, including ulnar deviation, hyperextension of PIP joint with flexion of DIP joint (swan-neck deformity), and PIP flexion with DIP hyperextension (boutonnière deformity). Rheumatoid nodules (bumps under the skin in areas of pressure, such as the back of the elbows) may be seen.

C. Diagnostic tests

1. Eighty-five percent have positive rheumatoid factor, usually IgM reactive against IgG. Usually increased erythrocyte sedimentation rate (ESR), with moderate anemia and sometimes positive antinuclear antibody (ANA).

2. X-ray shows periarticular osteoporosis, juxta-articular erosions, commonly subluxation of upper cervical spine (atlantoaxial joint).

III. Differential diagnosis. The differential diagnosis of progressive polyarthritis includes, in addition to RA, degenerative joint disease, the seronegative spondyloarthropathies (rarer conditions like ankylosing spondylitis and Reiter's syndrome), connective tissue diseases, hypothyroidism, gout, and pseudogout.

IV. Pathophysiology

A. Etiology is unknown, most probably autoimmune; 3:1 female to male predominance. Peak onset occurs at age 20–45. Risk factors include family history, histocompatibility locus antigen (HLA) DW4.

B. Typical pathology involves inflammation of the synovial membrane followed by hypertrophy and proliferation of the cells lining the synovial membrane (called pannus tissue), which erode into the soft tissue of the joint. Microscopic findings include the rheumatoid nodule, a focus of central necrosis surrounded by a palisade of connective tissue cells and granulation tissue.

C. **Complications** of RA can include amyloid deposits, Felty's syndrome (splenomegaly and neutropenia accompanying the arthropathy), Sjögren's syndrome (lymphocytic infiltration of the lacrimal and salivary glands), and other severe systemic vasculitides.

 ## OSTEOARTHRITIS (DEGENERATIVE JOINT DISEASE)

I. **Definition.** A chronic, progressive, noninflammatory osteoarthropathy primarily involving the articular cartilage.

II. **Clinical manifestations**

A. **History.** Onset is insidious, with stiffness, pain, crepitus. Symptoms precipitated by activity and relieved by rest. Minimal systemic involvement. Usually affects DIP and PIP joints in hand, as well as thumb, hip, knee, cervical and lumbar spine. May follow joint trauma.

B. **Physical exam.** Diminished range of motion, crepitation, and pain seen in interphalangeal and large weight-bearing joints. Look especially at hand for bony deformities: Heberden's nodes (DIP) and Bouchard's nodes (PIP).

C. **Diagnostic tests**

1. Serum tests, including rheumatoid factor, ESR, are usually normal.

2. X-ray shows narrowed joint space, increased subchondral bone density, osteophytes.

III. **Differential diagnosis.** Can be differentiated from RA by pattern of joint involvement, lack of systemic manifestations, normal lab tests, and characteristic x-ray findings.

IV. **Pathophysiology**

A. Persistent wear, trauma, aging, and obesity all contribute to this disease.

B. Classic pathology involves erosion of articular cartilage, osteophyte (bone spur) formation, and synovial hypertrophy with minimal inflammation.

SYSTEMIC LUPUS ERYTHEMATOSUS

I. **Definition.** An inflammatory autoimmune disease characterized by multiple organ involvement, joint symptoms, rash, and a positive ANA test.

II. **Clinical manifestations**

A. **History and physical exam.** SLE can affect nearly every organ system. A useful mnemonic to help you remember the American College of Rheumatology's 11 diagnostic criteria (of which 4 are needed to make the diagnosis) is "**Rina Hoaps, M.D.**" (**R**enal, **i**mmunologic, **n**eurologic, **A**NA positivity, **h**ematologic, **o**ral ulcers, **a**rthritis, **p**hotosensitivity, **s**erositis-pleuritis or carditis, **m**alar rash, **d**iscoid rash).

1. **Systemic:** fatigue, malaise, weight loss, fever, lymphadenopathy.

2. **Skin:** malar (butterfly) rash, discoid rash, photosensitivity, oral ulcers.

3. **Arthritis:** usually symmetric and nonerosive, involving hands, wrists, and knees.

4. **Renal:** ranges from mild proteinuria to renal failure. Nephrotic syndrome and rapidly progressive glomerulonephritis are common.

5. **Neurologic:** seizures, neuropathies, migraines, and behavioral and cognitive disturbances such as psychosis are all seen.

6. **Cardiac:** pericarditis, Libman-Sacks endocarditis (valvular lesions).

7. **Pulmonary:** pleuritis, tachypnea, cough, pneumonitis, small bilateral exudates.

8. **Gastrointestinal:** nausea, vomiting, anorexia, abdominal pain, hepatosplenomegaly.

B. **Lab findings.** Normochromic normocytic anemia, leukopenia, thrombocytopenia, increased ESR, false-positive serologic test for syphilis, increased serum globulin, positive Coombs' test, lowered complement, +LE cells, +ANA (autoantibodies to nucleic acids and ribonucleoprotein).

III. **Differential diagnosis.** SLE must be differentiated from discoid lupus (discoid rash with no other systemic disease), RA, and drug-induced lupus syndrome (seen with hydralazine, phenytoin, and procainamide).

IV. **Pathophysiology**

A. The vast majority of patients are young to middle-aged women. Prevalence is approximately 1:2000 people, with 8:1 female to male ratio. High twin concordance, with increased risk to people with HLA DR2 and DR3.

B. Etiology is unclear, but there is some evidence for defective suppressor T cells allowing overactive B cells to produce antibodies. Viral infection may contribute to disease induction in susceptible hosts.

SCLERODERMA

I. **Definition.** A chronic debilitating disease, affecting connective tissue in multiple organ systems. Also known as progressive systemic sclerosis (PSS), it has a 4% female to male ratio in terms of prevalence.

A. **CREST** variant of scleroderma: patients with **c**alcinosis, **R**aynaud's, **e**sophageal involvement, **s**clerodactyly, and **t**elangiectasias; thought to have a more benign course.

B. There are two forms of localized scleroderma without systemic effects:

1. **Morphea,** with localized skin lesions of scleroderma that heal completely.

2. **Linear,** which appears as isolated lines of sclerotic skin on the extremities in children.

II. **Clinical manifestations**

A. **History and physical exam.** Like SLE, scleroderma affects nearly every organ system.

1. **Skin:** first, changes are usually symmetric; painless swelling of hands, with tightened, thickened skin. Later trunk, face ("purse-string mouth"), and more proximal extremities become involved. Also seen are telangiectasic skin rashes and subcutaneous calcinosis.

2. **Raynaud's phenomenon** is seen in 90% of patients with scleroderma. It is a cold-related vasospasm of vessels in the distal extremities that leads to cyanosis and blanching, possibly to infarction in severe cases.

3. **Joints:** Joint stiffness and polyarthritis are common.

4. **GI:** Decreased peristalsis in lower esophagus leads to reflux, esophagitis, and Barret's metaplasia, increasing the risk of malignancy. Duodenal hypermotility leads to bacterial overgrowth and malabsorption. Wide-mouth colonic diverticula are also seen.

5. **Pulmonary.** Fibrosis leads to restrictive lung disease. Pulmonary vascular involvement can lead to pulmonary hypertension and cor pulmonale.

6. **Cardiac:** Myocardial fibrosis can lead to congestive heart failure and arrhythmias. Pericarditis can lead, rarely, to cardiac tamponade.

7. **Renal:** Can lead to progressive renal insufficiency, proteinuria and malignant hypertension.

B. Diagnostic tests

1. Increased ESR, decreased complement, increased ANA. Antibodies with nucleolar staining pattern are almost exclusively seen in scleroderma.

2. **X-ray** can show resorption of tufts of the distal phalanges, radius, ulna, ribs, and mandible.

III. Pathophysiology. Autoimmune disease with unknown etiology.

TEMPORAL ARTERITIS (GIANT CELL ARTERITIS)

I. Definition. A large-vessel vasculitis that affects branches of the carotid artery.

II. Clinical manifestations

A. History. Affects patients more than 50 years old almost exclusively. Presents with headache, jaw claudication, altered vision, fatigue, extremity stiffness, myalgias, fever, and weight loss.

B. Physical exam. Vision changes, including sudden loss of vision in one eye, prominent and tender temporal arteries.

C. Diagnostic test. Elevated ESR. Definitive diagnosis is made with temporal artery biopsy, but many false-negatives occur due to segmental involvement of the involved vessel.

III. Differential diagnosis. As many of the presenting signs and symptoms of temporal arteritis—such as headache, fever, and myalgias—are very nonspecific, the differential is usually huge. Temporal arteritis should especially be considered in any elderly patient with typical symptoms and an elevated ESR. It is an important diagnosis to make, as high-dose steroids given promptly can save a patient's vision.

IV. Pathophysiology. Many feel that temporal arteritis and polymyalgia rheumatica (a syndrome of symmetric proximal muscle pain and stiffness) are ends of the same disease spectrum, as many patients with one syndrome also display signs of the other.

CHAPTER 23

Neurologic Diseases

M y message to medical students for hospital clerkships is usually quite straightforward. Never underestimate the value of listening carefully, asking questions, being punctual, showing respect for your patients and teachers, and being honest and sincere. If you combine these simple dictums with an earnest and genuine desire to further your medical education and enhance your ability to care for others, there is no limit to how much you can achieve as a physician. I have seen this proven time and time again.

Humayun J. Chaudhry, D.O., FACP

After graduating from New York University and the New York College of Osteopathic Medicine (NYCOM) of New York Institute of Technology, Dr. Chaudhry completed an internal medicine residency at Winthrop-University Hospital, Mineola, New York, where he served as Chief Resident. He has Master's degrees from NYU and Harvard School of Public Health and is currently Assistant Dean for Pre-Clinical Education and Chairman and Clinical Associate Professor of Medicine at NYCOM. Dr. Chaudhry is also a flight surgeon in the United States Air Force Reserve and Medical Operations Flight Commander of 514th Aeromedical Staging Squadron, McGuire Air For Base, New Jersey.

SEIZURE DISORDER (EPILEPSY)

I. **Definition.** A group of disorders characterized by paroxysmal transitory changes in mental status and motor activity. There are two general types of seizures: **focal,** which are limited to one part of the brain, and **generalized,** which are more global in scope.

II. **Clinical manifestations.** Different types of seizures exhibit different clinical findings.

A. **Focal seizures**

1. **Motor:** Premonitory aura precedes focal convulsion, and consciousness is often retained. In **Jacksonian** epilepsy, there is a characteristic "march" of motor events through the body as the seizure slowly spreads through different areas of the cortex.

2. **Sensory:** flashing lights, tingling numbness are reported without motor events. Electroencephalogram (EEG) often shows discharge in the parietal and occipital lobes.

3. **Temporal lobe:** characterized by automatisms, emotional distress, hallucinations, autonomic dysfunctions, and complex behavioral changes such as hyperreligiosity.

B. Generalized seizures

1. **Grand mal** (tonic-clonic). Usually a sequence of tonic-clonic contractions, loss of bowel and bladder control, flaccid coma, postictal confusion. No aura or focality.

2. **Petit mal** (absence). Brief blank spells, myoclonic jerks, akinetic seizures. Most common in children. Three-per-second spike-and-wave morphology on EEG.

III. Pathophysiology

A. Initial events in the seizure cycle are unclear. A group of neurons begin firing synchronously, often recruiting neighboring groups. Seizures may be precipitated by drugs, hypoxia, hypoglycemia, sensory stimulation, trauma, or intracranial masses.

B. Focal seizures tend to be caused by local conditions, such as tumors and trauma, while generalized seizures are usually idiopathic, toxic, or metabolic.

COMA

I. Definition. A state of unconsciousness from which the patient cannot be aroused.

II. Clinical manifestations

A. **Physical exam** of patient should include vital signs, pain responses, careful inspection (note **Battle's** sign, the discoloration of skin behind the ear associated with skull fractures), pupillary and respiratory patterns, passive motion and limb-drop-maneuvers to search for hemiparesis, decerebrate or decorticate rigidity, nuchal rigidity, "doll's head" maneuver, ice-water caloric response.

B. **Diagnostic tests** should include: complete blood count (CBC), urinalysis (U/A), arterial blood gases (ABG), electrocardiogram (ECG), electrolytes, blood alcohol and toxicology levels, liver and kidney function tests, glucose level, prothrombin (PT) and activated partial thromboplastin time (PTT), and, if indicated, EEG, lumbar puncture (LP), computed tomography (CT) scan, and magnetic resonance imaging (MRI).

III. Differential diagnosis and pathophysiology. Principal question is etiology of coma.

A. **Intracranial etiologies** include trauma, vascular disease, tumors, central nervous system infections, seizure disorders, increased intracranial pressure.

B. **Extracranial etiologies** include shock (including post-MI), metabolic disorders (hypoglycemia, hepatic disturbances, acidosis, electrolyte disturbances), drug effects, systemic trauma (hyperthermia and hypothermia, electric shock, anaphylaxis).

C. A useful mnemonic to remember is **AEIOU TIPS:**

Alcoholism
Encephalopathy
Insulin excess or deficiency
Opiates and other drugs
Uremia and metabolic disorders
Trauma
Infection
Psychiatric disorders
Syncope

 CEREBROVASCULAR DISORDERS (STROKE AND TRANSIENT ISCHEMIC ATTACK)

 I. Definition. Acute derangement in neurologic function due to inadequate cerebral circulation. A **transient ischemic attack** (TIA) is any acute neurologic impairment that clears within 24 hours.

 II. Clinical manifestations. Premonitory signs may include headache, dizziness, confusion. Actual symptoms depend on structures affected by loss of circulation. A classic TIA sign is **amaurosis fugax,** described as "a shade coming down over one eye." Strokes may also be associated with vomiting, convulsions, fever, nuchal rigidity, or changed mental status.

III. Differential diagnosis. Common signs and symptoms associated with occlusion of particular arteries include:

 A. Middle cerebral artery (MCA). Contralateral hemiparesis (arm and face more than leg), numbness, homonymous hemianopsia, aphasias, apraxia.

 B. Anterior cerebral artery (ACA). Contralateral hemiplegia (maximal in leg), grasp and suck reflexes, incontinence.

 C. Posterior cerebral artery (PCA). Contralateral hemisensory loss, hemianopsia, visual and memory defects.

 D. Internal carotid artery. Variable; may be silent or similar to MCA stroke with profound changes in mental status. Upper extremity Sx are common.

 E. Vertebrobasilar artery. May overlap with PCA stroke; ipsilateral cranial nerve problems; contralateral or bilateral motor, sensory, cerebellar signs; staggering gait, ataxia, dysphagia, confusion. See Fig. 23–1 for a diagram of the circle of Willis.

IV. Pathophysiology. Strokes are caused by one of three basic disease processes.

 A. Thrombosis. Atheromatous thrombosis often involves large arteries, especially the carotid, vertebral, and basilar. **Hypertensive** thrombosis often affects small arteries within the brain itself.

 B. Embolism. Emboli can consist of calcific atherosclerotic plaques, fat, air, and the like. Although emboli often occur in "showers," they may affect individual cortical arteries, causing isolated defects that appear and resolve suddenly.

 C. Hemorrhage. Often occurs secondary to trauma, rupture of congenital aneurysms, arteriovenous malformations, tumors, intracranial hypertensive ruptures.

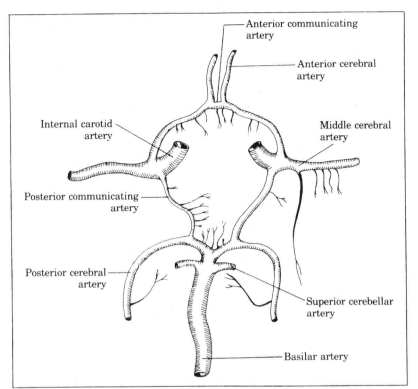

Fig. 23-1. The origins of the central arteries of the brain from the Circle of Willis.

MENINGITIS

I. **Definition.** Inflammation of the meninges of the brain or spinal cord, most often due to pneumococcus, *Neisseria meningitidis, Haemophilus influenzae,* mumps, Coxsackie virus, or echovirus.

II. **Clinical manifestations**

A. **History.** Seen most commonly in children, the elderly, and others with lowered immunity. Presents with headache, fever, chills, lethargy, vomiting, confusion, convulsions.

B. **Physical exam.** Nuchal rigidity, **Kernig's sign** (passive resistance to knee extension from flexed thigh position), **Brudzinski's sign** (neck flexion resulting in involuntary knee flexion in supine patient). Meningococcal meningitis is often associated with petechial mucous membrane and skin rashes.

C. **Diagnostic tests.** Increased peripheral white blood cell (WBC) count. Cerebrospinal fluid (CSF) findings vary by etiology (see Table 23–1 for details).

TABLE 23-1. Differential diagnosis on basis of CSF fluid

Disease type	CSF cell count	Predominant-cell type in CSF	Glucose (mg/100 ml)	Protein (mg/100 ml)
Normal	<5	Mononuclear	Two-thirds serum level or ~75	<40
Bacterial Meningitis	10–100,000	PMN	5–50	100–1,000
Viral				
Early phase	50–500	PMN	40–75	50–100
Late phase	20–200	Mononuclear	Normal	<100
Tuberculosis	20–1,000	Mononuclear	20–80	50–1,000
Fungal (usually)				
cryptococcus	25–500	Mononuclear	20–40	25–500

PMN = polymorphonuclear leukocyte.

III. Differential diagnosis. CSF findings can help differentiate etiological agents. See Table 23–1.

IV. Pathophysiology

 A. Entry may be through surgical or traumatic wound, or through inhaled droplets. Gram-positive meningitis may follow an infection of the lungs, middle ear, or sinuses.

 B. Infection in subarachnoid space → inflammatory reaction in pia, arachnoid, and CSF → accumulation of pus or toxin → damage to nerve roots, choroid plexuses, microvasculature, and interference with CSF flow leading to hydrocephalus.

CHAPTER **24**

Endocrine Diseases

The complaint I hear most often about doctors is that they will not talk to their patients adequately. A friendly and sincere interest in a patient's problem breaks the ice. Keep your appearance such that a patient will trust you. ("If he doesn't button up his shirt, how will he sew up my head?") Explain every move of the physical examination before it is done. Be courteous, respectful, and confidential. Show continued interest while in contact with the patient. Reappear frequently and at predictable times. Be reachable.

John Shillito, Jr., M.D., FACS

A graduate of Harvard College and Harvard Medical School, Dr. Shillito completed a surgical internship and residency at the Peter Bent Brigham Hospital, Boston, followed by a neurosurgical residency at Children's Hospital, Boston. He has served as Acting Chief of Neurosurgery at Children's Hospital, where the Shillito Fellowship in Pediatric Neurosurgery is named in his honor, and Professor of Surgery at Harvard Medical School. He has also served as President of the Congress of Neurological Surgeons.

 DIABETES MELLITUS

I. Definition. A group of chronic systemic diseases caused by insufficient insulin action, due either to a decreased level of insulin production (type 1) or to peripheral resistance to its effects (type 2), manifested by hyperglycemia.

  A. Type 1 diabetes (previously referred to as ketosis-prone, juvenile-onset, insulin dependent, or IDDM) tends to occur in younger individuals.

  B. Type 2 diabetes (previously referred to as non-insulin dependent diabetes mellitus, or NIDDM) is the most common type of diabetes (more than 90% of all cases of diabetes) and was also known as maturity-onset, late-onset, or adult-onset diabetes. Type 2 diabetes is becoming more prevalent in adolescents. Maturity-onset diabetes of youth (MODY) is associated with specific genetic mutations.

  C. Other types of diabetes are associated with genetic defects, pancreatic disease, medications (e.g., glucocorticoids, pentamidine, protease inhibitors), endocrinopathies (e.g., acromegaly, Cushing's syndrome), or pregnancy (also known as gestational diabetes).

  D. Impaired fasting glucose is defined as an early stage of persistent hyperglycemia (fasting plasma glucose between 110–125 mg/dl). **Impaired glucose tolerance** is defined as plasma glucose between 140–199 mg/dl 2 hours after a glucose load. While both are considered risk factors for the development of type 2 diabetes, abnormal glucose metabolism itself confers a significant risk for cardiovascular disease.

II. Clinical manifestations

A. **History and physical exam.** Classic triad of symptoms: **polyphagia, polyuria**, and **polydipsia.** Additional factors:

1. **Type 1**: age usually less than 30 years at onset. Onset is usually severe and rapidly progressive, with lassitude and weight loss. Other symptoms include blurred vision, leg cramps, and vomiting. May present in diabetic ketoacidosis (DKA); see p 292.

2. **Type 2**: common historical clues are: obesity, prior reactive hypoglycemia, history of recurrent soft tissue or fungal infections, women with vaginitis, and women whose children's birth weight is > 9 lbs. Onset is slow; often presents on screening blood or urine tests without symptoms. A skin finding, acanthosis nigricans, may be present (see COLOR PLATES.)

B. **Lab findings.** Diagnosis of diabetes mellitus (DM) can be made in an adult if one of three criteria are met.

1. Fasting plasma glucose of 126 mg/dl or greater, confirmed with a repeat test.

2. Random plasma glucose > 200 mg/dl and typical signs and symptoms of diabetes.

3. Plasma glucose > 200 mg/dl at 2 hours after ingestion of 75 gm of glucose (called an **oral glucose tolerance test**).

   Urine glucose correlates poorly with plasma glucose, and is no longer used in diagnosis or monitoring of diabetes mellitus. Hemoglobin A_1C levels should be used to measure degree of glycemic control over the previous 2–3 months.

III. Pathophysiology. Usual pathophysiology varies by type.

A. **Type 1**: significantly decreased or absent insulin production from pancreatic cells, thus decreased serum insulin levels. Autoimmune etiology is likely.

B. **Type 2**: insulin resistance due to defective insulin signalling in target cells. Insulin levels may be normal or somewhat increased, but inadequate to overcome the insulin resistance.

C. **Complications.** Acute and chronic complications of diabetes mellitus may be preventable. Progression of chronic complications may be slowed or halted completely.

1. **Diabetic ketoacidosis (DKA).** Seen more often in type 1 than type 2 diabetics, when lack of insulin causes a chain of events leading to metabolism of triglycerides, resulting in accumulation of ketoacids in the blood. Patients present with weakness, polyuria, polydipsia, **Kussmaul's respirations** (rapid, deep breathing), blurred vision, fruity-smelling breath, abdominal pain, and vomiting. Dehydration is significant. Stupor or coma indicates severe DKA. Common precipitants of DKA include infection, pregnancy, failure to keep to an insulin regimen, and myocardial infarction.

2. **Hyperosmolar hyperglycemic state.** Seen mainly in elderly patients with type 2 diabetes, severe dehydration and extremely high blood sugars (sometimes more than 2,000 mg/dl). Ketones may be present due to inanition, but generally do not contribute to acidosis. Can be triggered by myocardial infarction, stroke, infection, GI hemorrhage, some drugs (e.g., glucocorticoids), and stress due to surgery. Presents with a prodrome of polyuria and polydipsia, progressing to mental status changes ranging from confusion to stupor to coma. Can present with stroke, seizures, or with other neurologic signs.

3. **Cardiovascular complications.** Diabetes is so strongly linked with increased atherogenesis through a variety of factors, and increases the risk of heart disease by a factor of two in men and three in women, that any diabetic can be presumed to have some degree of underlying heart disease. Also, due to neuropathy of the cardiac nerves, many diabetics do not exhibit the characteristic symptoms of MI and thus can have silent infarctions.

4. **Neuropathy.** Many presentations, including: bilateral symmetrical sensory deficits, usually seen in a stocking and glove distribution; painful peripheral neuropathy, often described as burning in quality, tends to be worse at night; mononeuropathy; and impotence and gastroparesis due to involvement of autonomic system.

5. **Retinopathy.** If glucose is not controlled, diabetics develop proliferative and/or nonproliferative retinopathy within 20 years of onset of their disease (or within 20 years after onset of puberty). Retinal edema and exudates as well as neovascularization can be seen on ophthalmologic exam. Periodic eye screening (yearly or more frequently if needed) should be done for all diabetics, as laser photocoagulation can slow progression of some retinopathy.

6. **Renal failure.** A major problem in both types of diabetes, if poorly controlled. Presenting about 15 years after onset of diabetes (or 15 years after onset of puberty in type 1 diabetes). Kidney biopsies of diabetics show Kimmelstiel-Wilson lesions (nodular glomerulosclerosis) and diffuse hyaline thickening of glomerular basement membrane. Tight blood sugar control, blood pressure control (particularly with angiotensin converting enzyme [ACE] inhibitors or angiotensin receptor blockers [ARBs]), and low protein diet may prevent or slow renal deterioration.

 HYPERTHYROIDISM (THYROTOXICOSIS)

I. **Definition.** Clinical syndrome resulting from excess thyroid hormone.

II. **Clinical manifestations**

A. **History and physical exam.** Findings are outlined by organ system in Table 24–1.

B. **Lab findings.** Elevated levels of thyroxine (T4), Free T4, and triiodothyronine (T3). Suppressed thyroid stimulating hormone **(TSH).**

TABLE 24-1. Signs and symptoms of thyrotoxicosis

System	History	Physical exam
Constitutional	Fatigue, hyperactivity, insomnia, heat intolerance, ↑ appetite, weight loss	Hyperkinetism, tremulousness
Vital signs	N/A	Tachycardia, tachypnea, pyrexia, wide pulse pressure
Integument	Sweating, ↑ hair growth, pruritus, occasional urticaria	Warm, moist, fine hair; pretibial myxedema*; onycholysis; hyperpigmentation
Eyes*	Visual disturbance	Lid lag, stare, proptosis,* inflammation, ophthalmoplegia (upward gaze affected first), chemosis, periorbital edema
Neck	Neck mass	Goiter, lymphadenopathy
Cardiovascular	Palpitations, dyspnea	Hyperdynamic precordium, arrhythmias (new onset of atrial fibrillation or tachycardia)
Gastrointestinal	Increasing frequency of bowel movements, diarrhea	Active bowel sounds, splenomegaly*
Genitourinary	Nocturia, oligomenorrhea	N/A
Neuromuscular	Muscle weakness, tremor	Proximal muscle weakness, tremor, brisk deep tendon reflexes
Psychological	Emotional lability, nervousness	N/A

*Specifically characteristic of Graves' disease.

III. Differential diagnosis and pathophysiology. There are several common etiologies of hyperthyroidism.

    A. Graves' disease. TSH-like immunoglobulins stimulate a rise in thyroid hormone.

    B. Toxic multinodular goiter. Multiple autonomous areas of thyroid tissue lead to increased thyroid hormone production.

    C. Toxic adenoma. Overproduction of thyroid hormone by a single ("hot") nodule.

    D. Other less common causes include: thyroiditis, TSH-producing pituitary adenoma, trophoblastic tumors, iatrogenic or factitious exogenous thyroid hormone ingestion, and thyroid carcinoma.

HYPOTHYROIDISM

I. Definition. A multi-organ syndrome resulting from inadequate levels of thyroid hormone.

II. Clinical manifestations

A. History. Patients complain of feeling cold, lethargic, and depressed. Also constipation, myalgias, arthralgias, weight gain with no increased appetite, difficulty losing weight, and women may experience alteration in menses. Friends or family may note a bizarre sense of humor or frank psychosis.

B. Physical exam

1. Cool, coarse, rough, dry skin, with brittle hair and alopecia. Thinning of hair in the lateral third of the eyebrows (**Queen Anne's sign**) is frequently seen.

2. Periorbital edema and nonpitting puffiness (myxedema) throughout the body.

3. Bradycardia and delayed relaxation phase of deep tendon reflexes.

C. Diagnostic tests. Elevated TSH with low or low normal T4 and/or T3 are diagnostic of hypothyroidism. Anemia of multifactorial etiology is present in about one-fourth of patients. Low serum sodium, elevated protein in cerebrospinal fluid, low-grade proteinuria and moderately elevated serum cholesterol and creatine kinase are sometimes seen as well. Electrocardiogram (ECG) shows low voltage throughout.

III. Differential diagnosis and pathophysiology

A. Hashimoto's thyroiditis is the most common cause of hypothyroidism in the United States, and is an autoimmune attack on primarily thyroglobulin and thyroid peroxidase. Most commonly affects women 20 to 60 years old and presents with nontender, diffusely enlarged thyroid gland.

B. Iatrogenic hypothyroidism is seen in patients treated with I–131 (for thyrotoxicosis), thyroidectomy, or high-dose external radiation; and psychiatric patients taking lithium.

C. Iodine itself can inhibit the glandular release of thyroid hormone, and thus high doses of iodine can cause hypothyroidism (called the Wolff-Chaikoff effect). Can be seen in patients who have received a high dye load for radiologic procedures.

IV. Complications. The most serious complication of hypothyroidism is **myxedema coma**, usually brought on by concurrent illness. The risk of myxedema coma is not related to levels of circulating thyroid hormone or to replacement status.

HYPERCORTISOLISM (CUSHING'S SYNDROME)

I. Definition. Metabolic disease caused by glucocorticoid excess.

II. Clinical manifestations

A. History. Weakness, oligomenorrhea, easy bruising, and mental status changes.

B. Physical exam. Hypertension, purpura, abdominal striae, and muscle atrophy; characteristic habitus: central obesity with a "buffalo hump."

C. Diagnostic findings

1. Positive overnight dexamethasone suppression test (failure to suppress am cortisol).

2. Increased 24 hour urinary free cortisol.

3. Osteopenia on x-ray.

III. Differential diagnosis. There are four major causes of hypercortisolism:

A. Iatrogenic excess of any of several glucocorticoids.

B. Pituitary hyperfunction/adenoma **(Cushing's disease).**

C. Ectopic adrenocorticotropic hormone (ACTH) syndrome (causing **bilateral adrenal hyperplasia**).

D. Unilateral autonomous adrenal hypersecretion (**adrenal adenoma** or **carcinoma**).

IV. Pathophysiology of signs and symptoms (approximate frequency shown in parentheses).

A. Impaired glucose tolerance test (94%). Gluconeogenic effect of cortisol.

B. Central (truncal) obesity (88%). Increased lipid mobilization, redistribution of adipose stores.

C. Hypertension (82%). From accompanying mineralocorticoid activity, seen especially in ectopic ACTH syndrome, K^+ wasting.

D. Oligomenorrhea (72%). Along with decreased fertility and virilism (hirsutism), caused by androgen excess.

E. Osteoporosis (58%). Antagonism of $1,25(OH)_2$ vitamin D and inhibition of bone cell activation.

F. Purpura and striae (42%) and **muscle atrophy and weakness** (36%). Caused by catabolic effects of steroids.

HYPOCORTISOLISM (ADDISON'S DISEASE)

I. Definition. Syndrome consisting of many nonspecific symptoms caused by adrenal cortical insufficiency.

II. Clinical manifestations

A. History. Fatigue, weakness, weight loss, anorexia, irritability, sleeplessness.

B. Physical exam. Hypotension, hyperpigmentation of skin, loss of sexual hair in women.

C. Diagnostic tests. Most common screening test is a high-dose **corticotropin stimulation test**: if, 60 minutes after administration of synthetic ACTH, serum cortisol remains below 18 ug/dl, adrenal insufficiency is indicated. Baseline ACTH levels are generally elevated. Reduced serum sodium, increased potassium and BUN, and eosinophilia are seen in many but not all patients. Computed tomography (CT) may show small, noncalcified adrenals; adrenal enlargement; or normal-size adrenal glands.

III. Differential diagnosis. Hypocortisolism is seen in syndromes of polyglandular failure. Thus you should look for thyroiditis, DM, pernicious anemia, and hypoparathyroidism in these patients.

IV. Pathophysiology

    A. Causes of primary adrenal insufficiency may be autoimmune, infectious, congenital, chemical, ischemic, hemorrhagic, or infiltrative. Specific causes include infections or neoplasms associated with human immunodeficiency virus (HIV) disease, tuberculosis, tumors, and such drugs as etomidate and ketoconazole.

    B. In patients with hypocortisolism, even very minor illnesses can trigger an **Addisonian crisis,** in which they present with shock, fever, nausea and vomiting, hyperthermia, hypoglycemia, hyponatremia, and hyperkalemia. This is a medical emergency that requires immediate administration of IV glucose, saline, and hydrocortisone, as well as treatment of the underlying causes.

HYPERCALCEMIA

  I. Definition. An elevation of ionized calcium in serum.

  II. Clinical manifestations

    A. History. Many variable and nonspecific symptoms, generally related to neurologic and neuromuscular function; these include somnolence, apathy, memory loss, mental disturbances, irritability, stupor-coma (c/w acute, pronounced hypercalcemia), and proximal muscle weakness.

    B. Physical exam. Findings on exam are rarely helpful. Some associated findings are band keratopathy, hypertension, hypotonia, and reduced deep tendon reflexes.

    C. Diagnostic tests

      1. Chemistry. Calcium levels should be evaluated after correction for amount of serum albumin present. Since albumin binds calcium, the effective (ionized) calcium level is related to albumin concentration. Thus for every 1.0-mg decrease in albumin (normal = 4 mg/dl), you should add 0.8 mg/dl to the calcium level to get the actual calcium concentration. The reverse is true for hyperalbuminemia. For example:

      If **serum calcium** = 7.5 mg/dl and **albumin** = 2.0 mg/dl (decreased by 2 mg/dl), then the **corrected calcium** = 7.5 + 2(0.8) = 9.1 mg/dl.

      Or, if **serum calcium** = 11.0 mg/dl and **albumin** = 5.0 mg/dl (increased by 1 mg/dl), then the **corrected calcium** = 11.0 − 1(0.8) = 10.2 mg/dl.

      2. ECG can show a shortened Q-T interval, atrial arrythmias and various atrioventricular (AV) blocks.

      3. X-ray indicates soft tissue calcifications.

  III. Differential diagnosis. Causes include: malignancy (most frequent cause in hospital populations), primary hyperparathyroidism (most frequent in general population), sarcoidosis, vitamin D intoxication, thyrotoxicosis, milk-alkali syndrome, adrenal insufficiency, immobilization, vitamin A intoxication, and pheochromocytoma.

IV. Pathophysiology

A. Malignancies can cause hypercalcemia by several different mechanisms:

1. **Multiple myeloma.** Cytokine production and osteolytic bone disease are the most common mechanisms. May also be caused by hyperalbuminemia or immunoglobulins with increased binding capacity for calcium, both of which would result in falsely elevated serum calcium, but normal ionized calcium.

2. **Bone metastases** (e.g., from breast cancer). Direct bone invasion, but increased calcium probably due to local mediator production (e.g. cytokines, prostaglandins).

3. **Squamous cell lung cancer, renal cell cancer.** Due to production of parathyroid hormone related protein (PTHrP), which is distinct from intact PTH on bioassay and may be measured separately.

4. **Lymphoma.** Excess production of $1,25(OH)_2$ vitamin D, causing increased intestinal calcium absorption and bone resorption.

B. In **primary hyperparathyroidism**, autonomous production of PTH causes increased calcium. The interaction between the two most important regulators of calcium metabolism, **PTH** and **$1,25(OH)_2$ vitamin D**, is depicted below:

$$\uparrow \text{ renal phosphorus excretion}$$

$$PTH \rightarrow \quad \uparrow 1,25(OH)_2D \text{ production} \rightarrow \uparrow \text{ intestinal } Ca^{2+} \text{ mobilization}$$

$$\uparrow \text{ bone mobilization of } Ca^{2+} \text{ [probably synergistic with } 1,25(OH)_2D]$$

CHAPTER **25**

Hematologic Diseases

The first and most important thing is to touch the patient. And I don't mean shaking their hand as an introduction but comforting them and holding their hand when they are in pain or sorrow, because patients are vulnerable. The second most important thing is that if you don't know what you're treating, don't treat it and get some assistance.

Barbara Ross-Lee, D.O., Jr., M.S., FACOFP

Dr. Ross-Lee, a sister of singer Diana Ross, graduated from Wayne State University in Detroit and Michigan State University's College of Osteopathic Medicine, where she was appointed Chair of the Family Medicine Department, Associate Dean for Health Policy and, in 1993, as Dean. A member of the National Institutes of Health Advisory Committee on Research on Women's Health and President of the Association of Academic Health Centers, Dr. Ross-Lee currently serves as Dean of the New York College of Osteopathic Medicine and Vice President for Health Sciences and Medical Affairs at the New York Institute of Technology.

BLEEDING DISORDERS

I. **Definition.** Disorders of any element of the hemostatic system that result in an increased tendency to bleed. Dysfunction results from **abnormal hemostatic plug formation (platelet disorder)** or **clot formation (defect of the coagulation cascade).**

II. **Clinical manifestations**

A. **History and physical exam.** In general, in **platelet disorders** there will be a history of bruising or bleeding during the course of another serious illness or after drug ingestion; platelet disorders are rarely hereditary, and a lifelong history of bruising and bleeding is rare. In **coagulation disorders** there will be a lifelong history of easy bruising or bleeding, with a family history of bleeding in one or both sexes.

Platelet disorders result in skin and mucous membrane petechiae, purpura, and ecchymosis, whereas coagulation disorders typically result in deep tissue bleeding (hemarthrosis, subcutaneous and intramuscular hemorrhages, intracerebral hemorrhages).

B. **Diagnostic tests**

1. **Bleeding time.** Platelet aggregation at the site of vascular injury results in a **hemostatic plug** formation. This occurs prior to organized clotting. The bleeding time measures how long it takes a standardized

skin incision to stop bleeding. The bleeding time is prolonged in all platelet abnormalities but is normal in coagulation disorders.

2. **Prothrombin time (PT) and partial thromboplastin time (PTT).** Clot formation results from the activation of the **coagulation cascade.** The cascade involves sequences of plasma protein activations in two pathways. The **intrinsic pathway** begins with activation of factor XII, while the **extrinsic pathway** begins with exposure of plasma to tissue factor, which subsequently forms a complex with factor VII. Both pathways result in the activation of factor X, which then converts prothrombin to thrombin, which in turn converts fibrinogen to fibrin. Thrombin also activates factor XIII, which converts monomer fibrin to stabilized fibrin. See Fig. 25–1 for a diagram of the pathways.

   a. **PTT**, also known as the activated partial thromboplastin time (aPTT), measures the ability to form a fibrin clot by the intrinsic pathway. It therefore tests for all factors except factor VII.

   b. **PT** measures the ability to form a fibrin clot by the extrinsic pathway (see Fig. 25–1). A normal PT indicates normal levels of factor VII and those factors common to both the intrinsic and extrinsic pathways (V, X, thrombin, and fibrinogen).

III. **Differential diagnosis of common bleeding disorders**

A. **Platelet disorders**

   1. **Increased destruction**

      a. **Immune-mediated**

         (1) Drug-induced thrombocytopenia

         (2) Idiopathic thrombocytopenic purpura (ITP)

         (3) Transfusion reaction

         (4) Fetal-maternal incompatibility

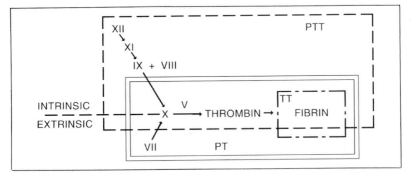

Fig. 25-1. Highly simplified scheme of the coagulation pathways. Shown are the factors involved in the intrinsic *(top)* and extrinsic *(bottom)* pathways. Also depicted by boxes are those aspects of the coagulation system tested by the three most common laboratory tests: thrombin time (TT); partial thromboplastin time (PTT); and prothrombin time (PT). (Modified from M. C. Fishman, et al.: Medicine, 3rd ed., Philadelphia: Lippincott Williams & Wilkins, 1991.)

(5) Vasculitis (e.g., systemic lupus erythematosus [SLE])

(6) Lymphoreticular disorders (e.g., chronic lymphocytic leukemia [CLL])

b. Non-immune mediated

(1) Prosthetic heart valves

(2) Thrombotic thrombocytopenic purpura (TTP)

(3) Sepsis

(4) Disseminated intravascular coagulation (DIC)

(5) Hemolytic-uremic syndrome

2. Decreased production

a. Abnormal marrow

(1) Marrow infiltration (e.g., leukemia, lymphoma)

(2) Marrow suppression

b. Inherited defect in production

(1) Wiskott-Aldrich syndrome

(2) May-Hegglin anomaly

c. Vitamin deficiencies

(1) B_{12}

(2) Folic acid

3. Platelet sequestration and pooling (e.g., splenomegaly)

4. Dilutional, secondary to massive transfusion

B. Defects of coagulation cascade

1. Inherited coagulation defects

a. Classic hemophilia (type A)

b. Christmas disease (type B)

c. Von Willebrand's disease

2. Acquired coagulation defects

a. DIC

b. Vitamin K deficiency or malabsorption

c. Hepatic failure

IV. Pathophysiology and clinical manifestations of specific bleeding disorders

A. Platelet disorders

1. ITP

a. Pathophysiology. Peripheral platelet destruction due to antiplatelet antibody; bone marrow examination reveals normal numbers of megakaryocytes.

b. Clinical manifestations. Platelets $< 50,000$, petechiae, purpura; predominantly affects pediatric population.

2. TTP

a. **Pathophysiology.** Unknown etiology; microangiopathic hemolytic anemia results in arteriolar occlusion and renal and neurologic dysfunction.

b. **Clinical manifestations.** Thrombocytopenic purpura, hemolytic anemia, acute renal failure, fluctuating neurologic signs (headache, seizure, acute psychosis), fever; fibrin split products usually present, suggesting DIC-like syndrome.

3. **Drug-induced thrombocytopenia**

a. **Pathophysiology.** Thrombocytopenia induced through marrow toxicity or platelet destruction. ETOH and thiazide diuretics suppress bone marrow production of megakaryocytes. Quinine, heparin, methyldopa, and sulfonamides induce an immunologic response that results in peripheral platelet destruction.

b. **Clinical manifestations.** Severe, sudden-onset thrombocytopenia and bleeding, which usually resolves after the offending agent is discontinued.

B. **Inherited coagulation defects**

1. **Classic hemophilia (type A)**

a. **Pathophysiology.** X-linked recessive gene causes either complete inability to produce factor VIII or production of a functionally inactive factor VIII.

b. **Clinical manifestations.** Episodic deep tissue bleeding (hemarthrosis, subcutaneous and intramuscular hemorrhages, intracerebral hemorrhages).

2. **Von Willebrand's disease**

a. **Pathophysiology.** Autosomal dominant inheritance. Disease caused by either a decrease in the amount of von Willebrand's factor (type I) or by synthesis of abnormal forms of the glycoprotein complex (types IIa and IIb). Von Willebrand's factor normally associates with factor VIII and stabilizes it; it is needed for platelet aggregation; and is needed for platelets to attach to injured vascular endothelium. All three functions are compromised in von Willebrand's disease.

b. **Clinical manifestations.** Normal platelet count, severe mucous membrane bleeding (epistaxis), easy bruising, and prolonged bleeding from wounds.

C. **Acquired coagulation defects**

1. **DIC**

a. **Pathophysiology.** Results from widespread activation of coagulation cascade leading to consumption of coagulation factors, prothrombin, and fibrinogen. Accompanying fibrinolysis yields high levels of fibrin split products (FSP), whose antihemostatic properties further enhance bleeding. Secondary to infection (bacterial sepsis), abnormal production or liberation of procoagulant tissue factors (tumors, fat emboli, necrotic tissue, massive acute hemolysis, obstetric catastrophe), and endothelial damage (shock, stroke, burns, acute glomerulonephritis, and Rocky Mountain spotted fever).

b. **Clinical manifestations.** Increased fibrin split products; microangiopathic hemolytic anemia; embolic and thrombotic phenomena; prolonged PT and PTT.

2. **Vitamin K deficiency or malabsorption**

a. **Pathophysiology.** Hepatocytes normal but unable to synthesize active form of factors II (prothrombin), VII, IX, X. Factor VII has the shortest half-life among the coagulation factors, and thus prolonged PT is the first evidence of vitamin K deficiency.

b. **Clinical manifestations.** Prolonged PT, same clinical picture as that for hemophilia.

3. **Hepatic failure**

a. **Pathophysiology.** Often secondary to ETOH.

b. **Clinical manifestations.** Hepatocytes damaged and unable to synthesize coagulation factors II, VII, IX, X; hypoalbuminemia; portal hypertension results in decreased platelets secondary to hypersplenism; same clinical picture as hemophilia.

ANEMIA

I. Definition. A reduction in the oxygen-carrying capacity of the blood resulting from a decreased concentration of hemoglobin. Anemia results from either **decreased RBC production** (deficiency of hematopoietic inputs or bone marrow failure) or **peripheral RBC destruction or loss** (hemolysis or hemorrhage).

II. Clinical manifestations

A. **History and physical exam.** For history, inquire about family and ethnic history, drug and toxic exposures, obstetric and menstrual history, external blood loss (gastrointestinal and genitourinary), dietary habits, and rapidity of onset. On physical exam, notice general appearance, vital signs (hypotension, tachycardia), skin (pallor of the conjunctivae, lips, oral mucosa, nail beds; jaundice, petechiae, purpura), mouth (glossitis), heart (listen for flow murmurs, prosthetic valves), abdomen (splenomegaly), rectum (examine stool for occult or gross blood), lymph nodes (infiltrative lesions, infections).

B. **Diagnostic tests**

1. **Hematocrit (Hct) and hemoglobin (Hgb).** Concentrations of circulating erythrocytes of Hct < 36 percent or Hgb < 12 gm/100 ml is considered anemic.

2. **Reticulocyte count.** Indicates whether an anemia is due to destruction or loss, or to inadequate production. An anemia with a low or normal reticulocyte count is thought to be due to inadequate production of RBCs in the bone marrow, while an anemia with a high reticulocyte count is thought to be due to RBC destruction or loss (see Fig. 10–1 for a summary of the diagnostic approach to anemia).

III. Differential diagnosis of anemia

A. Decreased RBC production

1. **Deficiency of hematopoietic inputs**
   a. Iron deficiency
   b. Folate deficiency
   c. B_{12} deficiency
   d. Thalassemia
   e. Anemia of chronic disease
   f. Sideroblastic anemia

2. **Bone marrow failure**
   a. Drug toxicity (myelosuppressive drugs, chloramphenicol, sulfonamides)
   b. Congenital defect (Fanconi's anemia)
   c. Infections (hepatitis C)
   d. Irradiation
   e. Neoplasm (leukemia)
   f. Toxins (benzene)
   g. Idiopathic

B. Peripheral RBC destruction or loss

1. **Acquired hemolysis**
   a. **Environmental factors**
      (1) Autoimmune: isohemagglutinins (transfusion reaction) or autoantibodies (warm and cold).
         (a) Idiopathic
         (b) Drugs (penicillin, quinidine, methyldopa)
         (c) Underlying disease (SLE, non-Hodgkin's lymphoma, CLL, mycoplasma)
      (2) Non-immune mediated
         (a) Microangiopathic (DIC, TTP, hemolytic-uremic syndrome, malignant hypertension)
         (b) Hypersplenism
         (c) Prosthetic cardiac valve
         (d) Burns
         (e) Infections (malaria)
         (f) Drugs (sulfonamides)
         (g) Toxins (heavy metals)
   b. **Membrane defects**
      (1) Paroxysmal nocturnal hemoglobinuria (PNH)
      (2) Spur-cell anemia
      (3) Wilson's disease

2. Congenital hemolysis

a. Defects of cell interior

(1) Hemoglobinopathies (sickle cell anemia, thalassemia)

(2) Enzymopathies (glucose-6-phosphate dehydrogenase, or G-6-P-D)

b. Membrane defects: hereditary spherocytosis, elliptocytosis

3. Hemorrhage. Usually acute gastrointestinal (GI) or genitourinary (GU) bleed.

IV. Clinical manifestations and pathophysiology of specific anemias

A. Anemias of decreased RBC production

1. Iron deficiency

a. History and physical exam. Pallor, fatigue, headaches, glossitis (smooth red tongue), angular cheilitis, koilonychia (spooning of the nails), pica, and tachycardia.

b. Diagnostic tests. Hypochromic microcytic smear (see COLOR PLATES); target cells; anisocytosis and poikilocytosis when severe; $\downarrow$ serum ferritin; absent or low serum iron; $\uparrow$ total iron binding capacity (TIBC); reticulocytes low or normal; $\downarrow$ Hct.

c. Pathophysiology. Depletion of iron stores (often due to blood loss), causing defective hemoglobin production.

2. Megaloblastic anemia

a. History and physical exam. Pallor, anorexia, glossitis; B_{12} deficiency causes neurologic dysfunction (symmetric paresthesias, loss of proprioception, ataxia, psychosis: "megaloblastic madness").

b. Diagnostic tests. Macrocytic blood smear, hypersegmented polymorphonuclear (PMN) cells (see COLOR PLATES), Howell-Jolly bodies, macro-ovalocytes, megablastic marrow with large erythrocyte and leukocyte precursors and abnormal megakaryocytes, low serum B_{12} or RBC folate levels; Schilling test may be useful in the diagnosis of pernicious anemia due to vitamin B_{12} deficiency, though a positive test for antibodies to intrinsic factor is specific for the diagnosis of pernicious anemia; reticulocyte count low, $\downarrow$ Hct; bone marrow biopsy is sometimes necessary to rule out myelodysplastic syndrome and other hematologic malignancies.

c. Pathophysiology. Faulty erythropoiesis due to $\downarrow$ nucleic acid synthesis, secondary to B_{12} or folate deficiency; B_{12} deficiency results from poor B_{12} intake over a long period of time, deficiency of gastric intrinsic factor (pernicious anemia), bacterial overgrowth, or loss of ileal function.

3. Thalassemias

a. History and physical exam. Pallor, fatigue, hepatosplenomegaly, facial bossing.

b. Diagnostic tests. Definitive diagnosis by Hgb electrophoresis, microcytic hypochromic blood smear, target cells, $\uparrow$ reticulocytes;

distinguish thalassemia smear from iron deficiency anemia smear by basophilic stippling and relatively higher Hct in thalassemia.

c. **Pathophysiology.** Hemoglobinopathy caused by unbalanced alpha- or beta-hemoglobin-chain synthesis, results in alpha-thalassemia or beta-thalassemia. Failure of the alpha- and beta-globin chains to match up reduces the hemoglobinization of erythroblasts to concentrations inadequate for survival, and leads to intracellular accumulations of unmatched chains, which aggregate as inclusion bodies. Most erythroblasts die in the marrow, a process called ineffective erythropoiesis, and those few that make it to the peripheral circulation are unable to slip through the splenic cords, due to the inclusion bodies, and are destroyed.

4. **Marrow aplasia**

   a. **History and physical exam.** Pallor, bleeding, lassitude.

   b. **Diagnostic tests.** Normochromic normocytic anemia on blood smear, pancytopenia, "dry," fatty, hypocellular marrow found on marrow aspiration.

   c. **Pathophysiology.** Depressed hematopoiesis due to drug toxicity in 50% of cases (myelosuppressive drugs, chloramphenicol, sulfonamides), congenital defects (Fanconi's anemia), infections (hepatitis C), irradiation, neoplasm (myelophthisis and myelofibrosis), toxins (benzene).

B. **Anemias of RBC destruction or loss.** The four most common causes of RBC destruction are **autoimmune hemolytic anemia, mechanical hemolysis, sickle cell anemia, and G-6-P-D deficiency.** Lab findings of all hemolytic anemias include elevated indirect bilirubin, decreased serum haptoglobin, elevated reticulocyte count, and decreased Hct. Following are the clinical manifestations and pathophysiology of selected **anemias of peripheral RBC destruction.**

   1. **Hereditary spherocytosis**

      a. **History and physical exam.** Pallor, splenomegaly, jaundice, gallstones, and malaise.

      b. **Diagnostic tests.** Spherocytes on blood smear, ↑ osmotic fragility of RBCs, hyperbilirubinemia, elevated mean corpuscular hemoglobin concentration (MCHC).

      c. **Pathophysiology.** Autosomal dominant defect in RBC spectrin causing deficit in surface area relative to volume. The low surface-to-volume ratio creates a slightly obese, rigid structure that lacks the suppleness necessary for traversing through the tight exits of the splenic cords. Stasis in the cords subjects red cells to deficiency of glucose, low pH, O_2 free radicals discharged by the cramped macrophages, and piecemeal loss of lipid bilayer. Each transit through the splenic cords results in ↓ surface area and ↑ rigidity. Eventually the small, unbending spherocyte gets lodged in the splenic cords and is hemolyzed.

2. **G-6-P-D deficiency**

   a. **History and physical exam.** Pallor; hemolysis is sudden and episodic; jaundice; history of sulfonamide ingestion.

   b. **Diagnostic tests.** Abnormal G-6-P-D assay, polychromatophilia, poikilocytosis.

   c. **Pathophysiology.** Intrinsic RBC defect of G-6-P-D deficiency results in an inability of the RBC to make the reducing agent NADPH. The RBC cannot handle oxidative stresses and hemolysis results. Sulfonamides are the most common oxidative stress to initiate hemolysis.

3. **Sickle cell anemia**

   a. **History and physical exam.** Pallor, fatigue, systolic ejection murmur; episodic **sickle cell crises** with fever, pain in back and joints, jaundice, vascular thrombosis, and microinfarction result in leg ulcers, functional asplenism, increased risk of aseptic necrosis of the femoral heads, and salmonella osteomyelitis; chronic hemolysis results in increased incidence of pigmented gallstones.

   b. **Diagnostic tests.** Definitive diagnosis by sickle test and Hgb electrophoresis; blood smear shows sickled cells (see COLOR PLATES), fragmented forms, target cells.

   c. **Pathophysiology.** Hemoglobinopathy caused by valine replacement of glutamate at the sixth position of the beta-hemoglobin chain. The altered hemoglobin, called hemoglobin S, has a strong tendency to form long crystalline aggregates when deoxygenated. These aggregates cause the RBC to assume the abnormal sickle shape. These sickled cells are then destroyed in the periphery. Intravascular sickling causes vascular sludging and thrombosis, which produces gradual but widespread tissue infarction.

4. **Autoimmune hemolytic anemias**

   a. **Warm-reacting antibodies**

      (1) **History and physical exam.** History of drug ingestion or underlying disease. Pallor, jaundice, hepatosplenomegaly, thrombophlebitis.

      (2) **Diagnostic tests.** Direct Coombs' test establishes the presence of bound immunoglobulin or complement on a patient's erythrocytes by demonstrating agglutination of the erythrocytes with either anti-immunoglobulin or anticomplement antibody. Blood smear shows spherocytes.

      (3) **Pathophysiology.** Most common of immune mediated hemolytic anemias. Warm-reacting antibodies have maximal effect above 31°C and are IgG antibodies. Thirty percent of autoimmune anemias are idiopathic, and 30 percent result from drug reactions. Drugs implicated include penicillin and quinidine. Penicillin attaches to the RBC membrane and serves as a hapten against which antibodies can be directed. Quinidine

stimulates the production of antibodies, and drug-antibody complexes attach non-specifically to the surface of RBCs, at which point the complement cascade is activated and hemolysis occurs. This is the most common mechanism of drug-induced hemolytic anemia. Underlying disease, such as infection (mycoplasma, Epstein-Barr virus) and lymphoproliferative disorders (chronic lymphocytic leukemia), have also been implicated in the formation of warm antibodies. Spherocytosis results from the ability of the IgG to opsonize the RBC and from partial phagocytosis by the reticuloendothelial system. Progressive loss of erythrocyte membrane renders it rigid and it assumes a spherical shape.

b. Cold-reacting antibodies

(1) History and physical exam. Pain and ulceration in chilled areas of the body, usually toes and fingers.

(2) Diagnostic tests. Diagnosis made by high titer of cold agglutinins (IgM) and low C_3.

(3) Pathophysiology. Cold-reacting antibodies have maximal effect below 31°C, are called cold agglutinins, and are IgM antibodies. Because IgM is multivalent, either hemolysis (due to complement activation) or agglutination of RBCs may dominate the clinical picture. Usually there is agglutination of RBCs resulting in vascular occlusion in the cold distal extremities. Hemolysis is highly variable, because although complement is activated, the cascade is interrupted when red cells coated with C_3 in the cool regions of the peripheral circulation return to the warm central regions where the warmed IgM rapidly dissociates and C_3 is inactivated. Cold-reacting antibodies can occur in patients with lymphoproliferative disease or infections (mycoplasma, falciparum malaria, Epstein-Barr virus), or they may be idiopathic.

LEUKEMIAS

I. Definition. A heterogeneous group of white blood cell (WBC) malignancies resulting in either a rapidly progressive accumulation of immature leukocytes **(acute leukemias)** or a somewhat more indolent overgrowth by relatively mature leukocytes **(chronic leukemias).**

II. Clinical manifestations and differential diagnosis

A. Acute leukemias

1. The **clinical features** of acute lymphocytic leukemia (ALL) and acute myelogenous leukemia (AML) are compared in Table 25–1.

2. Pathophysiology

a. ALL. CNS prophylaxis crucial; CNS and testicle are "sanctuaries" for leukemic cells. Most lymphoblasts are "null" cells; T-cell ALL has worse prognosis than null-cell ALL. At least 30–50 percent of patients have a chromosome abnormality in leukemic cells.

TABLE 25-1. Clinical manifestations of acute leukemias

	Acute lymphocytic leukemia	Acute myelogenous leukemia
History	Major childhood malignancy (rare in adults), recurrent infections, weakness, bleeding, anemia, lymphadenopathy	Exposure to radiation, chemicals, viruses; recurrent infection; weakness; bleeding; anemia; lymphadenopathy. AML is uncommon.
Physical exam	Pallor, fever, ecchymoses, adenopathy, hepatosplenomegaly	Similar to ALL, but less adenopathy and hepatosplenomegaly
Diagnostic tests	↑ WBC, ↑ lymphocytes (especially immature forms), anemia, ↓ platelets, ↑ uric acid	Anemia, ↓ platelets, moderately ↑ WBC (usually myeloblasts), ↑ uric acid, abnormal LFT; 50% of patients have Auer rods in myeloblasts (pathognomonic); peroxidase ⊕ cytoplasmic granules often found in malignant cells

    b. AML. DIC, leukostasis, and intracranial bleeds are common complications.

B. Chronic leukemias

    1. The **clinical features** of chronic lymphocytic leukemia (CLL) and chronic myelogenous leukemia (CML) are compared in Table 25–2.

    2. Pathophysiology

        a. CLL. Malignant cell usually a monoclonal B lymphocyte with defective IgG production; ↓ immune defense, so infection com-

TABLE 25-2. Clinical manifestations of chronic leukemias

	Chronic lymphocytic leukemia	Chronic myelogenous leukemia
History	Highest prevalence of any leukemia; old age (usually > 60), fatigue, weight loss, anorexia, pallor, fever, splenomegaly	2:1 male-female ratio; middle age, fatigue, weight loss, anorexia, pallor, fever, splenomegaly
Physical exam	Pallor, tachycardia, hepatosplenomegaly	Lymphadenopathy, hepatosplenomegaly
Diagnostic tests	Often extremely ↑ WBC (especially mature small lymphocytes)	↑ WBC, basophilia, mild anemia; 90% of patients have Philadelphia chromosome; usually low leukocyte alkaline phosphatase values

mon; hemolytic anemia a frequent complication. Mean survival after clinical onset is 7–10 years.

b. **CML.** Chronic disease usually lasts 2–5 years followed by a **blast crisis,** in which mature myelocytes are replaced by immature myeloblasts, promyeloblasts and/or lymphoblasts, with survival time of 6 months. Mean survival after diagnosis is 3–4 years.

III. Pathophysiology

A. **Cytokinetics** of leukemic cells involve slow, incomplete, or defective maturation; longer-than-average cell survival time; lack of control by normal hematopoietic feedback systems.

B. **Etiology** unknown; major speculations include viral agents, defective DNA repair, and oncogenes.

CHAPTER 26

Solid Tumors

The most important event in determining the success of cancer therapy is the initial management decision. *Treatment goals must be clearly defined.* If cure is the goal, then bold steps may be taken, but if palliation is the goal, then the treatment should be designed to relieve symptoms while producing as few as possible.

Samuel Hellman, M.D.

Dr. Hellman is the A.N. Pritzker Distinguished Service Professor of Radiation and Cellular Oncology at the Pritzker Medical School of the University of Chicago, where he has served as Dean. A graduate of the State University of New York School of Medicine in Syracuse, he completed training in general radiology and radiation therapy at Yale University. Known for advancing cancer treatment with his clinical research on malignant lymphomas and breast cancer, he has also served as Physician-in-Chief of the Memorial Sloan-Kettering Cancer Center in New York. He is the 2003 recipient of the American College of Radiology's highest award, the gold medal, and co-editor of Cancer: Principles and Practice of Oncology.

While cancer remains a major public health problem in the United States and in other developed countries, there is growing optimism in the field of oncology today with improvements in prevention, early detection, and treatment of many forms of cancer. Cancer statistics from 2003 show a continued decline in the death rate from all cancers combined and from each of the four major cancer sites. This chapter reviews those non-hematologic cancers that are responsible for the most deaths in American men and women (lung, breast, colorectal, esophageal, ovarian, prostate, and pancreatic) along with brain tumors and skin cancer. Fig. 26–1 and Fig. 26–2 show the incidence and mortality by site and gender. Table 26–1 gives the most common source of metastases to several organs.

LUNG CANCER

I. **Epidemiology.** Lung cancer accounts for 31% of cancer deaths in American men and 25% of cancer deaths in American women, making it the most common fatal cancer in the United States. Lung cancer surpassed breast cancer as the leading cause of cancer death in women in 1987. Approximately 172,000 Americans were expected to be diagnosed with lung cancer in 2003; over 90% of these people will die from this disease.

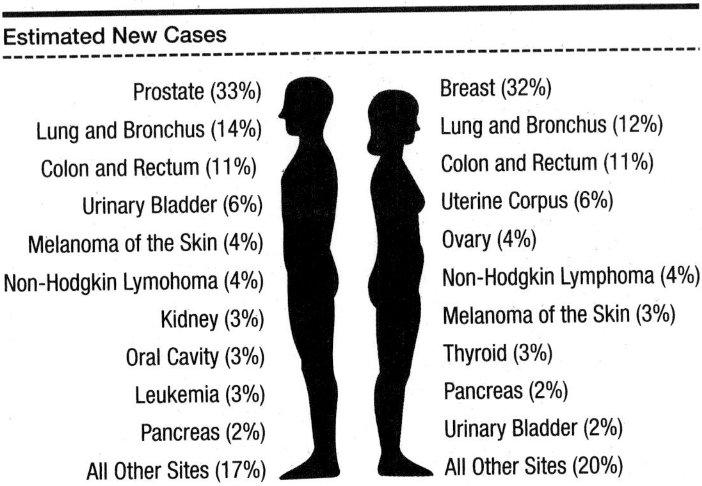

Estimated New Cases

Prostate (33%)	Breast (32%)
Lung and Bronchus (14%)	Lung and Bronchus (12%)
Colon and Rectum (11%)	Colon and Rectum (11%)
Urinary Bladder (6%)	Uterine Corpus (6%)
Melanoma of the Skin (4%)	Ovary (4%)
Non-Hodgkin Lymohoma (4%)	Non-Hodgkin Lymphoma (4%)
Kidney (3%)	Melanoma of the Skin (3%)
Oral Cavity (3%)	Thyroid (3%)
Leukemia (3%)	Pancreas (2%)
Pancreas (2%)	Urinary Bladder (2%)
All Other Sites (17%)	All Other Sites (20%)

Fig. 26–1. 2003 cancer incidence (estimated new cases) by site and sex (excluding basal and squamous cell skin cancers and in situ carcinomas except urinary bladder). (Reproduced with permission from American Cancer Society's Department of Epidemiology and Statistics, *Ca: A Cancer Journal for Clinicians,* 53(1):9, 2003.)

Estimated Deaths

Lung and Bronchus (31%)	Lung and Bronchus (25%)
Prostate (10%)	Breast (15%)
Colon and Rectum (10%)	Colon and Rectum (11%)
Pancreas (5%)	Pancreas (6%)
Non-Hodgkin Lymphoma (4%)	Ovary (5%)
Leukemia (4%)	Non-Hodgkin Lymphoma (4%)
Esophagus (4%)	Leukemia (4%)
Liver (3%)	Uterine Corpus (3%)
Urinary Bladder (3%)	Brain (2%)
Kidney (3%)	Multiple Myeloma (2%)
All Other Sites (22%)	All Other Sites (23%)

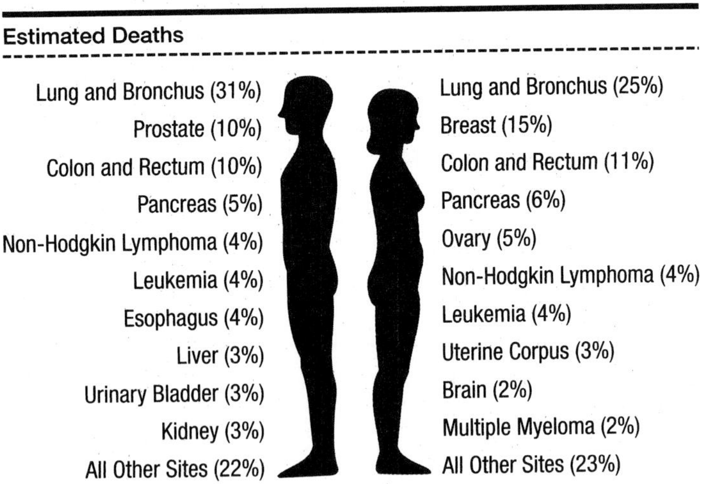

Fig. 26–2. 2003 cancer deaths (estimated) by site and sex (excluding basal and squamous cell skin cancers and in situ carcinomas except urinary bladder). (Reproduced with permission from American Cancer Society's Department of Epidemiology and Statistics, *Ca: A Cancer Journal for Clinicians,* 53(1):9, 2003.)

TABLE 26-1.   The most common sources of metastases

Metastases	Common primary tumors
Bone	Breast, lung, prostate, thyroid, kidney
Brain	Lung, breast, melanoma, GU tract, colon
Liver	Colon, stomach, pancreas, breast, lymphoma
Lung	Breast, colon, kidney, testis, stomach

II. Clinical manifestations and diagnosis

A. History. Most patients present with weight loss and symptoms related to local involvement of the tumor, including cough, dyspnea, hemoptysis, increased sputum production, bronchorrhea, and chest pain. Partial obstruction of a bronchus may lead to wheezing, while complete obstruction of a bronchus may lead to a post-obstructive pneumonia. Compression of the superior vena cava may lead to facial and upper extremity swelling. Bone pain, right upper quadrant (RUQ) pain, and a change in mental status may signify metastatic disease.

B. Physical exam. A thin or wasted general appearance, crackles or wheezing may be detected on auscultation of the lungs, dullness to percussion may signify a malignant pleural effusion. The triad of ptosis, myosis, and anhydrosis (**Horner's syndrome**) strongly suggests the presence of an apical tumor invading the brachial plexus. Hoarseness suggests involvement of the recurrent laryngeal nerve. Bone tenderness, RUQ abdominal tenderness, and neurologic changes may signify metastatic disease. Gynecomastia is a paraneoplastic syndrome seen in large cell lung cancer; hypertrophic pulmonary osteoarthropathy (digital clubbing) is especially associated with adenocarcinoma (see COLOR PLATES).

C. Risk factors. Cigarettes, asbestos (especially in combination with cigarettes), radiation, arsenic, industrial chemicals (e.g., nickel, chromate).

D. Diagnostic tests. Chest roentgenography (CXR) may reveal a pulmonary mass with or without hilar involvement and with or without cavitation. Sputum cytology is a minimally invasive diagnostic approach, although the false negative rate may be high in peripheral lesions. Cytological examination of a pleural effusion is a more invasive means of determining malignancy. Bronchoscopy allows for direct visualization as well as biopsy of suspicious lesions. Computed tomography (CT) of the chest may be used in conjunction with percutaneous needle aspiration to evaluate peripheral lesions. CT is also helpful in determining extent of disease. In addition, abnormal liver function tests (LFTs) suggest hepatic metastases, hypercalcemia suggests either bone involvement or parathyroid hormone related-protein activation and hyponatremia suggests presence of the syndrome of inappropriate antidiuretic hormone (SIADH).

E. Screening. Early detection of lung cancer in the absence of symptoms in the general population via CXR has not yet been shown to improve survival. However, alternative methods for screening are currently under investigation.

III. Differential diagnosis. One of the most helpful means of differentiating benign from malignant pulmonary lesions is the careful inspection of an old CXR. Benign lesions are usually smaller, have well-defined borders, have central calcification, and are present in people less than 40 years of age. In addition, nodules with doubling times less than 10 days or greater than 450 days are usually benign.

IV. Pathophysiology. Lung cancer is classified as either small cell or non-small cell carcinoma.

A. Small cell lung cancer accounts for about one-quarter of all lung cancers; it is extremely aggressive and has the greatest tendency to metastasize early. In fact, 80% of small cell cancer patients have metastases at diagnosis. CXR usually reveals a central lesion without cavitation. The paraneoplastic syndromes of small cell cancer include SIADH, ectopic adrenocorticotropic hormone (ACTH) production (Cushing's syndrome), and Lambert-Eaton syndrome.

B. Non-small cell lung cancer

1. **Squamous cell cancer** accounts for about one-third of lung cancers. In contrast to small cell cancer, squamous cell cancer typically does not metastasize early. CXR usually reveals a central lesion that often cavitates. Hypercalcemia is the paraneoplastic syndrome commonly associated with squamous cell cancer.

2. **Adenocarcinoma** accounts for about one-quarter of lung cancers. This type of cancer typically metastasizes early, often to the brain, adrenal glands, and bones. CXR often reveals a peripheral lesion with or without cavitation. Hypertrophic pulmonary osteoarthropathy (digital clubbing) is the paraneoplastic syndrome that is especially associated with adenocarcinoma of the lung.

3. **Large cell cancer** accounts for about one-fifth of lung cancers. CXR usually shows a peripheral lesion with a tendency to cavitate. Gynecomastia is the paraneoplastic syndrome most often associated with large cell lung cancer.

C. Metastases can occur via direct extension, lymphatic or hematogenous spread to the central nervous system, adrenal glands, bone, and liver.

BREAST CANCER

I. Epidemiology. Breast cancer is the most common malignant neoplasm found in American women. In 2003, 211,000 new cases of breast cancer were expected to be diagnosed and approximately 40,000 people were expected to die from the disease. The American Cancer Society estimates that the average American woman has a one in eight chance of developing breast cancer in her lifetime. It is estimated that 1,300 men will develop breast cancer in 2003, and about 400 men will die from the disease.

II. Clinical manifestations and diagnosis

A. History. A painless breast mass is noticed in up to 75% of cases. Other symptoms include nipple discharge, skin changes over breast tissue, and weight loss.

    B. Physical exam. In addition to a breast mass, findings may include erythema, dimpling, ulceration or thickening of the overlying breast skin and nipple, axillary and supraclavicular adenopathy, signs of hypercalcemia, and edema of the ipsilateral arm.

    C. Risk factors include increasing age, personal or family history of breast cancer, increased breast density, early menarche, nulliparity or late first pregnancy, obesity after menopause, radiation exposure before age 30, high fat intake, alcohol ingestion, and possibly recent use of oral contraceptives or estrogens. Positive BRCA1 and BRCA2 markers account for approximately 5% of all cases of breast cancer.

    D. Diagnostic tests. If a suspicious breast mass is found, the first diagnostic test to perform is a mammogram, which might reveal irregular clusters of microcalcifications or a breast density with irregular borders. An ultrasound of the mass can then be performed to determine whether the lesion is cystic or solid. Cystic lesions are virtually always benign. Ultrasound cannot distinguish between benign and malignant solid tumors; therefore, if a solid tumor is found, a biopsy is the next step. **A biopsy should be performed to evaluate any suspicious mass, even if the mammogram is negative.** A CXR, bone scan, and LFTs may be helpful in determining metastatic disease. A carcinoembryonic antigen (CEA) titer may be elevated, but is not specific for breast cancer.

    E. Screening. All adult women should perform monthly breast self-exams. A yearly breast exam should be performed by a physician in all women over age 40. Asymptomatic women greater than 50 years should receive an annual screening mammogram as well as a breast exam. In this age group, screening mammography has been shown to reduce mortality by 25%. Screening women with mammography between 40 and 50 years is controversial but the American Cancer Society recommends annual screening mammography in all women starting at age 40. For women less than 35 years, screening mammography is not helpful because of the increased density of the breast. High-risk patients, however, can be screened periodically after age 35 years.

III. Differential diagnosis. Breast carcinoma must be differentiated from benign breast masses, which include polycystic breast disease and fibrocystic changes (fibroadenomas). Greater than 90% of breast masses are benign. In contrast to malignancy, benign conditions are often well delineated and mobile, without signs of retraction.

IV. Pathophysiology

    A. Infiltrating ductal carcinoma accounts for 80% of breast cancer and is usually unilateral. **Invasive lobular carcinoma** accounts for 10% of breast cancer and tends to be bilateral. There are two types of **carcinoma in situ** (CIS), or non-invasive cancer. Lobular CIS itself does not evolve into invasive carcinoma, but it is a marker for the development of invasive disease. Ductal CIS itself evolves into invasive carcinoma.

    B. Staging and prognosis are shown in Table 26–2.

    C. Metastasis can occur via direct extension, lymphatic or hematogenous spread to the bone, lung, and liver.

TABLE 26-2. Clinical stage vs. survival rate for breast cancer

Stage	Description	5 yr Survival
I	Tumor < 2 cm	98%
IIA	Tumor 2–5 cm; axillary nodes negative	88%
IIB	Tumor 2–5 cm and axillary nodes positive; tumor > 5 cm and axillary nodes negative	76%
IIIA	Tumor of any size that has spread to the axillary nodes and axillary tissues	56%
IIIB	Tumor of any size that has attached itself to the chest wall, and has spread to the pectoral lymph nodes	49%
IV	Distant metastases	16%

Statistics from the American Cancer Society.

COLORECTAL CARCINOMA

I. **Epidemiology.** Colorectal cancer is the third most common cause of cancer deaths in both men and women in the United States. In 2003, an estimated 147,500 new cases of colorectal cancer were expected to be diagnosed, and approximately 57,100 people were expected to die of the disease. The male to female ratio is even; 90% of those who develop colorectal cancer are over 50. The lifetime risk of developing colorectal cancer is approximately 6%. Recently, mortality has been decreasing, perhaps because of improved screening techniques.

II. **Clinical manifestations and diagnosis**

A. **History.** Constipation, diarrhea, change in stool frequency, size, or color, abdominal pain, tenesmus, weight loss, fatigue, hemorrhoids, and blood per rectum are frequent presenting symptoms.

B. **Physical exam.** Stool positive for occult blood (guaiac positive stool), a mass found on rectal exam, or an abdominal mass are common findings.

C. **Risk factors** include age greater than 50 years, history of ulcerative colitis, familial polyposis, Gardner's syndrome, family history of colonic cancer, personal history of adenomatous polyps, low-fiber diets, obesity, low physical activity, smoking, daily red meat ingestion, and greater than one alcoholic drink per day.

D. **Screening.** For low or average risk patients, current screening recommendations include yearly digital rectal exams, fecal occult blood testing (FOBT), flexible sigmoidoscopy every five years, double contrast barium enema every five years, or colonoscopy every 10 years beginning age 50. The American Cancer Society recommends combining flexible sigmoidoscopy with fecal occult blood testing to improve screening. For high risk patients, colonoscopy is recommended more often. In 2002, an American Cancer Society advisory group concluded that while CT colonography (virtual colonoscopy), capsule video endoscopy, and stool tests for DNA mutations are promising new techniques, there is insufficient evidence at this time to recommend any of these tests for routine screening for colorectal cancer.

E. Diagnostic tests. Colonoscopy allows for direct visualization of the lumen of the colon as well as the ability to biopsy suspicious lesions. Microcytic anemia secondary to chronic gastrointestinal blood loss is common. Abnormal LFTs are suggestive of metastases to the liver; an abnormal CXR suggests metastases to the lungs. CT imaging is helpful in identifying metastatic lesions. Although nonspecific and not suitable for initial diagnosis, CEA is the marker of choice for monitoring the progression of colorectal cancer.

III. Differential diagnosis. In patients who present with gastrointestinal blood loss, the differential diagnosis includes inflammatory bowel disease (ulcerative colitis or Crohn's disease), diverticular disease, Osler-Weber-Rendu syndrome, foreign bodies, polyps, metastatic disease, intestinal lymphomas, and Kaposi's sarcoma. In patients who present with intestinal obstruction, causes other than malignancy include adhesions, peritonitis, inflammatory bowel disease, fecal impaction, and strangulated bowel.

IV. Pathophysiology

A. Ninety-eight percent of all cancers in the colon and rectum are **adenocarcinomas.**

B. Adenomatous polyps are precursor lesions for invasive colorectal carcinoma. The risk that a polyp is malignant is correlated with its size, histologic architecture, and the severity of epithelial dysplasia. Cancer is rare in tubular adenomas less than 1 cm in diameter. The risk of cancer is high (~ 40%) in sessile villous adenomas greater than 4 cm in diameter.

C. Staging and prognosis are shown in Table 26–3.

D. Metastasis. Colorectal tumors may spread by direct extension into adjacent structures as well as by metastasis through blood vessels and lymphatics. Common metastatic sites include the regional lymph nodes, liver, lung, bone, and brain.

ESOPHAGEAL CANCER

I. Epidemiology. Esophageal cancer represents 4% of cancer deaths in American men. It is the fifth most common non-hematological cancer death in this population, with approximately 10,000 deaths expected due to esophageal cancer in 2003.

II. Clinical manifestations and diagnosis

A. History. Common presenting symptoms include weight loss and dysphagia initially to solids and later to both solids and liquids. Other symptoms include aspiration pneumonia, substernal chest pain, and hoarseness due to impingement of the recurrent laryngeal nerve. Gastrointestinal blood loss is usually occult, but may be massive if the tumor erodes into the aorta. Early cancer is often asymptomatic.

TABLE 26-3. Staging and prognosis of colorectal cancer

TMN	Classification Dukes	Modified Astor-Coller	Description	5-year Survival
I	A	A	Lesion limited to mucosa; nodes negative	85–95%
		B_1	Extension of lesion through mucosa but still within bowel wall; nodes negative	
II	B	B_2	Extension through the entire bowel wall (including serosa); nodes negative	60–80%
III	C	C_1	Lesion limited to bowel wall; nodes positive	30–60%
		C_2	Extension of lesion through entire bowel wall (including serosa); nodes positive	
IV		D	Distant metastases	< 5%

Adapted from Macdonald JS. Adjuvant therapy for colon cancer. *CA Cancer J Clin.* 1999; 49(4):202–219.

B. **Physical exam.** Thin or wasted general appearance, crackles on ausculta- tion of the lungs, guaiac positive stool. Alternatively, the physical exami- nation may be normal.

C. **Risk factors.** Tobacco and alcohol abuse, lye ingestion, radiation, long- term stasis (achalasia), long-standing gastroesophageal reflux disease (GERD) leading to Barrett's esophagus.

D. **Diagnostic tests.** An upper GI series with barium contrast might show a filling defect in the esophageal lumen. Endoscopy allows for direct visual- ization of the esophageal lumen and biopsy of suspicious lesions. CT may be helpful in evaluating the extent of the tumor as well as involvement of other organs. Fecal occult blood testing is often positive. A microcytic ane- mia secondary to chronic gastrointestinal blood loss is common.

E. **Screening.** There are currently no screening recommendations for detect- ing esophageal cancer in the United States.

III. **Differential diagnosis.** Weight loss and dysphagia are also seen with esophageal webs and rings, strictures, esophageal spasm, scleroderma, and achalasia.

IV. **Pathophysiology**

A. Esophageal cancer is approximately evenly divided into squamous cell carcinoma and adenocarcinoma. As a general rule, the proximal 2/3 of the esophagus is the typical site for squamous cell carcinoma, while the distal 1/3 of the esophagus is the typical site for adenocarcinoma.

B. Columnar metaplasia of the distal esophagus occurs due to chronic acid reflux. This metaplasia is referred to as Barrett's esophagus. Barrett's esophagus is a major risk factor for the development of esophageal adenocarcinoma. The incidence of esophageal adenocarcinoma is increasing.

C. Metastasis. Because the esophagus has no serosal lining, the tumor can metastasize early to the regional lymph nodes, liver, lungs, and kidneys.

OVARIAN CANCER

I. Epidemiology. Ovarian cancer causes more deaths in the United States than any other gynecologic cancer. It is the second most common gynecologic malignancy behind uterine cancer. In 2003 approximately 25,000 American women were estimated to develop ovarian cancer, and about 14,500 were expected to die from this disease.

II. Clinical manifestations and diagnosis

A. History. Early symptoms tend to be non-specific, including vague abdominal pain, bloating, early satiety, and weight loss. Unfortunately, these non-specific symptoms tend to delay diagnosis. Later symptoms include increased abdominal girth.

B. Physical exam. Adnexal or pelvic masses, lymphadenopathy, and ascites.

C. Risk factors include increasing age, nulliparity, late menopause, history of pelvic radiation, history of breast cancer, family history of breast or ovarian cancer, and a positive BRCA 1 or BRCA 2 status. Oral contraceptive use, one full-term pregnancy, early menarche, and breast feeding appear to reduce the risk of ovarian cancer.

D. Diagnostic tests. Abdominal and transvaginal ultrasound as well as abdominal CT can all be useful in assessing an adnexal mass as well as in detecting ascites. CA-125 is often elevated in ovarian cancer, but is a non-specific marker.

E. Screening. Although there is no currently effective screening regimen, regularly scheduled pelvic examination remains an important tool for detecting ovarian cancer.

III. Differential diagnosis. Ovarian cysts, non-malignant ovarian tumors, tubal pregnancy, tumors of the abdominal wall, rectal cancer, pancreatic cancer.

IV. Pathophysiology

A. Epithelial-derived tumors account for approximately 85% of ovarian cancers and are more common in post-menopausal white women.

B. Germ cell tumors account for just 5% of ovarian cancers and are more common in young women.

C. Metastasis. Ovarian carcinoma can spread by local extension, lymphatic invasion, intraperitoneal implantation, hematogenous dissemination, and transdiaphragmatic passage. Intraperitoneal dissemination is characteristic of ovarian cancer. Distant metastasis sites include the liver, lung, brain, or the lymph nodes of the neck.

PROSTATE CANCER

I. Epidemiology. In 2003 approximately 221,000 American men were estimated to develop prostate cancer, and about 30,000 were expected to die from this disease. African-American men are twice as likely to die of prostate cancer. More than 30% of men over 70 have microscopic prostate cancer on autopsy.

II. Clinical manifestations and diagnosis

    A. History. The patient is usually asymptomatic early in the course of disease. Common presenting symptoms include weak or interrupted urine flow, inability to urinate, difficulty starting or stopping flow, increased urinary frequency, nocturia, hematuria, dysuria, and pyuria. In addition, the patient may present with severe bone pain due to metastases as well as weight loss.

    B. Physical exam. A firm, nodular, irregular prostate may be palpated on digital rectal exam (DRE). A finding of bone tenderness and lethargy (from hypercalcemia) is very suggestive of bone metastases.

    C. Risk factors include increasing age, black ethnicity, family history of prostate cancer, a diet high in animal fat, vasectomy, and increased serum testosterone level.

    D. Diagnostic tests. Once the suspicion of prostate cancer has been raised, a trans-rectal ultrasound or a pelvic CT can be performed to characterize the lesion and determine the presence of metastatic disease. A bone scan might be useful to evaluate bone pain. A calcium level might be helpful in evaluating lethargy, or a change in mental status. Prostate specific antigen may be used to detect recurrence of prostate cancer.

    E. Screening. Although controversial, the current preferred method of screening includes yearly digital rectal exams starting at age 40; after 50, yearly digital rectal exams and prostate specific antigen (PSA) levels should be performed after potential benefits (improved survival) and consequences (unnecessary invasive testing and potential complications of surgery when PSA levels are falsely elevated) are explained to patients.

III. Differential diagnosis. Benign prostatic hypertrophy, prostatitis, prostatic calculi.

IV. Pathophysiology

    A. Approximately 95% of all prostate cancers are adenocarcinomas.

    B. Grading is particularly helpful in the evaluation of prostate cancer because there is a good correlation between the degree of differentiation and prognosis. The Gleason Score is the most widely used grading system. Grade 1 represents a very well-differentiated tumor; Grade 5 represents a poorly-differentiated tumor. Tumors that are poorly differentiated connote a poorer prognosis.

    C. Metastases. The bones and lungs are common sites for metastatic prostate cancer.

 PANCREATIC CANCER

I. Epidemiology. Pancreatic cancer is the second most common gastrointestinal tumor after colorectal cancer. Approximately 30,000 new cases were expected in 2003, with about an equal number of deaths. Pancreatic cancer is almost universally fatal.

II. Clinical manifestations and diagnosis

A. History. Pancreatic cancer may present with an insidious onset of vague symptoms or with no symptoms at all. Dull epigastric pain that radiates to the back, anorexia, nausea, vomiting, diarrhea, malaise, weight loss, and depression are common presenting complaints. Pain may be relieved by bending forward, assuming the fetal position, or by taking aspirin. If the tumor develops in the vicinity of the common bile duct, the resulting biliary obstruction may lead to yellowing of the skin and sclera.

B. Physical exam. A palpable abdominal mass, migratory thrombophlebitis (Trousseau's sign), a palpable, non-tender gallbladder (Courvoisier's sign), signs consistent with hypercalcemia or Cushing's syndrome and guaiac positive stool are possible physical exam findings.

C. Risk factors include increasing age, cigarette and cigar smoking, obesity, physical inactivity, chronic pancreatitis, diabetes, and cirrhosis.

D. Diagnostic tests. Elevated CA 19–9 and CEA levels have a sensitivity of 80% and 40% in pancreatic cancer, respectively. Alkaline phosphatase and bilirubin may be elevated secondary to biliary obstruction. In most cases, diagnosis can be made by imaging the pancreas via ultrasound, abdominal CT, or endoscopic retrograde cholangiopancreatography (ERCP). Abdominal CT is the most widely used modality because it is non-invasive; ERCP, however, is the most sensitive for detection of pancreatic cancer because it allows for biopsy.

E. Screening. There are currently no screening recommendations to detect early pancreatic cancer.

III. Differential diagnosis. Gallbladder cancer, gastric neoplasm, gastric ulcers, acute and chronic pancreatitis.

IV. Pathophysiology

A. Adenocarcinomas arising from the exocrine pancreas comprise 95% of all pancreatic cancers.

B. The remaining 5% of tumors arise from the endocrine pancreas and include insulinomas, gastrinomas, and glucagonomas.

C. Metastasis. Pancreatic cancer typically first metastasizes to regional lymph nodes, then to the liver and lung.

 BRAIN TUMORS

I. Epidemiology. Primary brain cancers occur in approximately 11 people per 100,000 per year. About 90% of primary brain tumors occur in adults, roughly around age 60.

II. Clinical manifestations and diagnosis

A. History. Increased intracranial pressure is manifested as headache, ataxia, seizures, vomiting, change in mental status, and weakness. Specific symptoms relate to localized effects of the tumor on the brain. These vary according to the site and size of the tumor, and may include focal seizures, weakness, personality changes, and visual changes.

B. Physical exam. Papilledema, hemiplegia, hemiparesis, cerebellar signs, and cranial nerve signs are possible physical findings.

C. Risk factors. The only definitively proven risk factor for the development of brain tumors is radiation. However, intense exposure to vinyl chloride, lead, and certain pesticides has also been linked with the development of this disease.

D. Diagnostic tests. Magnetic resonance imaging (MRI) with contrast is the preferred modality to image brain tumors.

E. Screening. There are currently no screening recommendations to detect brain tumors.

III. **Differential diagnosis.** An expanding intracranial lesion may also represent granulomatous disease, parasitic cystic disease, hemorrhage, aneurysm, or abscess.

IV. **Pathophysiology**

A. Common adult brain tumors include meningiomas, gliomas, and astrocytomas.

B. Metastasis. Most primary brain tumors do not metastasize outside the cranium. Metastases to the brain are seen in patients with adenocarcinoma of the lung, colon, or breast as well as in patients with malignant melanoma.

 SKIN CANCER

I. **Epidemiology.** The incidence and mortality from cutaneous malignant melanoma have increased rapidly in the last few decades. In 2003, about 54,200 persons will have new diagnoses of melanoma, and 7,600 will die from the disease. The incidence of the other two skin cancers, basal cell carcinoma (BCC) and squamous cell carcinoma (SCC) is estimated to be >1 million new cases per year.

II. **Clinical manifestations and diagnosis**

A. History and risk factors. Sun exposure, sunlamps, tanning beds, insufficient use of sunscreen to block ultraviolet (UV) exposure.

B. Physican exam. SCC (see COLOR PLATES) usually appears on sun-exposed skin of fair-skinned adults and may develop in an actinic keratosis. It usually grows more quickly than a basal cell carcinoma, is firmer, and looks redder. BCC (see COLOR PLATES), though malignant grows slowly and seldom metastasizes. It usually appears on the face of fair-skinned adults. An initial translucent nodule spreads, leaving a depressed center and a firm, elevated border. Telangiectatic vessels are sometime visisble.

C. Diagnostic tests. Skin biopsy

D. Screening. While there are currently no screening recommendations to detect skin cancers, the American Cancer Society recommends patient eduction concerning sun avoidance and sunscreen use.

III. **Differential diagnosis.** Actinic keratosis, Kaposi's sarcoma.

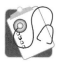

CHAPTER **27**

HIV Disease and AIDS

Shortly after graduating from medical school, I met up with my professor of tropical medicine, the aging but wise Dr. DeRevis. "With all your years of experience," I asked, "what advice could you give me to become the best physician possible?" His answer shocked me. He didn't relate his experiences with the great Dr. Koch, nor did he mention the years he spent fighting tropical disease during the building of the Panama Canal. He took my arm and simply said, "Be a patient." Decades later, I still realize the wisdom and insight of his advice. Experience the passage of renal calculi and you know what the patient means by severe pain. Wait for the pathologist's report on a biopsy of your breast and you know what makes a patient anxious. You will spend a wonderful lifetime filled with devotion to the art you have chosen. Just remember to try to put yourself in your patient's shoes and "be a patient."

Sidney Simon, D.O., FAAAI, FACOI

A 1950 graduate of the Philadelphia College of Osteopathy, Dr. Simon is Professor of Medicine at the New York College of Osteopathic Medicine of the New York Institute of Technology, where he has taught every graduate of the school and serves as the Division Chief of Allergy, Immunology and Rheumatology in the Department of Medicine. Active in private practice, he is a Fellow of the American Academy of Allergy and Immunology and a 1999 recipient of the Attending of the Year award by the New York Chapter of the American College of Osteopathic Internists.

I. Definitions

A. Human immunodeficiency virus (HIV) is an RNA retrovirus that invades and destroys CD_4^+ T cells. It is the virus responsible for acquired immunodeficiency syndrome (AIDS). There are two genetically related forms of HIV: HIV-1 (the most common type in the United States) and HIV-2 (the most common type in West Africa). The HIV-1 genome contains the *gag* gene (which encodes the core proteins, p24 and p18), the *pol* gene (which encodes the reverse transcriptase enzyme), and the *env* gene (which encodes the envelope glycoproteins, gp120 and gp41).

B. Acquired immunodeficiency syndrome (AIDS) encompasses a spectrum of diseases caused by cellular and humoral immune dysfunction resulting from HIV infection. More specifically, AIDS is defined as either a CD_4^+ T cell count less than 200 cells/uL or the development of one of the AIDS defining illnesses (see sections VI through XI).

II. Diagnostic tests

A. Enzyme-linked immunosorbent assay (ELISA) is an assay that detects the presence of IgG antibodies to HIV in the serum or oral fluids. With a sensitivity greater than 99%, ELISA is an **excellent screening test** for HIV. Of note, antibodies to HIV usually develop about 6 to 12 weeks after exposure.

B. Western blot is an assay that detects the presence of antibodies to specific HIV *proteins* (as opposed to antibodies to the virus itself). With a specificity greater than 99%, a Western blot is an excellent test to confirm a positive ELISA. Of note, antibodies to HIV proteins also usually develop about 6 to 12 weeks after exposure.

C. HIV RNA PCR is a technique that amplifies viral RNA. It is the earliest means of detecting HIV infection since the virus rapidly replicates in acute disease prior to the development of antibodies. In addition to diagnosis, HIV RNA PCR is used to measure the level of viremia, (i.e., the copies of HIV per mL), a quantity referred to as the **viral load.** Viral load is used to predict disease progression and guides the initiation and alteration of treatment regimens. The target viral load in a patient taking **highly active anti-retroviral treatment (HAART)** is an undetectable level.

D. p24 Antigen test can detect the actual p24 protein on the viral capsid about two weeks after exposure. While the test is very specific, it lacks the sensitivity of PCR.

E. CD_4^+ T cell count is useful in determining a patient's current immunologic status once HIV has been diagnosed. While it is less reliable than the viral load in predicting progression of disease, it is helpful in guiding prophylactic treatment.

III. Epidemiology

A. Worldwide

1. The worldwide prevalence of HIV-infected adults is estimated to be 41 million.

2. The worldwide prevalence of HIV-infected women is roughly 19 million (close to 50% of adult cases).

3. Approximately 4.2 million adults (and 800,000 children) acquired HIV in 2002.

4. Approximately 3 million adults (and 600,000 children) died from HIV in 2002.

B. United States

1. The CDC (Centers for Disease Control and Prevention, Atlanta, Georgia) estimates that about 1 million Americans are infected with HIV.

2. The yearly incidence of HIV-infection in the United States is estimated to be around 40,000. About 70% of these cases are men.

3. Of the men, 60% contracted HIV from homosexual intercourse, 25% contracted HIV from intravenous drug use, and 15% contracted HIV from heterosexual intercourse.

4. Of the 12,000 new cases of HIV in women, 75% contracted HIV

from heterosexual intercourse, and 25% contracted HIV from intravenous drug use.

IV. Risk factors

A. Unprotected vaginal, anal, or oral intercourse. The presence of genital ulceration strongly facilitates transmission of HIV, as does vaginal intercourse during menses.

B. Intravenous drug use. Needle transmission is responsible for roughly 25% of AIDS cases in the United States. Syringe and needle exchange programs have been shown to decrease the spread of HIV in this population.

C. Blood transfusions. The risk of acquiring HIV through blood transfusions is currently 1 in 153,000 for each unit of blood transfused. Prior to April 1985, blood products were not uniformly screened. As a result, populations that frequently require blood products (i.e., patients with hemophilia or myelodysplastic syndrome) were often infected through transfusion.

D. Occupational exposure. The risk of HIV infection after a needle stick injury depends on many factors, including the depth of the wound, the caliber of the needle, and the level of viremia in the contaminated fluid. The overall risk of seroconversion is 0.3%. In comparison, the risk of acquiring hepatitis C is 3% and the risk of acquiring hepatitis B is 30% after needle stick injury.

E. Vertical transmission. It is estimated that 7–39% of infants born to HIV-infected mothers become infected; the risk of vertical transmission increases with the level of viremia in the mother.

V. Natural history of HIV

A. Acute infection. When HIV initially enters the bloodstream, rapid viral replication ensues. This intense viremia is thought to correlate with a mild to severe **mononucleosis-like illness** that typically lasts 1–2 weeks. Symptoms commonly include fever, malaise, anorexia, myalgia, arthralgia, pharyngitis, lymphadenopathy, and a maculopapular rash that usually affects the trunk and face. Less common symptoms include polyneuropathy, neuritis, and odynophagia. On direct questioning, at least half of HIV-infected patients report a history of a flu-like illness prior to seroconversion. Once antibodies to HIV develop, the level of viremia is dramatically reduced, although replication continues in lymphoid tissue. Most patients are unaware that they have become infected.

B. Asymptomatic phase. The asymptomatic phase lasts on average 10 years after seroconversion. However, only 20% of HIV-infected patients are entirely asymptomatic. About 60% of HIV-infected patients experience enlarged lymph nodes, resulting from active viral replication in lymphoid tissue. The syndrome of persistent generalized lymphadenopathy (PGL) is defined as the presence of two or more extrainguinal sites of lymphadenopathy for a minimum of 3 to 6 months. In addition, because of the dysregulation of the humoral immunity, many HIV-infected patients develop recurrent bacterial pneumonias (commonly from encapsulated organisms like *Streptococcus pneumoniae* and *Haemophilus influenzae*).

Early evaluation of an HIV-infected patient includes a thorough **history** of sexually transmitted diseases, exposure to hepatitis B, hepatitis C and tuberculosis, immunosuppressive therapy (i.e., corticosteroids), immunizations, current sexual practices (number of partners and whether "safe sex" is practiced), and the use of intravenous drugs.

A comprehensive **physical examination** should be performed, with an emphasis on the dermatologic exam since many common conditions (including herpes simplex, herpes zoster, staphylococcal folliculitis, bacillary angiomatosis, molluscum contagiosum, seborrheic dermatitis, and candidiasis) can be treated effectively.

A baseline **laboratory evaluation** includes a complete blood count (CBC), serologies (for hepatitis B, hepatitis C, and syphilis), toxoplasma antibody, PPD placement as well as a CD_4^+ T cell count, and viral load determination. CD_4^+ T cell count and viral load should be repeated every 6 months in patients whose CD_4^+ T cell counts are above 600 cells/uL and every 3 months in those whose CD_4^+ T cell counts are below 600 cells/uL. A Papanicolaou smear looking for cervical dysplasia must be performed in all HIV-infected women every 6 to 12 months. Ophthalmologic exam screening for CMV retinitis is recommended every 6 months after the CD_4^+ T cell count falls below 100 cells/uL.

In addition, every HIV-infected patient must receive the pneumococcal vaccine; the value of the influenza vaccine is controversial since it has not been shown to reduce mortality. In those patients who are HepBsAg (-) and HepBsAb(-), the hepatitis B vaccination series should be administered. Live, attenuated viruses such as polio, typhoid, yellow fever **should not** be given to HIV-infected individuals.

C. **Symptomatic phase.** The symptomatic phase of HIV disease correlates with a dramatic decrease in CD_4^+ T cell count and an increase in viral load. It usually occurs about 10 years after seroconversion, although presentations are highly variable. As a generalization, if a patient's absolute CD_4^+ T cell count is greater than 500 cells/uL (or CD_4^+ T cell count % > 29%), new symptoms are very likely to be due to non HIV-associated illnesses. However, once a patient's absolute CD_4^+ T cell count falls below 200 cells/uL (or CD_4^+ T cell count % < 14%), new symptoms are probably due to HIV-associated illnesses. It should be stressed that not every HIV-associated illness conforms to this generalization; herpes zoster, for example, can be found in patients with CD_4^+ T cell counts over 500 cells/uL. Symptomatic HIV-infected patients are frequently afflicted not only with HIV-associated illness, but very often with AIDS-defining illnesses (see sections VI through XI).

The importance of an excellent doctor-patient relationship, especially during the symptomatic phase of HIV disease, cannot be overemphasized. Prompt, frequent and careful evaluations, routine prophylaxis, early diagnosis, and directed treatment are mainstays for successfully managing the symptomatic HIV-infected patient.

VI. AIDS-defining fungal illnesses

A. *Pneumocystis carinii*

1. **Definition.** *P. carinii* is a fungus endemic throughout the world whose natural habitat is the lung. *P. carinii* pneumonia (PCP) is the

most common opportunistic infection in AIDS patients. Those patients with an absolute CD_4^+ T cell count less than 200 cells/uL are most susceptible, especially if they are not receiving prophylaxis.

2. **History.** Patients typically complain of fever, night sweats, weight loss, fatigue, non-productive cough, and shortness of breath with exertion that starts gradually and may last weeks.

3. **Physical exam.** Physical findings include tachypnea, tachycardia, hypoxia, and cyanosis. Lung auscultation is often normal.

4. **Diagnostic data.** Arterial blood gas analysis demonstrates hypoxia, an increased alveolar-arterial (A-a) gradient, and a respiratory alkalosis. LDH is elevated. CXR often shows bilateral diffuse interstitial infiltrates and may show a pneumothorax. Fiberoptic bronchoscopy and bronchoalveolar lavage (BAL) with silver staining or immunofluorescence is about 95% sensitive and is the mainstay of diagnosis.

B. *Candida*

1. **Definition.** *Candida albicans*, the most important species of *Candida*, is an oval budding yeast that is part of the normal flora of the respiratory, gastrointestinal, and female genital tracts. Those patients with an absolute CD_4^+ T cell count less than 500 cells/uL are most susceptible to oral candidiasis, while esophageal candidiasis most commonly occurs in patients with an absolute CD_4^+ T cell count less than 100 cells/uL.

2. **History.** Common symptoms include painless, white lesions involving the mouth, tongue, or vagina, painful fissuring at the corners of the mouth, dysphagia, substernal chest pain, odynophagia, vaginal discharge, and pruritus and occasionally dysuria and dyspareunia. Hematogenous candidiasis can seed virtually any tissue and may manifest as fever, difficulty breathing, change in mental status, and orbital pain and blurry vision (suggestive of retinal abscesses).

3. **Physical exam.** Findings include confluent fever, white plaques in the oropharynx and vagina, "cotton wool patches" on ophthalmologic examination, cheilitis, meningeal signs, a murmur (suggesting endocarditis), tender joints (suggesting arthritis), pulmonary crackles, and abdominal tenderness (suggesting hepatic or splenic involvement).

4. **Diagnostic data.** The diagnosis of superficial candidiasis can be made by demonstrating pseudohyphae on a wet smear. The diagnosis of disseminated disease rests on culture and biopsy specimens. Serological tests are not useful.

C. *Cryptococcus neoformans*

1. **Definition.** *C. neoformans* is a ubiquitous, oval, budding yeast that usually grows in soil containing bird feces. Human infection results from inhalation. It is the leading cause of meningitis in AIDS patients. Those patients with an absolute CD_4^+ T cell count less than 100 cells/uL are most susceptible.

2. **History.** Common presenting symptoms include fever, nausea, vomiting, altered mental status, and headache. Seizures are infrequently reported. Although less commonly a cause of pulmonary disease, some patients present with fever, non-productive cough, and dyspnea.

3. **Physical exam.** Findings may include fever, tachypnea, hypoxia, altered sensorium, meningeal signs (stiff neck, presence of Kernig's and Brudzinski's signs), focal neurologic signs, and bilateral pulmonary crackles.

4. **Diagnostic data.** India ink preparation of CSF shows budding yeast with a surrounding wide capsule. High titers of cryptococcal capsular antigen in the CSF are also diagnostic. A definitive diagnosis is made by culturing the fungus. Multiple ring enhancing lesions on MRI suggest the presence of cryptococcomas. CXR may be significant for either diffuse or focal interstitial infiltrates.

D. *Histoplasma capsulatum*

1. **Definition.** *H. capsulatum* is a dimorphic fungus that is endemic to the Ohio and Mississippi River valleys and causes histoplasmosis. Human infection results from spore inhalation. Hematogenous dissemination occurs in those patients with an absolute CD_4^+ T cell count less than 200 cells/uL.

2. **History.** Most infections in the immune competent population are either asymptomatic or result in a self-limited respiratory illness. However, once the organism is disseminated, presenting symptoms may include fever, malaise, weight loss, myalgias, darkening of skin, papular rash, cough, dyspnea, hemoptysis, abdominal pain, enlarged lymph nodes, stiff neck, and pain in the oropharynx or nasal vestibule.

3. **Physical exam.** Depending on the sites of involvement, findings may include fever, orthostatic hypotension (suggestive of adrenal involvement), a rash containing multiple erythematous, scaling papules, diffuse crackles, murmur (suggesting endocarditis), hepatospenomegaly, lymphadenopathy, meningeal signs, and jaundice (suggestive of granulomatous hepatitis). In addition, ulceration in the mucous membranes of the mouth and nose is very common.

4. **Diagnostic data.** Pancytopenia suggests bone marrow involvement. CXR may show multiple nodules, alveolar infiltrates, cavities, and hilar adenopathy. Tissue biopsies or bone marrow aspirates will show oval yeast cells within macrophages.

E. *Coccidiodes immitis*

1. **Definition.** *C. immitis* is a spherical, non-budding yeast that is endemic to the southwestern United States and causes coccidioidomycosis. The organism is acquired by inhalation. Those patients with an absolute CD_4^+ T cell count less than 200 cells/uL are most susceptible to disseminated disease (while pulmonary involvement can occur in patients with an absolute CD_4^+ T cell count greater than 500 cells/uL).

2. **History.** Common presenting symptoms include fever, weight loss, cough, and shortness of breath. Less frequently, patients will complain of stiff neck and enlarging lymph nodes.

3. **Physical exam.** Depending on the sites of involvement, findings may include fever, tachypnea, hypoxia, crackles on lung auscultation, diffuse lymphadenopathy, and meningeal signs.

4. **Diagnostic data.** CXR most commonly reveals a diffuse reticulonodular pattern, although nodules, cavities, pleural effusions, hilar, and paratracheal lymphadenopathy are also sometimes present. To make the diagnosis, sputum and urine should be examined for *C. immitis* by wet smear and culture. Latex agglutination of CSF is helpful in diagnosing meningeal involvement.

VII. Defining bacterial illnesses

A. *Mycobacterium avium-intracellulare* complex (MAC)

1. **Definition.** MAC is an atypical mycobacterium that is found ubiquitously in the environment. It is diagnosed in approximately 40% of HIV-infected patients antemortem and around 80% of HIV-infected patients at autopsy. The presumed portals of entry are the respiratory and gastrointestinal tracts; however, the disease disseminates to other sites, including the bone marrow, skin, liver and lymph nodes. Those patients with an absolute CD_4^+ T cell count less than 75 cells/uL are most susceptible.

2. **History.** Common presenting symptoms include fever, weight loss, night sweats, fatigue, RUQ abdominal pain, shortness of breath, dyspnea on exertion, and diarrhea.

3. **Physical exam.** Findings may include fever, hypoxia, diaphoresis, crackles on chest auscultation, abdominal tenderness, hepatosplenomegaly, and lymphadenopathy.

4. **Diagnostic data.** Elevated alkaline phosphatase suggests hepatic involvement. CXR most commonly shows bilateral lower lobe interstitial infiltrates with or without hilar adenopathy. Bone marrow involvement is suggested by pancytopenia and confirmed by bone marrow biopsy, which often reveals large numbers of mycobacterium. Liver, intestinal, or lymph node biopsy can also make the diagnosis.

B. *Mycobacterium tuberculosis* (TB)

1. **Definition.** TB is an obligate aerobic mycobacterium that is transmitted via inhalation. Tuberculosis typically affects diabetics, the elderly, the urban poor, and, of course, the immunosuppressed. Those patients with an absolute CD_4^+ T cell count less than 200 cells/uL are most susceptible to disseminated disease, while pulmonary involvement can occur in patients with an absolute CD_4^+ T cell count greater than 500 cells/uL.

2. **History.** Primary tuberculous infection is usually asymptomatic. Most immunocompetent people confine the tubercle bacilli for years by forming granulomas. (The parenchymal lesion and the draining hilar lymph nodes are called a **Ghon complex**.) Reactivation tuberculosis occurs in the minority of patients who cannot contain the primary infection. Patients typically complain of fever, chills, weight loss, night sweats, non-productive chronic cough, and hemoptysis. Because nearly half of AIDS patients have extrapulmonary tuberculosis, the history is often significant for bone pain, enlarged cervical lymph nodes (**scrofula**), stiff neck, photophobia, and chronic diarrhea.

3. **Physical exam.** Findings include fever, hypotension (suggesting adrenal involvement), enlarged lymph nodes, tender bones, and a stiff neck. Lung findings are generally present only in extensive pulmonary disease.

4. **Diagnostic data.** CXR typically shows multinodular infiltration in the apical lobes with or without cavitation. CXR in miliary tuberculosis reveals uniformly distributed fine nodules throughout both lungs. Tubercle bacilli, or "red snappers," seen on sputum analysis cement the diagnosis, as do positive blood cultures. Of note, purified protein derivative (PPD) is often falsely negative in HIV-infected patients. In addition, in the HIV-infected population, a positive PPD is defined as an induration of greater than 5 mm.

C. *Salmonella*

1. **Definition.** *Salmonella choleraesuis* is a gram-negative rod that is introduced by the ingestion of contaminated food and water and is the most common cause of salmonella septicemia. Septicemia accounts for only 5–10 % of salmonella infections (the most common manifestations are enterocolitis and typhoid fever).

2. **History.** The septic course is indolent; symptoms begin with fever, but little or no enterocolitis. Bacteremia results in the seeding of many organs, most commonly the bone (causing osteomyelitis), lung (causing pneumonia), and the CNS (causing meningitis). In addition, previously damaged tissue (i.e., aneurysms or infarctions) is particularly susceptible to the development of metastatic abscesses.

3. **Physical exam.** Depending on the site of involvement, findings may include fever, hypoxia, bone tenderness, meningeal signs, and dullness to percussion on chest examination.

4. **Diagnostic data.** Diagnosis rests on isolation of the organism from blood, CSF, joint aspirate, or stool.

VIII. AIDS-defining viral illnesses

A. **Cytomegalovirus (CMV)**

1. **Definition.** CMV is a member of the human herpesvirus family and causes multi-system disease in immunocompromised hosts. It has a worldwide distribution and is found in saliva, milk, semen, cervical secretions, urine, and feces. Those patients with an absolute CD_4^+ T cell count less than 100 cells/uL are most susceptible.

2. **History.** Patients with CMV retinitis complain of painless, progressive loss of vision in both eyes. Those with CMV esophagitis most often present with substernal chest pain and odynophagia. CMV colitis is marked by abdominal pain, weight loss, and non-bloody diarrhea. Patients with CMV pneumonitis complain of shortness of breath and a non-productive cough.

3. **Physical exam.** Patients may be thin, febrile, tachypneic, and hypoxic. Hypotension should raise the suspicion of CMV adrenalitis. Ophthalomologic exam reveals perivascular hemorrhage and exudates in the retina. Abdominal exam may reveal tenderness or distention. Pulmonary exam may be significant for crackles.

4. **Diagnostic data.** Pancytopenia suggests bone marrow infiltration. CXR shows bilateral interstitial infiltrates, beginning in the periphery and spreading centrally. Endoscopy may show ulcerative lesions in any region of the GI tract. Because virtually every HIV-infected patient has antibodies to CMV, proving the diagnosis of clinically significant CMV can be difficult. A four-fold rise in antibody titer is very suggestive. Biopsy is diagnostic and classically shows intranuclear inclusion bodies with an "owl's eye" appearance.

B. **Herpes simplex virus (HSV)**

1. **Definition.** HSV is another member of the human herpesvirus family. It is distributed worldwide, spread by direct contact of infected secretions, and is found exclusively in humans. There are two subtypes of HSV: HSV-1 is found mostly in saliva, while HSV-2 is found in secretions of the genitourinary tract. However, either subtype can cause oral or genital lesions. Like other members of the human herpesvirus family, HSV may reactivate after years of latency in sensory ganglia. About 90% of Americans have antibody to HSV-1 by the fifth decade. Those patients with an absolute CD_4^+ T cell count less than 200 cells/uL are most susceptible.

2. **History.** The majority of patients infected with primary HSV are asymptomatic. Primary orofacial HSV infection can manifest as fever, malaise, anorexia, myalgias, swollen neck glands as well as pain in the oral cavity, tongue, lips, and gingiva. Primary genital HSV infection can manifest as fever, malaise, anorexia, and myalgias in addition to dysuria, vaginal or urethral discharge, inguinal lymphadenopathy, and painful genital or anal lesions. Patients with HSV encephalitis may present with fever, seizures, and an altered sensorium. Those with HSV esophagitis may complain of odynophagia, dysphagia, substernal pain, and weight loss. HSV pneumonitis is marked by respiratory compromise.

3. **Physical exam.** Depending on the site of involvement, the patient may be febrile or tachypneic. Dermatologic exam for primary HSV infection is typically significant for multiple vesicular, pustular, or ulcerative lesions on an erythematous base. HSV infection of the finger is called **herpetic whitlow.** Tender cervical or inguinal lymphadenopathy is common. An altered mental status, RUQ tenderness (suggestive of HSV hepatitis), orthostatic hypotension (suggestive of HSV adrenalitis), decreased visual fields (suggestive of HSV chorioretinitis), and crackles on chest examination can be found in cases of disseminated disease.

4. **Diagnostic data.** Rapid diagnosis from a skin lesion can be made using a Tzanck smear in which multinucleated giant cells are visualized. HSV PCR is another means of making the diagnosis. The CSF in HSV encephalitis may contain up to 1,000 white blood cells (with a lymphocytic predominance), moderately high protein, and an increased number of red blood cells.

C. **Progressive multifocal leukoencephalopathy (PML)**

1. **Definition.** PML is a fatal demyelinating disease of the white matter

caused by the JC virus, a human papilloma virus. Those patients with an absolute CD_4^+ T cell count less than 100 cells/uL are most susceptible.

2. **History.** Typical presenting symptoms include ataxia, aphasia, progressive dementia, visual impairment, seizures, hemiparesis, and sensory deficits that develop over days to weeks.

3. **Physical exam.** Findings vary depending on the site of white matter involvement. Patients are generally afebrile with a variable level of consciousness.

4. **Diagnostic data.** An MRI scan will usually reveal multiple enhanced white matter lesions and is diagnostic for PML. Importantly, these lesions do not enhance on CT scan. Brain biopsy is typically not performed.

IX. AIDS-defining protozoal illnesses

A. *Toxoplasma gondii*

1. **Definition.** *T. gondii* is the most common secondary CNS infectious agent in AIDS patients. Infection occurs worldwide; up to 50% of Americans have antibodies, indicating latent infection. The domestic cat is the definitive host; infection in humans starts with ingestion of cysts in undercooked meat or contamination with cat feces. Primary infection occurs early in life and is generally asymptomatic. In immunocompetent hosts, the organisms are contained as cysts within tissues. Once cell-mediated immunity is impaired, the infection tends to reactivate. Those patients with an absolute CD_4^+ T cell count less than 100 cells/uL are most susceptible.

2. **History.** Common presenting symptoms include fever, progressive headaches, new-onset seizures, aphasia, alterations in mental status, and changes in motor or sensory function.

3. **Physical exam.** Findings include fever, changes in sensorium, and focal neurologic deficits.

4. **Diagnostic data.** CT scan with contrast usually demonstrates multiple ring-enhancing lesions as well as focal edema in the gray matter. Although rarely performed, definitive diagnosis is a brain biopsy.

B. *Isospora belli/Cryptosporidium*

1. **Definition.** *I. belli* and *Cryptosporidium* are acid-fast protozoae, which affect the gastrointestinal tract in immunocompromised patients. The organisms are acquired by fecal-oral transmission. Those patients with an absolute CD_4^+ T cell count less than 100 cells/uL are most susceptible to intractable disease.

2. **History.** Presentation varies from a self-limited or intermittent diarrheal illness to a severe life-threatening condition characterized by the production of copious non-bloody diarrhea, abdominal cramping, nausea, and vomiting.

3. **Physical exam.** In advanced disease, orthostasis and other signs of dehydration (dry mucous membranes, poor skin turgor) are evident. Abdominal exam may reveal generalized tenderness. Guaiac exam for occult blood is negative.

4. **Diagnostic data.** Large, oval acid-fast cysts seen on stool examination are consistent with isospora infection. Small, round acid-fast cysts are consistent with cryptosporidium infection.

X. AIDS-defining neoplastic illnesses

A. Kaposi's sarcoma (KS)

1. **Definition.** KS is a vascular neoplasia that primarily affects the skin, lymph nodes, gastrointestinal tract, and lungs. It is the most common AIDS-associated malignancy. KS has been linked to prior infection with human herpesvirus-8 (HHV-8) and it disproportionally affects homosexual men. Interestingly, while visceral KS usually develops in patients whose CD_4^+ T cell counts are less than 75 cells/uL, mucocutaneous KS is seen in patients whose CD_4^+ T cell counts are up to 500 cells/uL.

2. **History.** Patients with KS of the skin may complain of multiple "bruises" that often occur in sun-exposed areas as well as in regions that have experienced minor trauma (**Koebner's phenomenon**). These lesions are most often asymptomatic, although ulceration and bleeding may occur. Patients with KS of the gastrointestinal tract may complain of tarry-colored stool (indicative of GI bleeding), abdominal bloating or obstipation (indicative of GI obstruction), or yellowing of the skin and right upper quadrant (RUQ) abdominal pain (indicative of biliary KS). Those with KS of the lungs may complain of shortness of breath or hemoptysis.

3. **Physical exam.** Because of the vascular nature of the lesion and the presence of extravasated red blood cells, skin lesions may be reddish-purple or yellowish-brown (see COLOR PLATES). The lesions are almost always raised; they vary in size from a few millimeters to several centimeters, may be discrete or confluent, and may be accompanied by significant edema. Scleral or sublingual icterus, RUQ tenderness, dark urine and pale stool are seen in KS involving the biliary tree. Guaiac positive stool, abdominal distention, and decreased bowel sounds are found in KS involving the gastrointestinal tract. Diffuse crackles on lung auscultation and dullness to percussion are consistent with KS involving the lung.

4. **Diagnostic data.** CXR shows bilateral lower lobe infiltrates accompanied by pleural effusions in 70% of cases. Depending on the degree of GI blood loss, a microcytic anemia may be present. Elevated total and direct bilirubin levels are consistent with obstructive jaundice. Biopsy makes the definitive diagnosis.

B. Non-Hodgkin's lymphoma

1. **Definition.** Lymphoma is a malignant neoplasm of cells native to lymphoid tissue. There are three main categories of lymphoma seen in HIV-infected patients: immunoblastic (60%), Burkitt's (20%), and primary CNS lymphoma (20%). About 90% are B-cell lymphomas and half contain Epstein-Barr virus DNA. Non-Hodgkin's lymphomas that do not involve the CNS generally occur in patients whose CD_4^+ T cell counts are less than 500 cells/uL, while CNS lym-

phomas typically develop in patients whose CD_4^+ T cell counts are less than 75 cells/uL.

2. **History.** Most patients will present with "B symptoms" (fever, chills, night sweats, and weight loss). Patients with primary CNS lymphoma typically present with headaches, seizures, and cranial nerve deficits. When the gastrointestinal tract is involved, patients may complain of odynophagia or abdominal pain. Bone marrow infiltration corresponds with fatigue. Pulmonary symptoms are less common.

3. **Physical exam.** Findings depend on the site of involvement, but may include fever, diaphoresis, focal neurologic deficits including cranial nerve abnormalities, lymphadenopathy, hepatosplenomegaly, abdominal tenderness, and crackles on pulmonary auscultation.

4. **Diagnostic data.** LDH is usually markedly elevated. Brain MRI or CT typically show up to three 3–5 cm ring-enhancing lesions that may occur in any location. Cytologic examination of the CSF may also lead to the diagnosis in those patients with leptomeningeal involvement. Lymph node or bone marrow biopsy is diagnostic.

C. Cervical/Anal cancer

1. **Definition.** Cancer of the cervix and anus starts as dysplasia of the epithelial cells and, if left unchecked, often progresses to invasive disease. It has been linked to prior infection with human papilloma virus (HPV). Approximately 60% of HIV-infected women and 40% of HIV-infected men have abnormal Papanicolaou smears.

2. **History.** The grand majority of patients are asymptomatic. Invasive carcinoma of the cervix is often heralded by irregular vaginal bleeding, painful coitus, and dysuria.

3. **Physical exam.** Usually normal to the naked eye, but colposcopy often uncovers an abnormal area.

4. **Diagnostic data.** Biopsy is required for confirmation.

XI. Other AIDS-defining conditions

A. HIV wasting syndrome

1. **Definition.** This clinical diagnosis is made in those HIV-infected patients who experience a combination of involuntary weight loss ($>10\%$ from baseline) plus either chronic diarrhea (at least two loose stools per day for 30 days) or chronic weakness and fever (intermittent or constant for more than 30 days) in the absence of other opportunistic infection or malignancy that could account for these symptoms. HIV wasting syndrome is thought to result from a direct effect of HIV. It is the most common AIDS-defining illness in Africa.

2. **History.** As the name suggests, patients present with at least a one-month history of constitutional symptoms including fever, weight loss, fatigue as well as diarrhea.

3. **Physical exam.** Findings are most notable for cachexia and possibly a fever and orthostatic hypotension.

4. **Laboratory data.** Along with a depressed CD_4^+ T cell count and an

elevated viral load, laboratory analysis would likely reveal anemia and hypoalbuminemia.

B. HIV dementia complex

1. **Definition.** This clinical diagnosis is made in those HIV-infected patients who experience a progressive decline in cognitive function. The HIV dementia complex is the initial AIDS-defining illness in about 10% of patients. Approximately two-thirds of HIV-infected patients will eventually develop clinically significant HIV dementia complex. Like HIV wasting syndrome, HIV dementia complex is thought to result from a direct effect of the virus.

2. **History.** Initially, patients may complain of difficulty concentrating and increased forgetfulness. Motor problems, including unsteady gait, poor balance, and difficulty with rapid alternating movements may subsequently develop. In its late stages, patients demonstrate only minimal intellectual and social comprehension. In addition, bowel and bladder incontinence is a complication of the late stage of this disease.

3. **Physical exam.** Findings vary depending on the severity of the disease. A Folstein Mini-Mental Status Score has been used as an objective means to assess disease progression. Increased muscle tone and brisk deep tendon reflexes are suggestive of spinal cord involvement. Paraplegia and incontinence are indicative of advanced disease.

4. **Diagnostic data.** Before a diagnosis of HIV dementia complex can be made, it is necessary to rule out other causes of cognitive decline, including infection (i.e., syphilis), neoplasm (i.e., CNS lymphoma), and toxic-metabolic alterations (i.e., hypothyroidism, vitamin B_{12}, and folate deficiencies). Lumbar puncture typically reveals increased cells and protein and is non-specific. CT and MRI show cerebral atrophy and ventricular dilatation.

PART IV

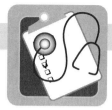

Complementary and Alternative Medicine

An increasing number of Americans from all socioeconomic and demographic backgrounds utilizes complementary and alternative medical (CAM) therapies, defined only a decade ago as interventions neither taught widely in medical schools nor generally available in hospitals. In response, managed care organizations have started to provide insurance coverage for some of these therapies, hospitals have begun to establish centers of complementary medicine for clinical care and research, and medical schools have begun offering courses on the subject.

Complementary medicine includes therapies used together with conventional medicine and an example would be using aromatherapy to help lessen a patient's discomfort after heart surgery. **Alternative medicine** refers to therapies used in place of conventional medicine and an example would be using certain herbal supplements for lung cancer instead of undergoing chemotherapy recommended by a physician. **Integrative medicine** combines mainstream medicine and CAM therapies for which there exists scientific evidence of safety and efficacy.

Some complementary medicine modalities, as evidenced by a steadily growing body of basic and applied research, offer hope to patients unwilling or unable to tolerate conventional therapies for such afflictions as chronic pain. Other modalities are questionable, at best, if not dangerous when they only offer false hope and hasten morbidity when used without conventional care. We provide in the following chapter expanded descriptions of some of the most common CAM therapies, focusing especially upon those therapies that are supported by some degree of scientific evidence, ending with a listing of modalities for which there is at present insufficient scientific evidence. Additional related information can be found in Appendix G, which lists many commonly used herbal remedies and popular indications for their usage. Appendix D is a table of common drug-drug and drug-herb interactions. Osteopathic medicine, a form of conventional medicine, is described in Appendix H.

CHAPTER 28

Traditional and Evidence-Based CAM Therapies

> W hat patients really need you to do is heal them in entirety. I'm trying to find out what kind of impact energy healers, hypnotherapists, acupuncturists, and aromatherapists can have on heart surgery. I believe alternative therapies like these give patients a taste of the awareness they should have about their lives.
>
> *Mehmet Oz, M.D., MBA, FACS*
>
> *After receiving his undergraduate degree from Harvard University, Dr. Oz received his M.D. and M.B.A. degrees from the University of Pennsylvania and Wharton Business School. A pioneer in the development of cardiac assist devices, he is the Irving Associate Professor of Cardiac Surgery at Columbia University and founder of the Complementary Medicine Program at the Columbia-Presbyterian Medical Center of New York-Presbyterian Hospital. His 1999 book,* Healing from the Heart, *won the prestigious "Books for a Better America" award.*

I. **History and recent trends.** Use of complementary and alternative medicine (CAM) therapies by a large proportion of the U.S. population is not new and probably dates to the 1950s or earlier. A 1997 survey by Kessler showed that more than one-third of Americans reported using CAM therapies that year while two-thirds reported using at least one complementary medical therapy in their lifetime. Users of CAM therapies pay an estimated $21 billion a year, mostly out-of-pocket, for these services and make more visits to CAM providers than to primary care providers. Responding to this phenomenon and the interest of scientists and physicians to validate these unconventional options, The National Center for Complementary and Alternative Medicine at the National Institutes of Health was established by the Congress in 1992 and invests more than $50 million a year to investigate the safety and efficacy of some of these approaches.

CAM therapies include a broad range of health care practices, from massage therapies and herbal remedies to ancient Chinese or Indian (Ayurvedic) traditions, as well as such modalities as chiropractic, homeopathy, and acupuncture. Many of these practices are considered mainstream options for health care in many parts of the world and have existed for centuries, while many others lack the rigorous scientific evidence we have come to expect in the West to prove a therapy's efficacy.

II. Managing patients who utilize CAM therapies

A. **Background.** Surveys show most patients are reluctant to discuss their use of CAM therapies with their physicians. Even though 97% of CAM users report having a regular physician, more than 60% don't tell their physicians about their usage of CAM therapies. Possible reasons for this reluctance include: most physicians don't ask about CAM usage in the first place, many physicians aren't well versed about CAM therapies, or patients fear a negative reaction from their physicians if they mention they are utilizing unconventional therapies.

B. **Understanding users of CAM therapies.** Studies show that most patients use CAM therapies because they believe they are more effective than traditional medical care, because their clinical complaints are not perceived by them to be serious enough to require a doctor's visit, or because they don't want to rely on medications or surgery. Statistics also show that patients historically seek out CAM therapies most often for chronic conditions like back pain, arthritis, depression, headaches, and cancer. Asking questions about usage of CAM therapies in an **open-ended, nonjudgmental fashion** should encourage patients to be more forthcoming and free about discussing unconventional practices they may be exploring or using.

C. **Exercising caution.** Once patients who utilize CAM therapies are identified, great care must be taken to ensure that there are no potential interactions with the conventional care you or your health care team plan to institute, whether medical or surgical. Patients who take multiple medications, particularly the elderly, need to be monitored carefully for drug-herbal interactions and potential liver or kidney toxicity. While some information is generally available about the side effects of most unconventional treatments, much is not known about the side effects of many others. Physicians should be cautious of products sold by relatively new companies or products that contain multiple substances rather than a single herb product.

D. **Knowing your limitations.** There are dozens of CAM therapies available to the general public and it is impractical for physicians to learn them all. When in doubt about an unconventional therapy mentioned by a patient, it is prudent to get more information by looking it up on the internet at a reputable website (i.e., www.nlm.nih.gov/nccam/camonpubmed.html or www.ods.od.nih.gov), consulting with a trusted colleague with more experience, or contacting one of the many centers of complementary medicine that now exist at reputable hospitals around the country, such as the Center for Alternative Medicine Research at Beth Israel Deaconess Medical Center in Boston.

III. Common CAM therapies

A. **Acupuncture** is a form of traditional Chinese medicine that has been practiced for nearly 4,000 years. In 1993, the Food and Drug Administration estimated that Americans made up to 12 million visits a year to acupuncturists, spending more than $500 million.

1. **Philosophy.** Practitioners of acupuncture believe there are as many as 2,000 acupuncture points on the human body connected by 20 pathways called meridians. These meridians are said to conduct energy, or **qi** (pronounced "chi"), between the surface of the body and its internal

organs. Each point is further said to have a different effect on the qi that passes through it. Scientific theories as to how acupuncture works relate to its possible ability to block pain impulses from reaching the spinal cord or by stimulating release of endorphins or other pain-relieving opioids. Unlike hypodermic needles, acupuncture needles are solid, hair-thin, and not designed to cut the skin.

2. **Scientific evidence.** In 1997, a consensus statement released by the National Institutes of Health said that acupuncture could be useful by itself or in combination with other therapies to treat addiction, headaches, menstrual cramps, tennis elbow, fibromyalgia, myofascial pain, osteoarthritis, lower back pain, carpal tunnel syndrome, and bronchial asthma. A 2003 analysis of 30 randomized controlled trials of acupuncture efficacy for the treatment of migraines/headache and nausea/vomiting, however, found researchers often neglected to report adequately on important clinical details and frequently did not comment on the reliability, validity, and clinical significance of the outcome measures used in the trials, rendering critical appraisal of clinical efficacy difficult. A similar review of studies looking at acupuncture for the treatment of obesity found most trials to be descriptive in nature, of short duration (less than or equal to 12 weeks), and designed using nonstandard treatment protocols.

3. **Scope of practice.** As a component of traditional Chinese medicine, acupuncture is often complemented by treatment with Chinese herbal supplements and remedies. Some allopathic and osteopathic physicians have received training in acupuncture and offer it as part of a more holistic approach to their patient's care. Since the 1970s, schools of acupuncture have flourished throughout the United States (now numbering 53), and acupuncture is independently licensed as a health care modality in 37 states.

B. **Ayurvedic** medicine is a holistic system of health care originating in India 6,000 years ago that uses what is called a constitutional model of care. Its aim is to provide guidance regarding food and lifestyle so that healthy people can stay healthy and individuals with disease can improve their health. Its recommendations vary depending on the patient's lifestyle.

1. **Philosophy.** In Ayurveda ("Ayu" means life, "veda" means knowledge), each person is considered a unique individual made up of five primary elements: space, air, fire, water, and earth. These elements combine in various ways to form one of three doshas (Vata dosha, Pitta dosha, and Kapha dosha), whose ratios are said to vary in each individual. When any dosha is felt to be in excess, Ayurvedic practitioners will suggest specific lifestyle and nutritional guidelines to reduce the excess and restore the necessary balance.

2. **Scientific evidence.** While there are few randomized controlled trials, much basic and descriptive research has been done over the past few decades, particularly in India. A 2003 review of the literature found turmeric, a spice, to be safe in six human trials where it demonstrated some anti-inflammatory activity.

C. **Chiropractic** is perhaps the largest and best recognized of CAM therapies. Once considered a "deviant" practice, it has undergone steadily increasing acceptance, and there are expected to be 100,000 chiropractors in the United States by 2010.

1. **Philosophy.** Daniel Palmer is credited with founding the profession, which primarily focuses on spinal manipulation (one of the oldest healing methods known to man), and is said to have performed his first spinal "adjustment" in 1895. Palmer criticized the use of drugs and surgery as unnatural invasions of the body and focused on what he perceived as normalizing the function of the nervous system as the key to health. Many chiropractors today also provide physical therapies such as heat, cold, and rehabilitation methods.

2. **Scientific evidence.** Forty-three randomized trials of spinal manipulation for the treatment of acute, subacute, and chronic low back pain have been published in the medical literature. Thirty favored manipulation over the comparison treatments in at least a subgroup of patients, while the other 13 found no significant differences.

3. **Scope of practice.** All patients traditionally paid for chiropractic care out-of-pocket until Medicare included chiropractic services in the 1970s. Today, more than 50% of health maintenance organizations and more than 75% of private health insurance plans now offer chiropractic services. Most colleges of chiropractic in the United States are accredited by the Council on Chiropractic Education, an agency certified by the U.S. Department of Education, and offer four academic years of professional education after a baccalaureate degree before students can qualify for licensure.

D. **Homeopathy** was founded by the German physician, Samuel Hahnemann, in the late 19th century and it quickly spread throughout Europe before reaching the United States.

1. **Philosophy.** Homeopathy follows the principle of "like cures like" (called the "Principle of Similars"), which claims that a substance that produces a set of symptoms in a healthy person should be able in highly diluted doses (often to the point where very little of the original substance is likely to remain) to treat an identical symptom successfully in a sick person.

2. **Scientific evidence.** Even though the limit of molecular dilution (Avogadro's number) was not discovered until the latter part of Hahnemann's life, homeopaths by then had already reported throughout the world that dilutions lower than Avogadro's number produced clinical effects. It is this fact that has led many physicians, scientists, and skeptics to believe that homeopathy's effectiveness is perhaps a delusion. Some data—including randomized, controlled trials in children with diarrhea and adults with influenza—show modest treatment (but not prevention) benefits from homeopathic remedies and this appears to defy any contemporary rational basis. One 2002 randomized, controlled trial of homeopathic potencies of house dust mite found no benefit, on the other hand, in the treatment of patients with bronchial asthma.

3. **Scope of practice.** Boston University School of Medicine and New York Medical College began as homeopathic colleges of medicine before abandoning that philosophy. Homeopaths today can be licensed independently in only three states and use some conventional care in addition to homeopathic practice and other CAM therapies. Because they are extremely diluted and not felt to be harmful, homeopathic medications were allowed by the 1939 Pure Food and Drug Act and are available over the counter.

IV. Miscellaneous CAM therapies

A. **Aromatherapy** involves the use of essential oils (extracts or essences) from flowers, herbs, and trees to promote health and well-being.

B. **Bioelectromagnetic fields** involve use of invisible lines of force to promote health in therapies that have not been scientifically proven. Included are such therapies as pulsed fields, magnetic fields, and alternating or direct current fields.

C. **Massage** therapists manipulate muscle and connective tissue to enhance function of those tissues and promote relaxation and well-being.

D. **Naturopathic** practitioners (naturopaths) work with natural healing forces within the body, with a goal of helping the body heal from disease and attain better health. Practices include dietary modifications, massage, exercise, acupuncture, minor surgery, and various other interventions.

E. **Qi gong** is a component of traditional Chinese medicine that combines movement, meditation, and regulation of breathing to enhance the flow of vital energy in the body, improve blood circulation, and enhance immune function.

F. **Reiki** is a Japanese word meaning "universal life energy." It is based on the belief that when spiritual energy is channeled through a Reiki practitioner, the patient's spirit is healed, in turn healing the physical body.

G. **Therapeutic touch** is derived from an ancient technique called laying-on of hands and is based on the premise that it is the healing force of the therapist that affects the patient's recovery.

REFERENCES

Chainani-Wu N: Safety and anti-inflammatory activity of curcumin: a compound of turmeric (Curcuma longa). *J Altern Complement Med*, 9(1):161–168, 2003.

Chairman's Summary of the Conference: Education of Health Professionals in Complementary/Alternative Medicine, Josiah Macy, Jr. Foundation, New York, pp. 1–4, 2001.

Cooper RA, Stoflet SJ: Trends in the education and practice of alternative medicine clinicians. *Health Aff* (Millwood), 15:226–238, 1996.

Eisenberg DM, Kessler RC, Foster C, et al: Unconventional medicine in the United States. Prevalence, costs, and patterns of use. *N Engl J Med*, 328: 246–252, 1993.

Elorriaga CA, Hanna SE, Fargas-Babjak A: Reporting of clinical trials in randomized controlled trials of acupuncture for the treatment of migraine/headache and nausea/vomiting. *J Altern Complement Med*, 9(1):151–159, 2003.

Jones WB, Kaptchuk TJ, Linde K: A critical overview of homeopathy. *Ann Intern Med*, 138:393–399, 2003.

Kelly CK: How to help patients who use alternative medicine. *ACP-ASIM Observer*, Philadelphia, p. 4, 2001.

Kessler RC, Davis RB, Foster DF, et al.: Long-term trends in the use of complementary and alternative medical therapies in the United States. *Ann Intern Med*, 135:262–268, 2001.

Lacey JM, Tershakovec AM, Foster GD: Acupuncture for the treatment of obesity: a review of the evidence. *Int J Obes Relat Metab Disord*, 27(4):419–427, 2003.

Lewith GT, Watkins ME, Hyland ME, et al.: Use of ultramolecular potencies of allergen to treat asthmatic people allergic to house dust mite: double blind randomized controlled clinical trial. *B Med J*, 324:520–523, 2002.

Maddox J, Randi J, Stewart WW: "High-dilution" experiments a delusion. *Nature*, 334:287–291, 1998.

Meeker WC and Haldeman S: Chiropractic: a profession at the crossroads of mainstream and alternative medicine. *Ann Intern Med*, 136:216–227, 2002.

Moore J: *Chiropractic in America. The history of a medical alternative.* Baltimore: Johns Hopkins Univ Press, 1993.

Pelletier KR, Marie A, Krasner M, and Haskell WL: Current trends in the integration and reimbursement of complementary and alternative medicine by managed care, insurance carriers, and hospital providers. *Am J Health Promot*, 12:112–122, 1997.

Wardwell WI: *Chiropractic. History and Evolution of a New Profession*, St. Louis: Mosby-Year Book, 1992.

Wetzel MS, Eisenberg DM, and Kaptchuk TJ: Courses involving complementary and alternative medicine at US medical schools. *JAMA*, 280:784–787, 1998.

www.nccam.nih.gov

PART V

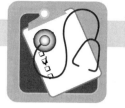

Appendices

Clinical Signs

While on the wards or in physicians' offices you will hear mentioned many clinical signs that have been named for the physicians who first described them or the phenomena they resemble. Following is a list of some of the most commonly mentioned signs. This list is meant to be used as a reference; however, we have starred (*) those signs that would be worth learning before you start seeing patients.

*   **Argyll Robertson pupil:** miotic pupil that responds normally to accommodation but not to light; associated with neurosyphilis.
    Austin-Flint murmur: a diastolic rumbling murmur heard best at the cardiac apex; associated with severe aortic regurgitation.
*   **Babinski reflex:** dorsiflexion of the big toe after stimulation of the lateral sole; associated with corticospinal tract lesions.
    Bagpipe sign: when patient cuts short a forced expiration while the stethoscope is on the chest, the sound of expelling air is heard to continue after his or her effort has ceased; associated with partial bronchial obstruction.
    Ballet's sign: external ophthalmoplegia, with loss of voluntary eye movements; the pupillary movements and reflex eye movements are intact; associated with Graves's disease and hysteria.
*   **Battle's sign:** discoloration in the line of the posterior auricular artery, the ecchymosis first appearing near the top of the mastoid process; associated with basilar skull fracture.
*   **Beck's triad:** distended neck veins, distant heart sounds, hypotension; associated with cardiac tamponade.
    Blumberg's sign: transient pain in the abdomen after approximated fingers pressed gently into abdominal wall are suddenly withdrawn—rebound tenderness; associated with peritoneal inflammation.
    Borsieri's sign: when fingernail is drawn along skin in early stages of scarlet fever, a white line is left that quickly turns red.
    Branham's bradycardia: bradycardia and augmentation of both systolic and diastolic arterial pressure after digital closure of an artery proximal to an arteriovenous fistula.
*   **Brudzinski's sign:** flexion of the hip and knee induced by flexion of the neck; associated with meningeal irritation.
    Carvallo's sign: an apical holosystolic murmur that becomes louder during inspiration and leaning forward; associated with tricuspid regurgitation.
*   **Chadwick's sign:** cyanosis of vaginal and cervical mucosa; associated with pregnancy.
*   **Charcot's triad:** nystagmus, intention tremor, staccato speech; associated with multiple sclerosis.
*   **Chvostek's sign:** facial muscle spasm induced by tapping on the facial nerve branches; associated with hypocalcemia.

* **Cheyne-Stokes respiration:** rhythmic cycles of deep and shallow respiration, often with apneic periods; associated with central nervous system respiratory center dysfunction.

Coppernail's sign: ecchymoses on the perineum, scrotum, or labia; associated with fracture of the pelvis.

Corrigan's pulse: an arterial pulse wave that rises suddenly and collapses abruptly; also known as a water hammer pulse; associated with severe aortic regurgitation.

* **Courvoisier's sign:** an enlarged nontender gallbladder; associated with carcinoma of the head of the pancreas.

* **Cullen's sign:** bluish discoloration of the umbilicus; associated with acute pancreatitis or hemoperitoneum, especially rupture of fallopian tube in ectopic pregnancy.

Dalrymple's sign: a peculiar staring appearance of the eyes caused by a widened palpebral fissure (lid retraction); associated with hyperthyroidism.

Delphian node: a lymph node that drains the thyroid gland and larynx and lies directly anterior to the cricothyroid ligament; associated with thyroid cancer, Hashimoto's thyroiditis, and laryngeal cancer.

De Musset's sign: anterior-posterior bobbing of the head that is synchronous with arterial pulsations; associated with severe aortic regurgitation.

* **Doll's eye sign:** dissociation between the movements of the head and eyes: as the head is raised the eyes are lowered, and as the head is lowered the eyes are raised; associated with global-diffuse disorders of the cerebrum.

* **Drawer sign:** supine patient flexes his or her knee and rests foot flat on table, and examiner sits on foot to anchor it; head of tibia is pulled toward the physician to test the anterior cruciate ligament, or pushed away from the physician to test the posterior cruciate ligament; movement of more than 1 cm is indicative of a torn cruciate ligament.

Duroziez' sign: a double to-and-fro murmur heard on auscultation of the femoral or brachial artery with firm pressure from a stethoscope; associated with severe aortic regurgitation.

Flag sign: dyspigmentation of the hair occurring as a band of light hair; seen in children who have recovered from kwashiorkor.

* **Fluid wave:** transmission across the abdomen of a wave induced by snapping the abdomen; associated with ascites.

Goldstein's sign: wide distance between the great toe and the adjoining toe; associated with cretinism and trisomy 21.

Gottron's sign/papules: cutaneous lesions consisting of symmetrical macular violaceous erythema, with or without edema, overlying the dorsal aspect of the interphalangeal joints of the hands, olecranon processes, patellas, and medial malleoli; pathognomonic of dermatomyositis.

* **Gowers' sign:** to stand from supine position, patient rolls to the prone position, kneels, and raises himself or herself to a standing position by pushing with the hands against shins, knees, and thighs; associated with pseudohypertrophic muscular dystrophy.

* **Grey Turner's sign:** discoloration of skin of lower abdomen and flanks, caused by massive nontraumatic ecchymoses; associated with hemorrhagic acute pancreatitis.

Grossman's sign: dilatation of the heart; associated with pulmonary tuberculosis.

* **Gunn's pupillary sign (Marcus Gunn pupil):** with patient's eye fixed at a distance and a straight light shining before the intact eye, a crisp bilateral contraction of the pupil is noted. On moving the light to the affected eye, both pupils will dilate for a short period. Then on return of the light to the intact eye, both pupils contract promptly and remain contracted; associated with damage to the optic nerve.

Hamman's sign: crunching sound in the precordium; associated with acute mediastinitis, pneumomediastinum, and pneumothorax.

Harlequin sign: in the newborn infant, reddening of the lower half of the laterally recumbent body and blanching of the upper half, due to a temporary vasomotor disturbance.

Hegar's sign: softening of the fundus of the uterus; associated with the first trimester of pregnancy.

Hoffmann's sign: flexion of the thumb and other fingers, induced by snapping of the index, middle, or ring finger; associated with corticospinal tract disease.

* **Homans' sign:** pain behind the knee, induced by dorsiflexion of the foot; associated with peripheral vascular disease, especially venous thrombosis in the calf.

* **Kehr's sign:** severe pain in the left upper quadrant, radiating to the top of the shoulder; associated with splenic rupture.

* **Kernig's sign:** inability to extend leg when sitting or lying with the thigh flexed on the abdomen; associated with meningeal irritation.

Knie's sign: unequal dilatation of the pupils; associated with Graves's disease.

* **Kussmaul's respiration:** paroxysmal air hunger; associated with acidosis, especially diabetic ketoacidosis.

Kussmaul's sign: paradoxical elevation of central venous pressure during inspiration; associated with constrictive pericarditis and severe congestive heart failure.

* **Levine sign:** clenching of the patient's fist over the sternum while describing chest discomfort; associated with angina.

Lhermitte's sign: development of sudden, transient, electric-like shocks spreading down the body when the patient flexes the head forward; associated with multiple sclerosis and cervical cord compression.

Lucas' sign: distention of the abdomen; associated with the early stages of rickets.

Ludloff's sign: sitting patient cannot flex the thigh; associated with avulsion of the lesser trochanter.

Marie's sign: tremor of the body or extremities; associated with Graves's disease.

Markle's sign: tenderness resulting from patient rising up on his or her toes, then suddenly relaxing so that the heels hit the floor and jar the whole body (jar tenderness); abdominal pain on walking is an equivalent test; associated with peritoneal irritation.

Mayne's sign: a diminution of 15 mm Hg in the diastolic pressure in the arm when it is elevated over the head, as compared with values taken when the arm is at heart level; associated with aortic regurgitation.

* **McBurney's sign:** tenderness at McBurney's point (located two-thirds of the distance from the umbilicus to the anterior-superior iliac spine); associated with appendicitis.

McMurray's sign: occurrence of a cartilage click during manipulation of the knee; associated with meniscal injury.

Müller's sign: pulsation of the uvula and redness of the tonsils and velum palati, occurring synchronously with the action of the heart; associated with severe aortic regurgitation.

* **Murphy's sign:** inspiratory arrest during midcycle of respiration by painful contact with fingers that are held under the liver border, where an inflamed gallbladder may descend upon them; associated with acute cholecystitis.

* **Obturator sign:** hypogastric or adductor pain elicited by passive internal rotation of the flexed thigh, due to contact between an inflammatory process and the internal obdurator muscle; associated with obdurator nerve irritation, often as a result of appendicitis.

* **Osler's node:** small, painful erythematous swellings in the skin of the hands and feet; associated with bacterial endocarditis.

* **Osler's sign:** radial or brachial artery distal to the blood pressure cuff on the arm remains palpable after inflation of the cuff above systolic blood pressure; associated with pseudohypertension due to arterial calcification and stiffness.

Pel-Ebstein fever: a relapsing fever characterized by periods of fever lasting days interspersed by equally long afebrile periods; associated with Hodgkin's disease.

Pemberton's sign: congestion of the face, cyanosis, and eventual discomfort induced by arm elevation; associated with a large substernal or retroclavicular goiter.

* **Psoas sign:** pain induced by hyperextension of the right thigh while lying on the left side; associated with appendicitis.

Quincke's sign: abnormally conspicuous capillary pulsations elicited by blanching a portion of the nailbed and then observing the pulsating border between the white and red color; associated with severe aortic regurgitation.

Radovici's sign: vigorous scratching or pricking of the thenar eminence causes a palomental primitive reflex, ipsilateral contraction of the muscles of the chin; associated with corticospinal tract disease, increased intracranial pressure, and latent tetany.

* **Romberg's sign:** unsteadiness or falling down when the eyes are closed and the feet are close together; associated with tabes dorsalis and labyrinthine disorders.

Romberg-Howship sign: pain down the medial aspect of the thigh to the knee due to obdurator nerve compression; associated with obturator hernias.

* **Rovsing's sign:** pressure over the left lower quadrant elicits pain in the right lower quadrant; associated with appendicitis.

Rumpel-Leede sign: development of petechiae on an arm distal to the application of positive pressure using a tourniquet or blood pressure cuff; associated with coagulopathies, scurvy, hypothyroidism, and Osler-Weber-Rendu syndrome.

* **Setting-sun sign:** downward deviation of the eyes so that each iris appears to "set" beneath the lower lid, with white sclera exposed between it and the upper lid; associated with increased intracranial pressure or irritation of the brainstem.

Shamroth's sign: the formation of a diamond-shaped window, its contour outlined by the bases of the nailbeds, when terminal phalanges of similar fingers are opposed back to back (especially the ring fingers); absence of the window is an indicator of clubbing and underlying respiratory disease.

Siegert's sign: pinky fingers are short and curved inward; associated with trisomy 21.

* **Sister Mary Joseph nodule:** a hard, dermal or subcutaneous umbilical nodule; associated with metastatic carcinoma.

Sisto's sign: constant inconsolable crying; associated with congenital syphilis in infancy.

Squire's sign: alternate contraction and dilatation of the pupil; associated with basilar meningitis.

Stellwag's sign: infrequent blinking, associated with thyrotoxicosis.

* **Tinel's sign:** tingling sensation felt from light percussion on the radial side of the palmaris longus tendon; associated with carpal tunnel syndrome.

Trendelenburg's sign: the falling of one buttock relative to the other because the muscles are not strong enough to sustain position when the femur is not engaged in the acetabulum; associated with dislocation of the hip.

Van Graefe's sign: the appearance of white sclera between the margin of the upper eyelid and corneal limbus (lid lag) as the patient looks downward; associated with hyperthyroidism.

Weber's sign: paralysis of the oculomotor nerve on one side and hemiplegia of the opposite side; associated with impending uncal herniation.

Westphal's sign: loss of knee jerk; associated with tabes dorsalis.

Whipple's triad: spontaneous hypoglycemia, central nervous or vasomotor system symptoms, relief of symptoms by the oral or intravenous administration of glucose; associated with insulin-producing tumors.

Williamson's sign: markedly diminished blood pressure in the leg as compared with that in the arm on the same side; associated with pneumothorax and pleural effusions.

Preventive Medicine Screening Recommendations

Every thoughtful physician recognizes that there is a distinct difference between carefully choosing screening tests for various maladies that are otherwise not recognizable on history and physical examination and indiscriminately ordering a battery of tests to look for the presence of disease. Screening tests are generally considered most useful when they are relatively inexpensive, easy and safe to perform, maintain a high sensitivity and specificity and are directed towards common diseases or conditions. The results should allow early intervention so that there is a positive impact on a patient's quality of life, morbidity, and mortality. It is prudent to have the patient actively involved in the decision-making for such testing, and this requires taking a few minutes to explain how the tests are run and what the results may mean before proceeding.

A number of medical specialty organizations (e.g., American College of Physicians), subspecialty societies (e.g., American Cancer Society), and national bodies comprised of prominent experts in the field of epidemiology and preventive medicine (e.g., United States Preventive Services Task Force) regularly review the world's evidence-based medical literature to develop and clarify cancer screening recommendations for physicians and other ancillary health care personnel to consider for their patients. The following list, current as of 2003, outlines the various positions and guidelines of these organizations for a number of common screening tests.

Type of Cancer	General Recommendation	Additional Screening Recommendations
Breast cancer	Breast examination by a physician every 1–2 years from age 40. Yearly mammography, from age 50–75. Monthly self-examination at midcycle.	ACS, ACOG: annual or biannual mammography and annual breast examination by a clinician from age 40–50.
Colorectal cancer	Annual fecal occult blood testing and flexible sigmoidoscopy every 3–5 years starting at age 50.	ACP: flexible sigmoidoscopy, colonoscopy, or double-contrast barium enema every 10 years from age 50–70.
Cervical cancer	Pap smear every 1–3 years, from start of sexual activity. Screening can be	More frequent screening for patients with risk factors including early onset of sexual

	stopped by age 65 if the examinations are consistently normal.	activity, multiple sex partners, low socio-economic status, or HIV infection.
Prostate cancer	Annual counselling about potential risks and benefits of screening with PSA and DRE so the patient can make an informed decision.	USPSTF: DRE and PSA are not recommended in asymptomatic men. ACS, AUA: yearly DRE and PSA starting at age 50, or age 40 in African-American men or men with a positive family history of prostate cancer.
Lung cancer	Screening with chest roentgenograph or sputum cytology is considered ineffective.	
Skin cancer	Complete skin inspection only for patients at high risk, patients with a family or personal history of skin cancer, or patients with a precursor lesion (e.g., dysplastic nevi).	ACS, AAD: periodic complete skin inspection by a clinician for all patients as well as monthly self-examination
Ovarian cancer	Careful examination of the uterine adnexa during annual pelvic examination.	ACP: counsel high-risk patients about the potential risks and benefits of lab screening with CA-125 and ultrasound.
Testicular cancer	Routine testicular examination only in high-risk patients: those with testicular atrophy, cryptorchidism, or orchiopexy.	ACS: testicular exam as part of the periodic health exam.

AAD-American Academy of Dermatology, ACOG-American College of Obstetricians and Gynecologists, ACP-American College of Physicians, ACS-American Cancer Society, AUA-American Urological Association, DRE-Digital rectal examination, PSA-Prostate-specific antigen, USPSTF: United States Preventive Services Task Force.

(Adapted with permission from Kutty K, Schapira RM, Ruiswyk JV, and Kochar MS. *Kochar's Concise Textbook of Medicine.* 4th ed. Lippincott Williams and Wilkins. 2003. pp. 23–24.)

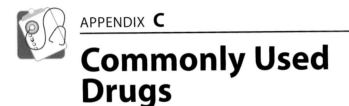

APPENDIX C

Commonly Used Drugs

Most of the patients you will see and manage will be taking several medications. This appendix is designed to serve as a quick guide to many of the most common medications you will encounter. Part one lists drugs by their chemical or generic name, and part two (beginning on page *369*) is a similar list sorted by trade name. Part three (beginning on page *383*) lists drugs by class, giving common indications and their mechanisms of action where known. Note that we have not included on this list any antineoplastic agents, a category of agents with their own unique indications, contraindications, efficacy, and mechanisms of action; instead we have listed those medications you are most likely to encounter in the inpatient and outpatient settings in the general population.

When a patient mentions a drug, look it up on the appropriate list, then turn to its drug class in part three to learn why it is probably being used and how it works. We do not mention here dosages or side effects; this is well covered in other sources (see, for instance, *Handbook of Commonly Prescribed Drugs*, 16th ed., by Digregorio and Babieri [Medical Surveillance, 2001]).

Part One: Drugs by Chemical/Generic Name

Chemical/ Generic name	Trade name	Drug class
Abacavir	Ziagen	Anti-HIV
Abacavir/Lamivudine/ Zidovudine	Trizivir	Anti-HIV
Abciximab	ReoPro	Antiplatelet
Acarbose	Precose	Antidiabetic
Acebutolol	Sectral	Antiarrhythmic
Acetazolamide	Diamox	Diuretic
Acetaminophen	Datril, Tempra, Tylenol	Nonopioid analgesic
Acyclovir	Zovirax	Antiviral
Albuterol	Proventil, Ventolin, Volmax	Antiasthmatic
Albuterol/Ipatropium	Combivent, Duoneb	Antiasthmatic
Alendronate	Fosamax	Antiosteoporosis
Allopurinol	Zyloprim	Antigout
Alprazolam	Xanax	Antianxiety
Alteplase	Activase	Thrombolytic
Amantidine	Symmetrel	Anti-influenza

Chemical/ Generic name	Trade name	Drug class
Amikacin	Amikin	Antibacterial
Amiloride	Midamor	Diuretic
Amiloride/HCTZ	Moduretic	Diuretic
Aminophylline	Aminophyllin	Antiasthmatic
Amiodarone	Cordarone, Pacerone	Antiarrhythmic
Amitriptyline	Elavil	Antidepressant
Amlodipine	Norvasc	Antihypertensive
Amlodipine and Benazepril	Lotrel	Antihypertensive
Amoxicillin	Amoxil, Trimox, Moxilin	Antibacterial
Amoxicillin and potassium clavulanate	Augmentin	Antibacterial
Amphetamine and dextroamphetamine	Adderall	Anti-ADHD
Amphoterocin B	Fungizone, Amphocin	Antifungal
Ampicillin	Amcill, Omnipen-N, Principen	Antibacterial
Ampicillin/sulbactam	Unasyn	Antibacterial
Amprenavir	Agenerase	Anti-HIV
Ardeparin	Normiflo	Anticoagulant
Aspirin	Bayer, Ecotrin	Nonopioid analgesic
Atenolol	Tenormin	Antihypertensive
Atenolol and chlorthalidone	Tenoretic	Antihypertensive
Atorvastatin	Lipitor	Cholesterol lowering
Atovaquone	Mepron	Antiprotozoal
Atropine and diphenoxylate	Lomotil	Antidiarrheal
Azithromycin	Zithromax	Antibacterial
Aztreonam	Azactam	Antibacterial
Baclofen	Lioresal	Antispastic
Beclomethasone	Beclovent, Beconase, Vancenase, Vanceril, Vanceril DS, Qvar	Antiasthmatic
Benazepril	Lotensin	Antihypertensive
Benazepril and amlodipine	Lotrel	Antihypertensive
Benazepril/HCTZ	Lotensin HCT	Antihypertensive
Bendroflumethiazide and nadolol	Corzide	Antihypertensive
Betaxolol	Kerlone	Antihypertensive
Bisacodyl	Dulcolax	Laxative
Bisoprolol	Zebeta	Antihypertensive
Bisoprolol/HCTZ	Ziac	Antihypertensive
Bitolterol	Tornalate	Antiasthmatic

Chemical/ Generic name	Trade name	Drug class
Bretylium	Bretylol	Antiarrhythmic
Bromocriptine	Bromocriptine	Antiparkinsonian
Budesonide	Pulmicort	Antiasthmatic
Bumetanide	Bumex	Diuretic
Bupropion	Wellbutrin, Wellbutrin SR	Antidepressant
Buspirone	BuSpar, Vanspar	Antianxiety
Calcitonin salmon	Miacalcin	Antiosteoporosis
Candesartan	Atacand	Antihypertensive
Candesartan/HCTZ	Atacand HCT	Antihypertensive
Captopril	Capoten	Antihypertensive
Captopril/HCTZ	Capozide	Antihypertensive
Carbamazepine	Tegretol, Tegretol XR, Carbatrol	Anticonvulsant
Carbenicillin	Geocillin, Geopen, Piopen	Antibacterial
Carbidopa/levodopa	Sinemet, Sinemet CR, Atamet	Antiparkinsonian
Carisoprodol	Soma	Muscle relaxant
Carteolol	Cartrol	Antihypertensive
Carvedilol	Coreg	Antihypertensive
Cefaclor	Ceclor	Antibacterial
Cefadroxil	Duricef	Antibacterial
Cefamandole	Mandol	Antibacterial
Cefepime	Maxipime	Antibacterial
Cefazolin	Ancef, Kefzol	Antibacterial
Cefdinir	Omnicef	Antibacterial
Cefixime	Suprax	Antibacterial
Cefotaxime	Claforan	Antibacterial
Cefotetan	Cefotan	Antibacterial
Cefoxitin	Mefoxin	Antibacterial
Cefpodoxime	Vantin	Antibacterial
Cefprozil	Cefzil	Antibacterial
Ceftazidime	Fortaz, Ceptaz, Tazicef	Antibacterial
Ceftibuten	Cedax	Antibacterial
Ceftizoxime	Cefizox	Antibacterial
Ceftriaxone	Rocephin	Antibacterial
Cefuroxime	Zinacef, Kefurox, Ceftin	Antibacterial
Celecoxib	Celebrex	Nonopioid analgesic
Cephalothin		Antibacterial
Cephalexin	Keflex, Bio-Cef	Antibacterial
Cephapirin	Cefadyl	Antibacterial
Cephradine	Velosef	Antibacterial

Chemical/ Generic name	Trade name	Drug class
Cetirizine	Zyrtec	Antihistamine
Chloral hydrate	Noctec	Sedative
Chloramphenicol	Chloromycetin	Antibacterial
Chlordiazepoxide	Librium	Antianxiety
Chlorothiazide	Diuril	Diuretic
Chlorpromazine	Thorazine	Antipsychotic
Chlorpropramide	Diabenese	Antidiabetic
Chlorthalidone	Thalitone	Diuretic
Cholestyramine	Questran, Questran Light, Prevalite	Cholesterol lowering
Cidofovir	Vistide	Antiviral
Cimetidine	Tagamet	Antiulcer
Ciprofloxacin	Cipro	Antibacterial
Citalopram	Celexa	Antidepressant
Clarithromycin	Biaxin	Antibacterial
Clindamycin	Cleocin	Antibacterial
Clofibrate		Cholesterol lowering
Clonazepam	Klonopin	Anticonvulsant
Clonidine	Catapres, Catapres-TTS	Antihypertensive
Clopidogrel	Plavix	Antiplatelet
Clorazepate	Tranxene	Antianxiety
Clotrimazole	Lotrimin, Mazole	Antifungal
Clotrimazole and Betamethasone	Lotrisone	Antifungal
Clozapine	Clozaril	Antipsychotic
Codeine		Opioid analgesic
Colchicine		Antigout
Colesevelam	WelChol	Cholesterol lowering
Colestipol	Colestid	Cholesterol lowering
Cortisone	Deltasone	Steroid
Cromolyn sodium	Intal, Nasalcrom, Opticrom	Antiasthmatic
Cyclobenzaprine	Flexeril	Muscle relaxant
Cyproheptadine	Periactin	Antihistamine
Dalfopristin and quinupristin	Synercid	Antibacterial
Dalteparin	Fragmin	Anticoagulant
Dantrolene sodium	Dantrium	Antispastic
Delavirdine	Rescriptor	Anti-HIV
Desipramine	Norpramin	Antidepressant
Desloratidine	Clarinex	Antihistamine
Desmopressin	DDAVP, Stimate	Hormone
Dexamethasone	Decadron	Steroid

Chemical/ Generic name	Trade name	Drug class
Diazepam	Valium, Diastat	Antianxiety
Diclofenac	Cataflam, Voltaren, Voltaren-XR	Nonopioid analgesic
Diclofenac and Misoprostol	Arthrotec	Nonopioid analgesic
Dicloxacillin	Dycell, Dynapen	Antibacterial
Didanosine	Videx, Videx EC	Anti-HIV
Digoxin	Lanoxicaps, Lanoxin, Digitek	Inotropic agent
Diltiazem	Cardizem, Cardizem CD, Cartia, Dilacor, Dilacor CR, Diltia, Tiazac	Antianginal
Diphenhydramine	Benadryl, Benolyn	Antihistamine
Diphenoxylate with atropine	Lomotil	Antidiarrheal
Dipyridamole	Persantine	Anticoagulant
Dirithromycin	Dynabac	Antibacterial
Disopyramide	Norpace, Norpace CR	Antiarrhythmic
Disulfiram	Antabuse	Antialcohol
Divalproex	Depakote	Anticonvulsant
Dobutamine	Dobutrex	Inotropic agent
Dofetilide	Tikosyn	Antiarrhythmic
Dopamine	Dopistat, Intopin	Inotropic agent
Doxazosin	Cardura	Antihypertensive
Doxepin	Atapin, Sinequan	Antidepressant
Doxycycline	Vibramycin, Vibra-Tabs	Antibacterial
Ducosate sodium	Colace	Laxative
Dyphylline	Lufyllin	Antiasthmatic
Ebtifibatide	Integrilin	Antiplatelet
Efavirenz	Sustiva	Anti-HIV
Enalapril	Vasotec	Antihypertensive
Enalapril/HCTZ	Vaseretic	Antihypertensive
Enalaprilat	Vasotec IV	Antihypertensive
Enoxaparin	Lovenox	Anticoagulant
Ephedrine		Inotropic agent
Epinephrine	Adrenalin	Inotropic agent
Eprosartan	Teveten	Antihypertensive
Erythromycin	E-Mycin, Erythrocin, Ilosone, Ery-Tab	Antibacterial
Esmolol	Brevibloc	Antiarrhythmic
Esomeprazole	Nexium	Antiulcer
Estradiol	Estrace	Hormone
Estrogen	Premarin	Hormone

Chemical/ Generic name	Trade name	Drug class
Estazolam	Prosom	Antianxiety
Ethacrynic Acid	Edecrin	Diuretic
Ethinyl Estradiol	Mircette	Contraceptive
Ethinyl Estradiol and Norethindrone	Necon 1/35	Contraceptive
Ethionamide	Trecator-SC	Antituberculous
Ethotoin	Preganone	Anticonvulsant
Ethosuximide	Zarontin	Anticonvulsant
Famcyclovir	Famvir	Antiviral
Famotidine	Pepcid	Antiulcer
Felbamate	Felbatol	Anticonvulsant
Felodipine	Plendil	Antihypertensive
Fenofibrate	Tricor	Cholesterol lowering
Fentanyl	Sublimaze	Opioid analgesic
Fexofenadine	Allegra	Antihistamine
Fexofenadine and Pseudoephedrine	Allegra-D	Antihistamine
Flecanide	Tambocor	Antiarrhythmic
Fluconazole	Diflucan	Antifungal
Flunisolide	Aerobid	Antiasthmatic
Fluoxetine	Prozac	Antidepressant
Fluphenazine	Permitil, Prolixin	Antipsychotic
Flurazepam	Dalmane	Antianxiety
Fluticasone	Flonase, Flovent	Antiasthmatic
Fluvastatin	Lescol, Lescol XL	Cholesterol lowering
Formoterol	Foradil	Antiasthmatic
Foscarnet	Foscavir	Antiviral
Fosinopril	Monopril	Antihypertensive
Fosphenytoin	Cerebyx	Anticonvulsant
Furosemide	Lasix, Furocot	Diuretic
Gabapentin	Neurontin	Anticonvulsant
Ganciclovir	Cytovene, Vitrasert	Antiviral
Gatifloxacin	Tequin	Antibacterial
Gemfibrozil	Lopid	Cholesterol lowering
Gentamycin	Garamycin	Antibacterial
Glargine Insulin	Lantus	Antidiabetic
Glimepiride	Amaryl	Antidiabetic
Glipizide	Glucotrol, Glucotrol XL	Antidiabetic
Glyburide	Diabeta, Micronase	Antidiabetic
Glyburide micronized	Glycron, Glynase, Pres-Tab	Antidiabetic

Chemical/ Generic name	Trade name	Drug class
Glyburide/metformin	Glucovance	Antidiabetic
Griseofulvin	Fulvicin, Grifulvin, Grisactin, Gris-PEG	Antifungal
Guanfacine	Tenex	Antihypertensive
Haloperidol	Haldol	Antipsychotic
Heparin sodium		Anticoagulant
Hydralazine	Apresoline	Antihypertensive
Hydrochlorothiazide	HydroDiuril, Hydrocot, Microzide, Oretic	Diuretic
Hydrocodone and Ibuprofen	Vicoprofen	Opioid analgesic
Hydrocortisone	Solu-Cortef	Steroid
Hydromorphone	Dilaudid	Opioid analgesic
Hydroxyzine	Atarax, Vistaril	Antihistamine
Hyoscyamine	Cytospaz, Levbid, Levsin, LuLev	Antispasmodic
Ibuprofen	Advil, Motrin	Nonopioid analgesic
Ibutilide	Corvert	Antiarrhythmic
Imipenem/cilastatin	Primaxin	Antibacterial
Imipramine	Tofranil	Antidepressant
Indapamide	Lozol	Diuretic
Indinavir	Crixivan	Anti-HIV
Insulin		Hormone
Ipratropium bromide	Atrovent	Antiasthmatic
Irbesartan	Avapro	Antihypertensive
Irbesartan/HCTZ	Avalide	Antihypertensive
Isoniazid	INH	Antituberculous
Isoniazid and pyrazinamide and rifampin	Rifater	Antituberculous
Isoniazid/rifampin	Rifamate	Antituberculous
Isosorbide dinitrate	Isordil, Diltrate-DR	Antianginal
Isosorbide mononitrate	Imdur, Ismo, Monoket	Antianginal
Isradipine	DynaCirc	Antihypertensive
Itraconazole	Sporanox	Antifungal
Ketoconazole	Nizoral	Antifungal
Labetolol	Normodyne	Antihypertensive
Lamivudine	Epivir	Anti-HIV
Lamivudine and zidovudine	Combivir	Anti-HIV
Lansoprazole	Prevacid	Antiulcer
Lactulose	Chronulac	Laxative
Latanoprost	Xalatan	Antiglaucoma

Chemical/ Generic name	Trade name	Drug class
Lepirudin	Refludan	Anticoagulant
Levalbuterol	Xopenex	Antiasthmatic
Levofloxacin	Levaquin	Antibacterial
Levonorgestrel	Mirena, Norplant System, Alesse, Levlite	Contraceptive
Levothyroxine	Synthroid, Levothyroid, Levoxyl	Hormone
Lidocaine	Xylocaine	Antiarrhythmic
Linezolid	Zyvox	Antibacterial
Lisinopril	Prinivil, Zestril	Antihypertensive
Lisinopril/HCTZ	Zestoretic, Prinzide	Antihypertensive
Lispro Insulin	Humalog	Antidiabetic
Lithium carbonate	Eskalith	Antimanic
Lomefloxacin	Maxaquin	Antibacterial
Loperamide	Imodium	Antidiarrheal
Lopinavir/Ritonavir	Kaletra	Anti-HIV
Loracarbef	Lorabid	Antibacterial
Loratidine	Claritin Reditabs	Antihistamine
Loratidine and Pseudoephedrine	Claritin-D	Antihistamine
Lorazepam	Ativan	Antianxiety
Losartan	Cozaar	Antihypertensive
Losartan/HCTZ	Hyzaar	Antihypertensive
Lovastatin	Mevacor	Cholesterol lowering
Loxapine	Loxitane	Antipsychotic
Meclizine	Antivert	Antihistamine
Medroxyprogesterone	Depo-Provera	Contraceptive
Meperidine	Demerol	Opioid analgesic
Meprobamate and aspirin	Equagesic	Muscle relaxant
Meropenem	Merrem	Antibacterial
Mesoridazine	Serentil	Antipsychotic
Metaproterenol	Alupent, Metaprel	Antiasthmatic
Metaraminol	Aramine	Inotropic agent
Metformin	Glucophage	Antidiabetic
Methadone	Dolophine	Opioid analgesic
Methicillin	Staphcillin	Antibacterial
Methimazole	Tapazole	Antithyroid
Methocarbamol	Robaxin	Muscle relaxant
Methsuximide	Celontin	Anticonvulsant
Methyclothiazide	Enduron	Diuretic
Methyldopa	Aldomet	Antihypertensive

Chemical/ Generic name	Trade name	Drug class
Methyldopa and chlorothiazide	Aldoclor	Antihypertensive
Methylphenidate	Ritalin, Concerta, Methylin	CNS stimulant
Methylprednisolone	Medrol, Depo-Medrol, Solu-Medrol	Steroid
Metoclopramide	Reglan	GI motility agent
Metolazone	Zaroxolyn, Mykrox	Diuretic
Metoprolol	Lopressor, Toprol-XL	Antihypertensive
Metronidazole	Flagyl	Antibacterial
Mezlocillin	Mezlin	Antibacterial
Miconazole	Monistat	Antifungal
Midazolam	Versed	Sedative
Midodrine	ProAmatine	Inotropic agent
Miglitol	Glyset	Antidiabetic
Milrinone	Primacor	Inotropic agent
Minocycline	Dynacin, Minocin, Vectrin	Antibacterial
Minoxidil	Loniten, Rogaine	Antihypertensive
Mirtazapine	Remeron	Antidepressant
Moexipril	Univasc	Antihypertensive
Moexipril/HCTZ	Uniretic	Antihypertensive
Molindone	Moban	Antipsychotic
Mometasone	Elocon, Nasonex	Steroid
Montelukast	Singulair	Antiasthmatic
Moxifloxacin	Avelox	Antibacterial
Mupirocin	Bactroban	Antibacterial
Moricizine	Ethmozine	Antiarrhythmic
Morphine		Opioid analgesic
Nabumetone	Relafen	Nonopioid analgesic
Nadolol	Corgard	Antianginal
Nafcillin	Nallpen	Antibacterial
Naproxen	Naprosyn	Nonopioid analgesic
Naratriptan	Amerge	Antimigraine
Nateglinide	Starlix	Antidiabetic
Nedocromil	Tilade	Antiasthmatic
Nefazodone	Serzone	Antidepressant
Nelfinavir	Viracept	Anti-HIV
Nevirapine	Viramune	Anti-HIV
Niacin	Niaspan, Nicolar	Cholesterol lowering
Nicardipine	Cardene, Cardene SR	Antianginal
Nifedipine	Procardia, Procardia XL, Adalat, Adalat CC	Antianginal

Chemical/ Generic name	Trade name	Drug class
Nisoldipine	Sular	Antihypertensive
Nitrofurantoin	Macrobid, Furadantin, Macrodantin	Antibacterial
Nitroglycerin		Antianginal
Nizatidine	Axid	Antiulcer
Norepinephrine	Levophed	Inotropic agent
Norfloxacin	Noroxin	Antibacterial
Norethindrone and Ethinyl Estradiol	Loestrin Fe 1/20	Contraceptive
Norgestimate/ Ethinyl Estradiol	Ortho Tri-Cyclen, Ortho-Cyclen, Ortho-Novum 7/7/7	Contraceptive
Norgestrel/Ethinyl Estradiol	Lo/Ovral	Contraceptive
L-Norgestrel/Ethinyl Estradiol	Triphasil	Contraceptive
Nortriptyline	Pamelor, Aventyl	Antidepressant
Nystatin	Micostatin, Nilstat	Antifungal
Ofloxacin	Floxin	Antibacterial
Olanzapine	Zyprexa, Zyprexa Zydis	Antipsychotic
Omeprazole	Prilosec	Antiulcer
Orlistat	Xenical	Antiobesity
Oseltamivir	Tamiflu	Anti-influenza
Oxacillin	Bactocill, Prostaphlin	Antibacterial
Oxazepam	Serax	Antianxiety
Oxybutinin	Ditropan, Ditropan XL	Antispasmodic
Oxycodone	Percocet, Percodan, Roxicet, Tylox, Endodan	Opioid analgesic
Oxytocin	Pitocin	Hormone
Palivizumab	Synagis	Antiviral
Pancrelipase	Cotazyme, Pancrease	Hormone
Pantoprazole	Protonix	Antiulcer
Paramethadione	Paradione	Anticonvulsant
Paroxetine	Paxil	Antidepressant
Penbutolol	Levatol	Antihypertensive
Penicillin G, V	Penicillin VK, Veetids	Antibacterial
Pentamidine	Pentam, Nebupent	Antiprotozoal
Perindopril	Aceon	Antihypertensive
Perphenazine	Trilafon	Antipsychotic
Phenelzine	Nardil	Antidepressant
Phenobarbital		Anticonvulsant
Phenylephrine	Neo-Synephrine	Inotropic agent

Chemical/ Generic name	Trade name	Drug class
Phenytoin	Dilantin	Anticonvulsant
Pindolol	Visken	Antihypertensive
Pioglitazone	Actos	Antidiabetic
Piperacillin	Pipracil	Antibacterial
Piperacillin and tazobactam	Zosyn	Antibacterial
Pirbuterol	Maxair	Antiasthmatic
Polythiazide	Renese	Diuretic
Potassium chloride	K-Dur, K-Lor	Potassium supplement
Pravastatin	Pravachol	Cholesterol lowering
Prazosin	Minipress	Antihypertensive
Prednisone		Steroid
Probenecid	Benemid	Antigout
Probenecid and colchicine	ColBENEMID	Antigout
Procainamide	Procan, Pronestyl, Procanbid	Antiarrhythmic
Prochlorperazine	Compazine	Antipsychotic, antiemetic
Promazine		Antipsychotic
Promethazine	Phenergan	Antihistamine
Propafenone	Rhythmol	Antiarrhythmic
Propranolol	Inderal, Inderal LA	Antihypertensive
Propanolol/HCTZ	Inderide, Inderide LA	Antihypertensive
Propoxyphene	Darvocet-N, Darvon-N, Dolene	Opioid analgesic
Pyrazinamide		Antituberculous
Quazepam	Doral	Antianxiety
Quetiapine	Seroquel	Antipsychotic
Quinapril	Accupril	Antihypertensive
Quinapril/HCTZ	Accuretic	Antihypertensive
Quinidine	Quinidex, Quiniglute	Antiarrhythmic
Rabeprazole	Aciphex	Antiulcer
Raloxifene	Evista	Hormone
Ramipril	Altace	Antihypertensive
Ranitidine	Zantac	Antiulcer
Repaglinide	Prandin	Antidiabetic
Reteplase	Retavase	Thrombolytic
Ribavirin	Virazole	Antiviral
Rifabutin	Mycobutin	Antibacterial
Rifampin	Rifadin, Rimactane	Antituberculous
Rifapentine	Priftin	Antituberculous

Chemical/ Generic name	Trade name	Drug class
Rimantidine	Flumadine	Anti-influenza
Risedronate	Actonel	Antiosteoporosis
Risperidone	Risperdal	Antipsychotic
Ritonavir	Norvir	Anti-HIV
Rizatriptan	Maxalt, Maxalt-MLT	Antimigraine
Rofecoxib	Vioxx	Nonopioid analgesic
Rosiglitazone	Avandia	Antidiabetic
Salmeterol	Serevent	Antiasthmatic
Saquinavir	Fortovase, Invirase	Anti-HIV
Secobarbital	Seconal	Sedative
Sertraline	Zoloft	Antidepressant
Sibutramine	Meridia	Antiobesity
Sildenafil	Viagra	Erectile stimulant
Simvastatin	Zocor	Cholesterol lowering
Sotalol	Betapace, Betapace AF	Antiarrhythmic
Sparfloxacin	Zagam	Antibacterial
Spironolactone	Aldactone	Diuretic
Spironolactone/HCTZ	Aldactazide	Diuretic
Stavudine	Zerit	Anti-HIV
Streptokinase	Kabikinase, Streptase	Thrombolytic
Streptomycin		Antituberculous
Sucralfate	Carafate	Antiulcer
Sulfadiazine		Antibacterial
Sulfamethoxazole	Gantanol	Antibacterial
Sulfisoxazole	Gantrisin	Antibacterial
Sumatriptan	Imitrex	Antimigraine
Tamoxifen	Nolvadex	Hormone
Tamsulosin	Flomax	Antiadrenergic
Telmisartan	Micardis	Antihypertensive
Telmisartan/HCTZ	Micardis HCT	Antihypertensive
Temazepam	Restoril	Antianxiety
Tenecteplase	TNKase	Thrombolytic
Terazosin	Hytrin	Antihypertensive
Terbinafine	Lamisil	Antifungal
Terbutaline	Brethine	Antiasthmatic
Tetracycline	Achromycin, Symycin	Antibacterial
Theophylline	Theo-Dur, Theolair, Theo-24, Resbid, Slo-Phyllin	Antiasthmatic
Thioridazine	Mellaril	Antipsychotic

Chemical/ Generic name	Trade name	Drug class
Thiothixene	Navane	Antipsychotic
Ticarcillin	Ticar	Antibacterial
Ticarcillin and clavulanate	Timentin	Antibacterial
Timolol	Blocadren, Timoptic	Antihypertensive
Timolol/HCTZ	Timolide	Antihypertensive
Tinzaparin	Innohep	Anticoagulant
Tirofiban	Aggrastat	Antiplatelet
Tobramycin	Nebcin, Tobradex	Antibacterial
Tocainide	Tonocard	Antiarrhythmic
Tolazamide	Tolinase	Antidiabetic
Tolbutamide	Tol-Tab, Orinase	Antidiabetic
Tolterodine	Detrol, Detrol LA	Antispasmodic
Torsemide	Demadex	Diuretic
Tramadol	Ultram	Nonopioid analgesic
Tramadol and Acetaminophen	Ultracet	Nonopioid analgesic
Trandolapril	Mavik	Antihypertensive
Trandolapril and verapamil	Tarka	Antihypertensive
Tranylcypromine	Parnate	Antidepressant
Triamcinolone	Azmacort	Antiasthmatic
Triamterene	Dyrenium	Diuretic
Triamterene/HCTZ	Dyazide, Maxzide	Diuretic
Triazolam	Halcion	Sedative
Trifluoperazine	Stelazine	Antipsychotic
Trimethoprim-sulfamethoxazole	Bactrim, Bactrim DS, Septra, Septra DS	Antibacterial
Trimetrexate	Neutrexin	Antiprotozoal
Urokinase	Abbokinase	Thrombolytic
Valacyclovir	Valtrex	Antiviral
Valganciclovir	Valcyte	Antiviral
Valproic acid	Depakene, Depakote	Anticonvulsant
Valsartan	Diovan	Antihypertensive
Valsartan/HCTZ	Diovan HCT	Antihypertensive
Vancomycin	Vancocin, Vancoled	Antibacterial
Vardenafil	Levitra	Erectile stimulant
Vasopressin	Pitressin	Hormone
Venlafaxine	Effexor, Effexor XR	Antidepressant
Verapamil	Calan, Calan SR, Isoptin SR, Verapamil SR, Covera-HS, Verelan, Verelan PM	Antiarrhythmic

Chemical/ Generic name	Trade name	Drug class
Vidarabine	Vera-A	Antiviral
Warfarin sodium	Coumadin	Anticoagulant
Yohimbine	Aphrodyne	Erectile stimulant
Zafirlukast	Accolate	Antiasthmatic
Zalcitabine	Hivid	Anti-HIV
Zaleplon	Sonata	Sedative
Zanamivir	Relenza	Anti-influenza
Zidovudine	Retrovir, AZT	Anti-HIV
Zileuton	Zyflo	Antiasthmatic
Ziprasidone	Geodon	Antipsychotic
Zolmitriptan	Zomig, Zomig-ZMT	Antimigraine
Zolpidem	Ambien	Sedative
Zonisamide	Zonegran	Anticonvulsant

Part Two: Drugs by Trade Name

Trade name	Chemical/Generic name	Drug class
Abbokinase	Urokinase	Thrombolytic
Accolate	Zafirlukast	Antiasthmatic
Accupril	Quinapril	Antihypertensive
Accuretic	Quinapril/HCTZ	Antihypertensive
Aceon	Perindopril	Antihypertensive
Achromycin	Tetracycline	Antibacterial
Aciphex	Rabeprazole	Antiulcer
Activase	Alteplase	Thrombolytic
Actonel	Risedronate	Antiosteoporosis
Actos	Pioglitazone	Antidiabetic
Adalat, Adalat CC	Nifedipine	Antihypertensive
Adderall	Amphetamine and dextroamphetamine	Anti-ADHD
Adrenalin	Epinephrine	Inotropic agent
Advil	Ibuprofen	Nonopioid analgesic
Aerobid	Flunisolide	Antiasthmatic
Agenerase	Amprenavir	Anti-HIV
Aggrastat	Tirofiban	Antiplatelet
Aldactazide	Spironolactone/HCTZ	Diuretic
Aldactone	Spironolactone	Diuretic
Aldoclor	Methyldopa and chlorothiazide	Antihypertensive
Aldomet	Methyldopa	Antihypertensive

Trade name	Chemical/Generic name	Drug class
Alesse	Levonorgestrel	Contraceptive
Allegra	Fexofenadine	Antihistamine
Allegra-D	Fexofenadine and pseudoephedrine	Antihistamine
Altace	Ramipril	Antihypertensive
Alupent	Metaproterenol	Antiasthmatic
Amaryl	Glimepiride	Antidiabetic
Ambien	Zolpidem	Sedative
Amcill	Ampicillin	Antibacterial
Amerge	Naratriptan	Antimigraine
Amikin	Amikacin	Antibacterial
Aminophyllin	Aminophylline	Antiasthmatic
Amoxil	Amoxicillin	Antibacterial
Amphocin	Amphotericin B	Antifungal
Ancef	Cefazolin	Antibacterial
Antabuse	Disulfiram	Antialcohol
Antivert	Meclizine	Antihistamine
Aphrodyne	Yohimbine	Erectile stimulant
Apresoline	Hydralazine	Antihypertensive
Aramine	Metaraminol	Inotropic agent
Arthrotec	Diclofenac and misoprostol	Nonopioid analgesic
Atacand	Candesartan	Antihypertensive
Atacand HCT	Candesartan/HCTZ	Antihypertensive
Atamet	Carbidopa/levodopa	Antiparkinsonian
Atapin	Doxepin	Antidepressant
Atarax	Hydroxyzine	Antihistamine
Ativan	Lorazepam	Antianxiety
Atrovent	Ipratropium bromide	Antiasthmatic
Augmentin	Amoxicillin/potassium clavulanate	Antibacterial
Avalide	Irbesartan/HCTZ	Antihypertensive
Avandia	Rosiglitazone	Antidiabetic
Avapro	Irbesartan	Antihypertensive
Avelox	Moxifloxacin	Antibacterial
Aventyl	Nortriptyline	Antidepressant
Axid	Nizatidine	Antiulcer
Azactam	Aztreonam	Antibacterial
Azmacort	Triamcinolone	Antiasthmatic
AZT, Retrovir	Ziduvodine	Antiviral
Bactocill	Oxacillin	Antibacterial
Bactrim, Bactrim DS	Trimethoprim-sulfamethoxazole	Antibacterial

Trade name	Chemical/Generic name	Drug class
Bactroban	Mupirocin	Antibacterial
Bayer	Aspirin	Nonopioid analgesic
Beclovent, Beconase	Beclomethasone	Antiasthmatic
Benadryl, Benolyn	Diphenhydramine	Antihistamine
Benemid	Probenecid	Antigout
Betapace, Betapace AF	Sotalol	Antiarrhythmic
Biaxin	Clarithromycin	Antibacterial
Bio-Cef	Cephalexin	Antibacterial
Blocadren	Timolol	Antihypertensive
Brethine	Terbutaline	Antiasthmatic
Bretylol	Bretylium	Antiarrhythmic
Brevibloc	Esmolol	Antiarrhythmic
Bromocriptine	Parlodel	Antiparkinsonian
Bumex	Bumetanide	Diuretic
BuSpar	Buspirone	Antianxiety
Calan, Calan SR	Verapamil	Antiarrhythmic
Capoten	Captopril	Antihypertensive
Capozide	Captopril/HCTZ	Antihypertensive
Carafate	Sucralfate	Antiulcer
Carbatrol	Carbamazepine	Anticonvulsant
Cardene, Cardene SR	Nicardipine	Antianginal
Cardizem, Cardizem CD, Cartia	Diltiazem	Antianginal
Cardura	Doxazosin	Antihypertensive
Cartrol	Carteolol	Antihypertensive
Cataflam	Diclofenac	Nonopioid analgesic
Catapres, Catapres-TTS	Clonidine	Antihypertensive
Ceclor	Cefaclor	Antibacterial
Cedax	Ceftibuten	Antibacterial
Cefadyl	Cephapirin	Antibacterial
Cefizox	Ceftizoxime	Antibacterial
Cefotan	Cefotetan	Antibacterial
Ceftin	Cefuroxime	Antibacterial
Cefzil	Cefprozil	Antibacterial
Celebrex	Celecoxib	Nonopioid analgesic
Celexa	Citalopram	Antidepressant
Celontin	Methsuximide	Anticonvulsant
Ceptaz	Ceftazidime	Antibacterial
Cerebyx	Fosphenytoin	Anticonvulsant
Chloromycetin	Chloramphenicol	Antibacterial
Chronulac	Lactulose	Laxative

Trade name	Chemical/Generic name	Drug class
Cipro	Ciprofloxacin	Antibacterial
Claforan	Cefotaxime	Antibacterial
Clarinex	Desloratidine	Antihistamine
Claritin	Loratidine	Antihistamine
Claritin-D	Loratidine and pseudoephedrine	Antihistamine
Cleocin	Clindamycin	Antibacterial
Clozaril	Clozapine	Antipsychotic
Colace	Ducosate sodium	Laxative
ColBENEMID	Probenecid and colchicine	Antigout
Colestid	Colestipol	Cholesterol lowering
Combivent	Albuterol and ipatropium	Antiasthmatic
Combivir	Lamivudine and zidovudine	Anti-HIV
Compazine	Prochlorperazine	Antipsychotic, antiemetic
Concerta	Methylphenidate	CNS Stimulant
Cordarone	Amiodarone	Antiarrhythmic
Coreg	Carvedilol	Antihypertensive
Corgard	Nadolol	Antihypertensive
Corvert	Ibutilide	Antiarrhythmic
Corzide	Bendroflumethiazide and nadolol	Antihypertensive
Covera-HS	Verapamil	Antiarrhythmic
Cotazyme	Pancrelipase	Hormone
Coumadin	Warfarin sodium	Anticoagulant
Cozaar	Losartan	Antihypertensive
Crixivan	Indinavir	Anti-HIV
Cytospaz	Hyoscyamine	Antispasmodic
Cytovene	Ganciclovir	Antiviral
Dalmane	Flurazepam	Antianxiety
Dantrium	Dantrolene sodium	Antispastic
Darvocet-N, Dolene, Darvon-N	Propoxyphene	Opioid analgesic
Datril	Acetaminophen	Nonopioid analgesic
DDAVP	Desmopressin	Hormone
Decadron	Dexamethasone	Steroid
Deltasone	Cortisone	Steroid
Demadex	Torsemide	Diuretic
Demerol	Meperidine	Opioid analgesic
Depakene, Depakote	Valproic acid	Anticonvulsant
Depo-Medrol	Methylprednisolone	Steroid
Depo-Provera	Medroxyprogesterone	Contraceptive

Trade name	Chemical/Generic name	Drug class
Detrol, Detrol LA	Tolterodine	Antispasmodic
Diabenese	Chlorpropramide	Antidiabetic
Diabeta	Glyburide	Antidiabetic
Diamox	Acetazolamide	Diuretic
Diastat	Diazepam	Antianxiety
Diflucan	Fluconazole	Antifungal
Digitek	Digoxin	Inotropic agent
Dilacor, Dilacor CR	Diltiazem	Antianginal
Dilantin	Phenytoin	Anticonvulsant
Dilaudid	Hydromorphone	Opioid analgesic
Diovan	Valsartan	Antihypertensive
Diovan HCT	Valsartan/HCTZ	Antihypertensive
Diltrate-DR	Isosorbide dinitrate	Antianginal
Ditropan, Ditropan XL	Oxybutinin	Antispasmodic
Diuril	Chlorothiazide	Diuretic
Dobutrex	Dobutamine	Inotropic agent
Dolene	Propoxyphene	Opioid analgesic
Dolophine	Methadone	Opioid analgesic
Dopistat	Dopamine	Inotropic agent
Doral	Quazepam	Antianxiety
Dulcolax	Bisacodyl	Laxative
Duoneb	Albuterol and ipatropium	Antiasthmatic
Duricef	Cefadroxil	Antibacterial
Dynacirc	Isradipine	Antihypertensive
Dyazide	Triamterene/HCTZ	Diuretic
Dycell, Dynapen	Dicloxacillin	Antibacterial
Dynabac	Dirithromycin	Antibacterial
Dynacin	Minocycline	Antibacterial
Dyrenium	Triamterene	Diuretic
E-Mycin	Erythromycin	Antibacterial
Ecotrin	Aspirin	Nonopioid analgesic
Edecrin	Ethacrynic acid	Diuretic
Effexor, Effexor XR	Venlafaxine	Antidepressant
Elavil, Endep	Amitriptyline	Antidepressant
Elocon	Mometasone	Steroid
Endodan	Oxycodone	Opioid analgesic
Enduron	Methyclothiazide	Diuretic
Epivir	Lamivudine	Anti-HIV
Equagesic	Meprobamate and aspirin	Muscle relaxant
Ery-Tab, Erythrocin	Erythromycin	Antibacterial
Eskalith	Lithium carbonate	Antimanic

Trade name	Chemical/Generic name	Drug class
Estrace	Estradiol	Hormone
Ethmozine	Moricizine	Antiarrhythmic
Evista	Raloxifene	Hormone
Famvir	Famcyclovir	Antiviral
Felbatol	Felbamate	Anticonvulsant
Flagyl	Metronidazole	Antibacterial
Flexeril	Cyclobenzaprine	Muscle relaxant
Flomax	Tamsulosin	Antiadrenergic
Flonase, Flovent	Fluticasone	Antiasthmatic
Floxin	Ofloxacin	Antibacterial
Flumadine	Rimantidine	Anti-influenza
Foradil	Formoterol	Antiasthmatic
Fortaz	Ceftazidime	Antibacterial
Fortovase	Saquinavir	Anti-HIV
Fosamax	Alendronate	Antiosteoporosis
Foscavir	Foscarnet	Antiviral
Fragmin	Dalteparin	Anticoagulant
Fulvicin	Griseofulvin	Antifungal
Fungizone	Amphoterocin B	Antifungal
Furadantin	Nitrofurantoin	Antibacterial
Furocot	Furosemide	Diuretic
Gantanol	Sulfamethoxazole	Antibacterial
Gantrisin	Sulfisoxazole	Antibacterial
Garamycin	Gentamycin	Antibacterial
Geocillin	Carbenicillin	Antibacterial
Geodon	Ziprasidone	Antipsychotic
Geopen	Carbenicillin	Antibacterial
Glucophage	Metformin	Antidiabetic
Glucotrol, Glucotrol XL	Glipizide	Antidiabetic
Glucovance	Glyburide and metformin	Antidiabetic
Glycron, Glynase	Glyburide micronized	Antidiabetic
Glyset	Miglitol	Antidiabetic
Grifulvin, Grisactin, Gris-PEG	Griseofulvin	Antifungal
Halcion	Triazolam	Sedative
Haldol	Haloperidol	Antipsychotic
Hivid	Zalcitabine	Anti-HIV
Humalog	Lispro insulin	Antidiabetic
Hydrocot, HydroDiuril	Hydrochlorothiazide	Diuretic
Hytrin	Terazosin	Antihypertensive
Hyzaar	Losartan/HCTZ	Antihypertensive
Ilosone	Erythromycin	Antibacterial

Trade name	Chemical/Generic name	Drug class
Imdur	Isosorbide dinitrate	Antianginal
Imitrex	Sumatriptan	Antimigraine
Imodium	Loperamide	Antidiarrheal
Inderal, Inderal LA	Propranolol	Antihypertensive
Inderide, Inderide LA	Propanolol/HCTZ	Antihypertensive
INH	Isoniazid	Antituberculous
Innohep	Tinzaparin	Anticoagulant
Intal	Cromolyn sodium	Antiasthmatic
Integrelin	Ebtifibatide	Antiplatelet
Intopin	Dopamine	Inotropic agent
Invirase	Saquinavir	Anti-HIV
Ismo	Isosorbide dinitrate	Antianginal
Isoptin, Isoptin SR	Verapamil	Antiarrhythmic
Isordil	Isosorbide dinitrate	Antianginal
K-Dur, K-Lor	Potassium chloride	Supplement
Kabikinase	Streptokinase	Thrombolytic
Kaletra	Lopinavir/ritonavir	Anti-HIV
Keflex	Cephalexin	Antibacterial
Kefurox	Cefuroxime	Antibacterial
Kefzol	Cefazolin	Antibacterial
Kerlone	Betaxolol	Antihypertensive
Klonopin	Clonazepam	Anticonvulsant
Lamisil	Terbinafine	Antifungal
Lanoxicaps, Lanoxin	Digoxin	Inotropic agent
Lantus	Glargine insulin	Antidiabetic
Larotid	Amoxicillin	Antibacterial
Lasix	Furosemide	Diuretic
Lescol, Lescol XL	Fluvastatin	Cholesterol lowering
Levaquin	Levofloxacin	Antibacterial
Levatol	Penbutolol	Antihypertensive
Levbid, Levsin, LuLev	Hyoscyamine	Antispasmodic
Levitra	Vardenafil	Erectile stimulant
Levlite	Levonorgestrel	Contraceptive
Levophed	Noepinephrine	Inotropic agent
Levothyroid, Levoxyl	Levothyroxine	Hormone
Librium	Chlordiazepoxide	Antianxiety
Lioresal	Baclofen	Antispastic
Lipitor	Atorvastatin	Cholesterol lowering
Loestrin Fe 1/20	Norethindrone and Ethinyl Estradiol	Contraceptive
Lomotil	Diphenoxylate with atropine	Antidiarrheal

Trade name	Chemical/Generic name	Drug class
Loniten	Minoxidil	Antihypertensive
Lo-Ovral	Norgestrel and Ethinyl Estradiol	Contraceptive
Lopid	Gemfibrozil	Cholesterol lowering
Lopressor	Metoprolol	Antihypertensive
Lorabid	Loracarbef	Antibacterial
Lotensin	Benazepril	Antihypertensive
Lotensin HCT	Benazepril/HCTZ	Antihypertensive
Lotrel	Amlodipine and benazepril	Antihypertensive
Lotrimin, Mazole	Clotrimazole	Antifungal
Lotrisone	Clotrimazole and betamethasone	Antifungal
Lovenox	Enoxaparin	Anticoagulant
Loxitane	Loxapine	Antipsychotic
Lozol	Indapamide	Diuretic
Lufyllln	Dyphylline	Antiasthmatic
Macrobid, Macrodantin	Nitrofurantoin	Antibacterial
Mandol	Cefamandole	Antibacterial
Mavik	Trandolapril	Anithypertensive
Maxair	Pirbuterol	Antiasthmatic
Maxalt, Maxalt-MLT	Rizatriptan	Antimigraine
Maxaquin	Lomefloxacin	Antibacterial
Maxipime	Cefepime	Antibacterial
Maxzide	Triamterene/HCTZ	Diuretic
Medrol	Methylprednisolone	Steroid
Mefoxin	Cefoxitin	Antibacterial
Mellaril	Thioridazine	Antipsychotic
Mepron	Atovaquone	Antiprotozoal
Meridia	Sibutramine	Antiobesity
Merrem	Meropenem	Antibacterial
Metaprel	Metaproterenol	Antiasthmatic
Methylin	Methylphenidate	CNS stimulant
Mevacor	Lovastatin	Cholesterol lowering
Mezlin	Mezlocillin	Antibacterial
Miacalcin	Calcitonin salmon	Antiosteoporosis
Micardis	Telmisartan	Antihypertensive
Micardis HCT	Telmisartan/HCTZ	Antihypertensive
Micronase	Glyburide	Antidiabetic
Microzide	Hydrochlorothiazide	Diuretic
Midamor	Amiloride	Diuretic
Minipress	Prazosin	Antihypertensive

Trade name	Chemical/Generic name	Drug class
Minocin	Minocycline	Antibacterial
Mircette	Ethinyl Estradiol	Contraceptive
Mirena	Levonorgestrel	Contraceptive
Moban	Molindone	Antipsychotic
Moduretic	Amiloride/HCTZ	Diuretic
Monistat	Miconazole	Antifungal
Monoket	Isosorbide dinitrate	Antianginal
Monopril	Fosinopril	Antihypertensive
Motrin	Ibuprofen	Nonopioid analgesic
Moxilin	Amoxicillin	Antibacterial
Mycobutin	Rifabutin	Antituberculous
Mycostatin	Nystatin	Antifungal
Mykrox	Metolazone	Diuretic
Nallpen	Nafcillin	Antibacterial
Naprosyn	Naproxen	Nonopioid analgesic
Nardil	Phenylzine	Antidepressant
Nasalcrom	Cromolyn sodium	Antiasthmatic
Nasonex	Mometasone	Steroid
Navane	Thiothixene	Antipsychotic
Nebcin	Tobramycin	Antibacterial
Nebupent	Pentamidine	Antiprotozoal
Necon 1/35	Ethinyl Estradiol and Norethindrone	Contraceptive
Neo-Synephrine	Phenylephrine	Inotropic agent
Neurontin	Gabapentin	Anticonvulsant
Neutrexin	Trimetrexate	Antiprotozoal
Nexium	Esomeprazole	Antiulcer
Niaspan	Niacin	Cholesterol lowering
Nicolar	Niacin	Cholesterol lowering
Nilstat	Nystatin	Antifungal
Nizoral	Ketoconazole	Antifungal
Noctec	Chloral hydrate	Sedative
Nolvadex	Tamoxifen	Hormone
Normiflo	Ardeparin	Anticoagulant
Normodyne	Labetolol	Antihypertensive
Noroxin	Norfloxacin	Antibacterial
Norpace, Norpace CR	Disopyramide	Antiarrhythmic
Norplant	Levonorgestrel	Contraceptive
Norpramin	Desipramine	Antidepressant
Norvasc	Amlodipine	Antihypertensive
Norvir	Ritonavir	Anti-HIV

Trade name	Chemical/Generic name	Drug class
Omnicef	Cefdinir	Antibacterial
Omnipen-N	Ampicillin	Antibacterial
Opticrom	Cromolyn sodium	Antiasthmatic
Oretic	Hydrochlorothiazide	Diuretic
Orinase	Tolbutamide	Antidiabetic
Ortho-Cyclen, Ortho Novum 7–7-7, Ortho Tri-Cyclen	Norgestimate and Ethinyl Estradiol	Contraceptive
Pamelor	Nortriptyline	Antidepressant
Pacerone	Amiodarone	Antiarrhythmic
Pancrease	Pancrelipase	Hormone
Paradione	Paramethadione	Anticonvulsant
Parlodel	Bromocriptine	Antiparkinsonian
Parnate	Tranylcypromine	Antidepressant
Paxil	Paroxitene	Antidepressant
Penicillin VK	Penicillin V	Antibacterial
Pentam	Pentamidine	Antiprotozoal
Pepcid	Famotidine	Antiulcer
Percocet, Percodan	Oxycodone	Opioid analgesic
Periactin	Cyproheptadine	Antihistamine
Permitil	Fluphenazine	Antipsychotic
Persantine	Dipyridamole	Anticoagulant
Phenergan	Promethazine	Antihistamine
Piopen	Carbenicillin	Antibacterial
Pipracil	Piperacillin	Antibacterial
Pitocin	Oxytocin	Hormone
Pitressin	Vasopressin	Hormone
Plavix	Clopidogrel	Antiplatelet
Plendil	Felodipine	Antihypertensive
Polymox	Amoxicillin	Antibacterial
Prandin	Repaglinide	Antidiabetic
Pravachol	Pravastatin	Cholesterol lowering
Precose	Acarbose	Antidiabetic
Preganone	Ethotoin	Anticonvulsant
Premarin	Estrogen	Hormone
Pres-Tab	Glyburide micronized	Antidiabetic
Prevacid	Lansoprazole	Antiulcer
Prevalite	Cholestyramine	Cholesterol lowering
Priftin	Rifapentine	Antituberculous
Prilosec	Omeprazole	Antiulcer
Primacor	Milrinone	Inotropic agent

Trade name	Chemical/Generic name	Drug class
Primaxin	Imipenem/cilastatin	Antibacterial
Principen	Ampicillin	Antibacterial
Prinivil	Lisinopril	Antihypertensive
Prinzide	Lisinopril/HCTZ	Antihypertensive
ProAmatine	Midodrine	Inotropic agent
Procan, Procanbid	Procainamide	Antiarrhythmic
Procardia, Procardia XL	Nifedipine	Antianginal
Prolixin	Fluphenazine	Antipsychotic
Pronestyl	Procainamide	Antiarrhythmic
Prosom	Estazolam	Antianxiety
Prostaphlin	Oxacillin	Antibacterial
Protonix	Pantoprazole	Antiulcer
Proventil	Albuterol	Antiasthmatic
Provera	Medroxyprogesterone	Hormone
Prozac	Fluoxetine	Antidepressant
Pulmicort	Budesonide	Antiasthmatic
Questran, Questran Light	Cholestyramine	Cholesterol lowering
Quinidex, Quiniglute	Quinidine	Antiarrhythmic
Qvar	Beclomethasone	Antiasthmatic
Refludan	Lepirudin	Anticoagulant
Reglan	Metoclopramide	GI motility agent
Relafen	Nabumetone	Nonopioid analgesic
Relenza	Zanamivir	Anti-influenza
Remeron	Mirtazipine	Antidepressant
Renese	Polythiazide	Diuretic
Reopro	Abciximab	Antiplatelet
Resbid	Theophylline	Antiasthmatic
Rescriptor	Delavirdine	Anti-HIV
Restoril	Temazepam	Antianxiety
Retavase	Reteplase	Thrombolytic
Retrovir, AZT	Ziduvodine	Antiviral
Rhythmol	Propafenone	Antiarrythmic
Rifadin	Rifampin	Antituberculous
Rifamate	Isoniazid/rifampin	Antituberculous
Rifater	Isoniazid and pyrazinamide	Antituberculous
Rimactane	Rifampin	Antituberculous
Risperdal	Risperidone	Antipsychotic
Ritalin	Methylphenidate	CNS stimulant
Robaxin	Methocarbamol	Muscle relaxant
Rocephin	Ceftriaxone	Antibacterial
Rogaine	Minoxidil	Antihypertensive

Trade name	Chemical/Generic name	Drug class
Roxicet	Oxycodone	Opioid analgesic
Seconal	Secobarbital	Sedative
Sectral	Acebutolol	Antiarrhythmic
Septra, Septra DS	Trimethoprim-sulfamethoxazole	Antibacterial
Serax	Oxazepam	Antianxiety
Serentil	Mesoridazine	Antipsychotic
Serevent	Salmeterol	Antiasthmatic
Seroquel	Quetiapine	Antipsychotic
Serzone	Nefazodone	Antidepressant
Sinemet, Sinemet CR	Carbidopa/levodopa	Antiparkinsonian
Sinequan	Doxepin	Antidepressant
Singulair	Montelukast	Antiasthmatic
Slo-Phyllin	Theophylline	Antiasthmatic
Solu-Cortof	Hydrocortisone	Steroid
Solu-Medrol	Methylprednisolone	Steroid
Soma	Carisoprodol	Muscle relaxant
Somophyllin	Aminophylline	Antiasthmatic
Sonata	Zaleplon	Sedative
Sporanox	Itraconazole	Antifungal
Staphcillin	Methicillin	Antibacterial
Starlix	Nateglinide	Antidiabetic
Stelazine	Trifluoperazine	Antipsychotic
Stimate	Desmopressin	Hormone
Streptase	Streptokinase	Thrombolytic
Sublimaze	Fentanyl	Opioid analgesic
Sular	Nisoldipine	Antihypertensive
Suprax	Cefixime	Antibacterial
Sustiva	Efavirenz	Anti-HIV
Symmetrel	Amantidine	Anti-influenza
Symycin	Tetracycline	Antibacterial
Synagis	Palivizumab	Antiviral
Synercid	Dalfopristin and quinupristin	Antibacterial
Synthroid	Levothyroxine	Hormone
Tagamet	Cimetidine	Antiulcer
Tambocor	Flecanide	Antiarrythmic
Tamiflu	Oseltamivir	Anti-influenza
Tapazole	Methimazole	Antithyroid
Tarka	Trandolapril/verapamil	Antihypertensive
Tazicef	Ceftazidime	Antibacterial

Trade name	Chemical/Generic name	Drug class
Tegretol, Tegretol XR	Carbamazapine	Anticonvulsant
Tempra	Acetaminophen	Nonopioid analgesic
Tenex	Guanfacine	Antihypertensive
Tenoretic	Atenolol and chlorthalidone	Antihypertensive
Tenormin	Atenolol	Antihypertensive
Tequin	Gatifloxacin	Antibacterial
Teveten	Eprosartan	Antihypertensive
Thalitone	Chlorthalidone	Diuretic
Theo-Dur, Theolair, Theo-24	Theophylline	Antiasthmatic
Thorazine	Chlorpromazine	Antipsychotic
Tiazac	Diltiazem	Antianginal
Ticar	Ticarcillin	Antibacterial
Tikosyn	Dofetilide	Antiarrhythmic
Tilade	Nedocromil	Antiasthmatic
Timentin	Ticarcillin and clavulanate	Antibacterial
Timolide	Timolol/HCTZ	Antihypertensive
Timoptic	Timolol	Antihypertensive
TNKase	Tenecteplase	Thrombolytic
Tobradex	Tobramycin	Antibacterial
Tofranil	Imipramine	Antidepressant
Tol-Tab	Tolbutamide	Antidiabetic
Tolinase	Tolazamide	Antidiabetic
Tonocard	Tocainide	Antiarrhythmic
Toprol XL	Metoprolol	Antihypertensive
Tornalate	Bitolterol	Antiasthmatic
Tranxene	Clorazepate	Antianxiety
Trecator-SC	Ethionamide	Antituberculous
Tricor	Fenofibrate	Cholesterol lowering
Trilafon	Perphenazine	Antipsychotic
Trimox	Amoxicillin	Antibacterial
Triphasil	L-Norgestrel and Ethinyl Estradiol	Contraceptive
Trizivir	Abacavir/lamivudine and zidovudine	Anti-HIV
Tylenol	Acetaminophen	Nonopioid analgesic
Tylox	Oxycodone	Opioid analgesic
Ultracet	Tramadol and acetaminophen	Nonopioid analgesic
Ultram	Tramadol	Nonopioid analgesic
Unasyn	Ampicillin/sulbactam	Antibacterial
Uniretic	Moexipril/HCTZ	Antihypertensive

Trade name	Chemical/Generic name	Drug class
Univasc	Moexipril	Antihypertensive
Valcyte	Valganciclovir	Antiviral
Valium	Diazepam	Antianxiety
Valtrex	Valacyclovir	Antiviral
Vancenase, Vanceril, Vanceril DS	Beclomethasone	Antiasthmatic
Vancocin, Vancoled	Vancomycin	Antibacterial
Vanspar	Buspirone	Antianxiety
Vantin	Cefpodoxime	Antibacterial
Vaseretic	Enalapril/HCTZ	Antihypertensive
Vasotec	Enalapril	Antihypertensive
Vectrin	Minocycline	Antibacterial
Veetids	Penicillin	Antibacterial
Velocef	Cephradine	Antibacterial
Ventolin	Albuterol	Antiasthmatic
Vera-A	Vidarabine	Antiviral
Verelan, Verelan PM	Verapamil	Antiarrhythmic
Versed	Midazolam	Sedative
Viagra	Sildenafil	Erectile stimulant
Vibramycin, Vibra-Tabs	Doxycycline	Antibacterial
Vicoprofen	Hydrocodone and ibuprofen	Opioid analgesic
Videx, Videx EC	Didanosine	Anti-HIV
Vioxx	Rofecoxib	Nonopioid analgesic
Viracept	Nelfinavir	Anti-HIV
Viramune	Nevirapine	Anti-HIV
Virazole	Ribavirin	Antiviral
Visken	Pindolol	Antihypertensive
Vistide	Cidofovir	Antiviral
Vistaril	Hydroxyzine	Antihistamine
Vitrasert	Ganciclovir	Antiviral
Volmax	Albuterol	Antiasthmatic
Voltaren, Voltaren-XR	Diclofenac	Nonopioid analgesic
WelChol	Colesevelam	Cholesterol lowering
Wellbutrin, Wellbutrin SR	Bupropion	Antidepressant
Xalatan	Latanoprost	Antiglaucoma
Xanax	Alprazolam	Antianxiety
Xenical	Orlistat	Antiobesity
Xopenex	Levalbuterol	Antiasthmatic
Xylocaine	Lidocaine	Antiarrhythmic

Trade name	Chemical/Generic name	Drug class
Zagam	Sparfloxacin	Antibacterial
Zantac	Ranitidine	Antiulcer
Zarontin	Ethosuximide	Anticonvulsant
Zaroxolyn	Metolazone	Diuretic
Zebeta	Bisoprolol	Antihypertensive
Zerit	Stavudine	Anti-HIV
Zestoretic	Lisinopril/HCTZ	Antihypertensive
Zestril	Lisinopril	Antihypertensive
Ziac	Bisoprolol/HCTZ	Antihypertensive
Ziagen	Abacavir	Anti-HIV
Zinacef	Cefuroxime	Antibacterial
Zithromax	Azithromycin	Antibacterial
Zocor	Simvastatin	Cholesterol lowering
Zoloft	Sertraline	Antidepressant
Zomig, Zomig-ZMT	Zolmitriptan	Antimigraine
Zonegran	Zonisamide	Anticonvulsant
Zosyn	Piperacillin and tazobactam	Antibacterial
Zovirax	Acyclovir	Antiviral
Zyflo	Zileuton	Antiasthmatic
Zyloprim	Allopurinol	Antigout
Zyprexa, Zyprexa Zydis	Olanzapine	Antipsychotic
Zyrtec	Cetirizine	Antihistamine
Zyvox	Linezolid	Antibacterial

Part Three: Drug Classes

A. Antialcohol. Indications: used to deter ethanol ingestion.

Acetaldehyde dehydrogenase blocker

Disulfiram (Antabuse)

Mechanism: inhibits acetaldehyde dehydrogenase, which leads to buildup of acetaldehyde after consumption of alcohol, causing nausea, vomiting, and headache.

B. Antianginal. Indications: to relieve angina pectoris (chest pain due to coronary artery spasm).

1. Calcium channel blockers

Diltiazem (Cardizem, Cardizem CD, Cartia, Dilacor, Dilacor CR, Tiazac)

Nicardipene (Cardene, Cardene SR)

Nifedipine (Procardia, Procardia XL)

Mechanism: reduces muscle contractility by blocking voltage-dependent calcium channels and thus decreasing intracellular calcium concentration.

2. **Nitrates**

   Nitroglycerin

   Isosorbide mononitrate

   Isosorbide dinitrate (Diltrate-DR, Ismo, Isordil, Monoket)

   Mechanism: releases nitric oxide in smooth muscle, increasing cGMP, leading to smooth muscle relaxation.

C. **Antianxiety**

   1. **Benzodiazepines**

      Alprazolam (Xanax)

      Chlordiazepoxide (Librium)

      Clorazepate (Tranxene)

      Diazepam (Valium, Diastat)

      Flurazepam (Dalmane)

      Lorazepam (Ativan)

      Oxazepam (Serax)

      Quazepam (Doral)

      Temazepam (Restoril)

      Mechanism: acts at a specific benzodiazepine receptor that is part of the GABA receptor—chloride ion channel complex found in many brain regions. Binding of benzodiazepines appears to facilitate inhibitory effects of GABA and glycine.

   2. **Azaspirone**

      Buspirone (BuSpar, Vanspar)

      Mechanism: partially blocks the serotonin 1A receptor, dose-dependently decreasing levels of serotonin and increasing those of dopamine and noradrenaline.

D. **Antiarrhythmic.** Indications: for treating abnormal cardiac rhythms (see Chap. 13).

   1. **Class I**

      Disopyramide (Norpace, Norpace CR)

      Flecanide (Tambocor)

      Lidocaine (Xylocaine)

      Moricizine (Ethmozine)

      Procainamide (Procan, Procanbid, Pronestyl)

      Propafenone (Rhythmol)

      Quinidine (Quinidex, Quiniglute)

      Tocainide (Tonocard)

      Mechanism: sodium channel blocker. Lidocaine is also frequently used as a local anesthetic.

2. **Class II**

Acebutolol (Sectral)

Esmolol (Brevibloc)

Mechanism: beta-adrenergic receptor blocker—suppresses abnormal pacemakers.

3. **Class III**

Amiodarone (Cordarone)

Bretylium (Bretylol)

Dofetilide (Tikosyn)

Ibutilide (Corvert)

Sotalol (Betapace, Betapace AF)

Mechanism: potassium channel blocker—prolongs the action potential and increases refractory period.

4 **Class IV**

Verapamil (Calan, Calan SR, Cover-HS, Isoptin, Isoptin SR, Verelan, Verelan PM)

Mechanism: calcium channel blocker—most effective in arrhythmias that involve calcium-dependent cardiac tissue, such as the atrioventricular node.

5. **Cardiac glycosides**

Digoxin (Digitek, Lanoxicaps, Lanoxin)

Mechanism: inhibits Na^+-K^+ ATPase of cell membrane, which increases intracellular sodium as well as calcium. Used in treating atrial fibrillation and also as a positive inotropic agent in cardiac failure.

E. **Antiasthmatics.** Indication: for the treatment of bronchial asthma.

1. **Inhaled corticosteroids**

Beclomethasone (Beclovent, Beconase, Vancenase, Vanceril, Vanceril DS, Qvar)

Budesonide (Pulmicort)

Flunisolide (Aerobid)

Fluticasone (Flonase, Flovent)

Triamcinolone (Azmacort)

Mechanism: decreases inflammation of airways, perhaps by blocking synthesis of arachadonic acid by phospholipase A2. Also used in severe asthma are systemic corticosteroids.

2. **Beta agonists**

Albuterol (Proventil, Ventolin, Volmax)

Bitolterol (Tornalate)

Formoterol (Foradil)

Isoetharine (Bronkosol)

Levalbuterol (Xopenex)

Metaproterenol (Alupent, Metaprel)

Pirbuterol (Maxair)

Salmeterol (Serevent)

Terbutaline (Brethine)

Mechanism: increases cAMP in smooth muscle cells, inducing muscle relaxation and bronchodilation.

3. **Leukotriene antagonists**

Montelukast (Singulair)

Zafirlukast (Accolate)

Mechanism: inhibits bronchoconstriction and bronchial hyperresponsiveness by competitively blocking leukotriene D4 and E4, components of slow-reacting substance of anaphylaxis (SRSA).

4. **Methylxanthines**

Aminophylline (Aminophyllin, Somophyllin)

Dyphylline (Lufyllin)

Theophylline (Resbid, Slo-Phyllin, Theo 24, Theo-Dur, Theolair)

Mechanism: causes bronchodilation, perhaps by inhibiting phosphodiesterase.

5. **Cromolyn**

Cromolyn sodium (Intal, Nasalcrom, Opticrom)

Mechanism: decreases the release of mediators such as histamines and leukotrienes from mast cells. Used more for prophylaxis than for treatment of asthma attacks.

6. **Muscarinic antagonist**

Ipratropium bromide (Atrovent)

Mechanism: blocks muscarinic acetylcholine receptors, preventing bronchoconstriction.

7. **Anti-inflammatory**

Nedocromil sodium (Tilade)

Mechanism: inhibits release of histamine and other mediators from mast cells.

8. **5-lipoxygenase inhibitor**

Zileuton (Zyflo)

Mechanism: blocks the enzyme that catalyzes the formation of leukotrienes from arachidonic acid, inhibiting bronchoconstriction.

F. **Antibacterial**

1. **Cell wall inhibitors**

   a. **Penicillins**

    (1) Limited spectrum
        Penicillin G, Pencillin VK (Veetids)
    (2) Broader spectrum
        Amoxicillin (Amoxil, Larotid, Moxilin, Polymox)
        Ampicillin (Amcill, Omnipen-N, Principen)
        Carbenicillin (Geopen, Geocillin, Piopen)
        Piperacillin (Pipracil)
        Ticarcillin (Ticar)
    (3) Beta-lactamase resistant
        Dicloxacillin (Dycell, Dynapen)
        Methicillin (Staphcillin)
        Mezlocillin (Mezlin)
        Nafcillin (Nallpen)
        Oxacillin (Bactocill, Prostaphlin)
    (4) Combinations
        Amoxicillin/potassium clavulanate (Augmentin)
        Ampicillin/sulbactam (Unasyn)
        Piperacillin/tazobactam (Zosyn)
        Ticarcillin/clavulanate (Timentin)

b. Cephalosporins
    (1) First generation: active against gram-positive, *E. coli*
        Cefadroxil (Duricef)
        Cefazolin (Ancef, Kefzol)
        Cephalexin (Keflex)
        Cephapirin (Cefadyl)
        Cephalexin (Bio-Cef, Keflex)
        Cephradine (Velocef)
    (2) Second generation: provides more gram negative coverage
        Cefaclor (Ceclor)
        Cefamandole (Mandol)
        Cefdinir (Omnicef)
        Cefotetan ((Cefotan)
        Cefoxitin (Mefoxin)
        Cefprozil (Cefzil)
        Cefuroxime (Ceftin, Kefurox, Zinacef)
        Loracarbef (Lorabid)
    (3) Third generation: crosses blood-brain barrier
        Cefixime (Suprax)
        Cefotaxime (Claforan)

Cefpodoxime (Vantin)

Ceftazidime (Ceptaz, Fortaz, Tazicef)

Ceftibuten (Cedax)

Ceftizoxime (Cefizox)

Ceftriaxone (Rocephin)

Mechanism: inhibits cell wall synthesis by preventing cross-linking of peptidoglycan chains.

(4) **Fourth generation: excellent aerobic gram-negative, gram-positive, and anaerobic coverage**

Cefepime (Maxipime)

2. **Protein synthesis inhibitors**

Aminoglycosides

Amikacin (Amikin)

Gentamycin (Garamycin)

Tobramycin (Nebcin, Tobradex)

Mechanism: binds to 30S ribosomal unit of bacteria, preventing the formation of an initiation complex. Ototoxicity and nephrotoxicity are dangerous side effects.

Chloramphenicol (Chloromycetin)

Mechanism: binds to 50S ribosomal unit of bacteria and inhibits peptidyltransferase.

Tetracycline (Achromycin, Symycin), Doxycycline (Vibramycin, Vibra-Tabs), and Minocycline (Dynacin, Minocin, Vectrin)

Mechanism: binds to 30S subunit of bacterial ribosomes, preventing the binding of aminoacyl tRNA to the ribosome.

3. **Fluoroquinolones**

Ciprofloxacin (Cipro)

Gatifloxacin (Tequin)

Levofloxacin (Levaquin)

Lomefloxacin (Maxaquin)

Moxifloxacin (Avelox)

Norfloxacin (Noroxin)

Ofloxacin (Floxin)

Sparfloxacin (Zagam)

Mechanism: blocks DNA gyrase.

4. **Macrolides**

Azithromycin (Zithromax)

Clarithromycin (Biaxin)

Dirithromycin (Dynabac)

Erythromycin (E-Mycin, Ery-Tab, Erythrocin, Ilosone)

Mechanism: binds to ribosomal sub-unit to prevent translocation.

5. Other commonly used antibacterials

Aztreonam (Azactam): inhibits cell wall synthesis.

Clindamycin (Cleocin): inhibits protein synthesis.

Imipenem/cilastatin (Primaxin), Merpenem (Merrem): inhibits cell wall synthesis.

Linezolid (Zyvox): inhibits bacterial protein synthesis.

Metronidazole (Flagyl): interferes with DNA synthesis; also antiprotozoal.

Mupirocin (Bactroban): inhibits bacterial protein synthesis.

Nitrofurantoin (Furadantin, Macrobid, Macrodantin): inactivates or alters bacterial ribosomal proteins.

Synercid (Dalfopristin and quinupristin): inhibits protein synthesis.

Trimethoprim-sulfamethoxazole (Bactrim, Bactrim DS, Septra, Septra DS): inhibits folic acid synthesis.

Vancomycin (Vancocin, Vancoled): inhibits cell wall synthesis.

G. Anticoagulant. Indications: prevention and treatment of venous thromboses, pulmonary emboli, acute arterial occlusions; prevention of emboli and occlusion in atrial fibrillation, atherosclerotic disease.

Ardeparin (Normiflo), Dalteparin (Fragmin), Enoxaparin (Lovenox), Tinzaparin (Innohep): inactivates factor Xa.

Dipyridamole (Persantine): decreases platelet aggregation.

Heparin sodium: binds to antithrombin III and blocks conversion of prethrombin to thrombin.

Lepirudin (Refludan): a thrombin-specific inhibitor used in the treatment of heparin-induced thrombocytopenia.

Warfarin sodium (Coumadin): inhibits vitamin K-dependent clotting factors (II, VII, IX, X).

H. Anticonvulsant. Indications: to stop the spread of aberrant electrical activity in the brain.

Carbamazapine (Carbatrol, Tegretol, Tegretol XR): for seizures refractory to other meds; blocks sodium channels.

Clonazepam (Klonopin): for petit mal, akinetic, myoclonic seizures; acts at benzodiazepine receptor.

Ethosuximide (Zarontin): for petit mal seizures; motor cortex depressant.

Felbamate (Felbatol): for generalized tonic-clonic and partial seizures.

Gabapentin (Neurontin): mechanism unknown.

Methsuximide (Celontin): for petit mal seizures refractory to other drugs; motor cortex depressant.

Phenobarbital: used most commonly for children; barbiturate.

Fosphenytoin (Cerebyx), Phenytoin (Dilantin): for grand mal, myoclonic seizures; blocks sodium channels.

Valproic acid (Depakene, Depakote): for absence seizures; mechanism unknown.

Zonisamide (Zonegran): a sulfonamide that blocks sodium channels.

I. Antidepressant

1. Tricyclics

Amitriptyline (Elavil, Endep)

Desipramine (Norpramin)

Doxepin (Atapin, Sinequan)

Imipramine (Tofranil)

Nortriptyline (Aventyl, Pamelor)

Mechanism: acutely inhibits reuptake of norepinephrine in the brain; however, the relationship of this mechanism to the clinical effect of the drug is not clear.

2. Selective serotonin reuptake inhibitors (SSRI)

Citalopram (Celexa)

Fluoxetine (Prozac)

Nefazodone (Serzone)

Paroxetine (Paxil)

Sertraline (Zoloft)

Venlafaxine (Effexor, Effexor XR)

Mechanism: acutely inhibits reuptake of serotonin (5-HT) in the brain; however, the relationship of this mechanism to the clinical effect of the drug is not clear.

3. Monoamine oxidase (MAO) inhibitors

Tranylcypromine (Parnate)

Mechanism: increases epinephrine, norepinephrine and serotonin throughout the nervous system.

4. Other anti-depressants

Bupropion (Wellbutrin, Wellbutrin SR): inhibits neuronal uptake of norepinephrine, serotonin, and dopamine.

Mirtazipine (Remeron): enhances central noradrenergic and serotenergic activity.

J. Antidiabetic. Indications: for type 2 diabetes mellitus, either alone or in combination with insulin.

1. Sulfonylureas

Chlorpromazine (Diabenese)

Glimepiride (Amaryl)

Glipizide (Glucotrol, Glucotrol XL)

Glyburide (Diabeta, Micronase)

Glyburide micronized (Glycron, Glynase, Pres-Tab)

Tolazamide (Tolinase)

Tolbutamide (Orinase, Tol-Tab)

Mechanism: these drugs stimulate the release of endogenous insulin from the pancreas. They may reduce glucagon release and increase the number of peripheral insulin receptors.

2. **Meglitinides**

   Nateglinide (Starlix)

   Repaglinide (Prandin)

   Mechanism: depolarizes pancreatic beta cells, producing calcium influx and insulin secretion.

3. **Biguanides**

   Metformin (Glucophage, Glucophage XR)

   Mechanism: decreases hepatic glucose production and intestinal glucose absorption.

4. **Thiazolidinediones**

   Pioglitazone (Actos)

   Rosiglitazone (Avandia)

   Mechanism: improves insulin sensitivity.

5. **Alpha-glucosidase inhibitors**

   Acarbose (Precose)

   Miglitol (Glyset)

   Mechanism: competitively and reversibly blocks pancreatic alpha-amylase and intestinal alpha-glucosidase hydrolase enzymes.

6. **Combination medications**

   Glyburide/Metformin (Glucovance)

K. **Antidiarrheal.** Indications: for the symptomatic relief of nonbloody diarrhea.

Diphenoxylate with atropine (Lomotil)

Loperamide (Imodium)

Mechanism: mild narcotics that slow intestinal transit time.

L. **Antifungal**

1. **Drugs for systemic mycoses**

   Amphotericin B (Fungizone): binds to ergosterol to change permeability of fungal membrane.

   Fluconazole (Diflucan): inhibits fungal demethylation.

   Ketoconazole (Nizoral): inhibits demethylation of lanosterol, decreasing ergosterol formation.

2. **Drugs for superficial infections**

   Clotrimazole (Lotrimin, Mazole), Clotrimazole/Betamethasone (Lotrisone): causes breakdown of cellular nucleic acids.

Griseofulvin (Fulvicin, Grifulvin, Grisactin, Gris-PEG): interferes with microtubule function.

Itraconazole (Sporanox): inhibits synthesis of ergosterol.

Miconazole (Monistat), Nystatin (Mycostatin, Nilstat): binds to ergosterol.

Terbinafine (Lamisil): inhibits squalene epoxidase, blocking ergosterol biosynthesis.

M. Antigout

Allopurinol (Zyloprim): inhibits xanthine oxidase to reduce the conversion of purines to uric acid.

Colchicine: inhibits microtubule assembly, thus inhibiting leukocyte migration and reducing inflammation.

Probenecid (Benemid): accelerates renal excretion of uric acid by competing for reabsorption in the renal tubule.

N. Antihistamine. Indications: differ for each drug.

Cetirizine (Zyrtec): for allergic rhinitis.

Cyproheptadine (Periactin): for allergic rhinitis.

Desloratadine (Clarinex): for allergic rhinitis.

Diphenhydramine (Benadryl, Benolyn): for allergic reactions: sedation and treatment of extrapyramidal reactions.

Fexofenadine (Allegra), Fexofenadine-Pseudoephedrine (Allegra-D): for allergic rhinitis.

Hydroxyzine (Atarax): for allergic reactions.

Loratidine (Claritin), Loratidine/Pseudoephedrine (Claritin-D): for allergic rhinitis.

Meclizine (Antivert): for vertigo.

Promethazine (Phenergan): for allergic reactions.

Mechanism: blockade of histamine receptors.

O. Antihypertensive

1. Angiotensin-converting enzyme inhibitors

Benazepril (Lotensin)

Captopril (Capoten)

Enalapril (Vasotec)

Fosinopril (Monopril)

Lisinopril (Prinivil, Zestril)

Moexipril (Univasc)

Perindopril (Aceon)

Quinapril (Accupril)

Ramipril (Altace)

Trandolapril (Mavik)

2. Angiotensin-receptor blockers

Candesartan (Atacand)

Eprosartan (Teveten)

Irbesartan (Avapro)

Losartan (Cozaar)

Telmisartan (Micardis)

Valsartan (Diovan)

3. **Beta-adrenergic receptor blockers**

Acebutolol (Sectral)

Atenolol (Tenormin)

Betaxolol (Kerlone)

Bisoprolol (Zebeta)

Carteolol (Cartrol)

Carvedilol (Coreg)

Esmolol (Brevibloc)

Labetolol (Normodyne)

Metoprolol (Lopressor, Toprol XL)

Nadolol (Corgard)

Penbutolol (Levatol)

Pindolol (Visken)

Propranolol (Inderal, Inderal LA)

Timolol (Blocadren, Timoptic)

4. **Calcium-channel blockers**

Amlodipine (Norvasc)

Diltiazem (Cardizem, Cardizem CD, Cartia, Dilacor, Dilacor CR)

Nifedipine (Adalat, Adalat CC, Procardia, Procardia XL)

Nisoldipine (Sular)

Verapamil (Calan, Calan SR, Covera-HS, Isoptin, Isoptin SR, Verelan, Verelan PM)

5. **Alpha-2 adrenergic agonists**

Clonidine (Catapres)

Guanfacine (Tenex)

Methyldopa (Aldomet)

6. **Alpha-1 adrenergic blockers**

Doxazosin (Cardura)

Prazosin (Minipress)

Terazosin (Hytrin)

7. **Vasodilators**

Hydralazine (Apresoline)

Minoxidil (Loniten, Rogaine): also used for baldness.

8. **Combination medications**

Amlodipine/Benazepril (Lotrel)

Atenolol/Chlorthalidone (Tenoretic)

Benazepril/HCTZ (Lotensin HCT)

Bisoprolol/HCTZ (Ziac)

Candesartan/HCTZ (Atacand HCT)

Captopril/HCTZ (Capozide)

Enalapril/HCTZ (Vaseretic)

Irbesartan/HCTZ (Avalide)

Lisinopril/HCTZ (Prinzide, Zestoretic)

Losartan/HCTZ (Hyzaar)

Methyldopa/Chlorothiazide (Aldoclor)

Nadolol/Bendroflumethiazide (Corzide)

Propanolol/HCTZ (Inderide, Inderide LA)

Quinapril/HCTZ (Accuretic)

Telmisartan/HCTZ (Micardis HCT)

Timolol/HCTZ (Timolide)

Trandolapril/Verapamil (Tarka)

Valsartan/HCTZ (Diovan HCT)

P. **Antimanic**

Lithium carbonate (Eskalith)

Mechanism: affects generation of phosphoinositides as second messengers, but actual mechanism of action is unknown.

Q. **Antimigraine agents**

Naratriptan (Amerge)

Rizatriptan (Maxalt, Maxalt-MLT)

Sumatriptan (Imitrex)

Mechanism: acts as agonist for vascular serotonin receptors that mediate vasoconstriction.

R. **Antiparkinsonian.** Indications: ameliorates the symptoms of Parkinson's disease.

Bromocriptine (Parlodel): partial dopamine-receptor agonist.

Carbidopa/Levodopa (Atamet, Sinemet): levodopa is a dopamine precursor; carbidopa inhibits its activation in the periphery so that more can be activated in the brain.

S. **Antiplatelet agents**

Tirofiban (Agrastat)

Ebtifibatide (Integrelin)

Mechanism: blocks platelet glycoprotein IIb/IIIa receptors, inhibiting platelet aggregation.

T. Antiprotozoal. Indications: mainly used for *Pneumocystitis carinii*, also trypanosomiasis.

Atovaquone (Mepron)

Trimetrexate (Neutrexin)

Pentamidine (Nebupent, Pentam)

Mechanism: unknown.

U. Antipsychotic. Indications: for relief of psychosis seen in many disorders, including schizophrenia, mania.

Chlorpromazine (Thorazine)

Clozapine (Clozaril)

Compazine (Prochlorperzine)

Fluphenazine (Permitil, Prolixin)

Haloperidol (Haldol)

Loxapine (Loxitane)

Mesoridazine (Serentil)

Molindone (Moban)

Olanzapine (Zyprexa, Zyprexa Zydis)

Perphenazine (Trilafon)

Promazine

Quetiapine (Seroquel)

Risperidone (Risperdal)

Thioridazine (Mellaril)

Thiothixene (Navane)

Trifluoperazine (Stelazine)

Ziprasidone (Geodon)

Mechanism: the drugs block dopamine receptors in the CNS, but the relationship between this and the clinical effects of the medications is unclear.

V. Antispasmodic. Indications: used in disorders with high skeletal muscle activity, such as cerebral palsy, multiple sclerosis, stroke.

Baclofen (Lioresal): inhibits muscle firing by acting at the GABA-B receptor in the spinal cord.

Dantrolene sodium (Dantrium): reduces release of calcium from sarcoplasmic reticulum of skeletal muscle cells.

Hyoscyamine (Levbid, Levsin, LuLev)

W. Antituberculous. Indication: for the treatment and secondary prevention of tuberculosis. Usually given in combination to prevent drug resistance.

Isoniazid (INH): inhibits cell wall synthesis.

Pyrazinamide: mechanism unknown.

Rifabutin (Mycobutin), Rifampin (Rifadin, Rimactane): inhibits DNA-dependent RNA polymerase.

Streptomycin: protein synthesis inhibitor.

X. Antiulcer. Indications: for the treatment of peptic ulcer disease.

1. H2 blockers

Cimetidine (Tagamet)

Famotidine (Pepcid)

Nizatidine (Axid)

Ranitidine (Zantac)

Mechanism: reduces acid secretion by blocking H2 (histamine) receptors in parietal cells.

2. Proton pump inhibitors

Esomeprazole (Nexium)

Lansoprazole (Prevacid)

Omeprazole (Prilosec)

Pantoprazole (Protonix)

Rabeprazole (Aciphex)

Mechanism: reduces acid secretion by blocking hydrogen-potassium ATPase pump.

3. Protective

Sucralfate (Carafate)

Mechanism: increases the tissue's resistance to acid.

Y. Antiviral

Acyclovir (Zovirax): for herpes viruses (e.g., HSV, EBV, VZV); a purine analog blocks DNA synthesis.

Famcyclovir (Famvir): for herpes simplex viruses types 1 and 2 and varicella zoster virus; a synthetic acyclic guanine derivative.

Foscarnet (Foscavir): for herpes simplex viruses types 1 and 2 and cytomegalovirus; selectively inhibits pyrophosphate binding site.

Ganciclovir (Cytovene, Vitrasert), Valganciclovir (Valcyte): for cytomegalovirus and herpes simplex viruses; a synthetic guanine derivative.

Palivizumab (Synagis): for respiratory syncytial virus; a monoclonal antibody.

Ribavirin (Virazole): for respiratory syncytial virus; mechanism unknown.

Vidarabine (Vera-A): for herpes simplex encephalitis; a purine analog—blocks DNA synthesis.

Zidovudine (AZT, Retrovir): for HIV; inhibits reverse transcriptase.

Z. Cholesterol lowering. Indications: for the lowering of serum cholesterol to decrease the risk of atherosclerotic disease.

1. Statins

Atorvastatin (Lipitor)

Fluvastatin (Lescol, Lescol XL)

Lovastatin (Mevacor)

Pravastatin (Pravachol)

Simvastatin (Zocor)

Mechanism: inhibits HMG-CoA reductase, decreasing cholesterol synthesis.

2. **Other medications**

Cholestyramine (Prevalite, Questran, Questran Light),

Colestipol (Colestid): binds bile acids in intestine.

Fenofibrate (Tricor), Gemfibrozil (Lopid): increases lipoprotein clearance.

Niacin (Niaspan, Nicolar): reduces VLDL secretion.

AA. **Diuretics.** Indications: to increase renal excretion of fluid, in situations such as edema, CHF, hypertension.

1. **Carbonic anhydrase inhibitors**

Acetazolamide (Diamox)

2. **Loop diuretics**

Bumetanide (Bumex)

Furosemide (Furocot, Lasix)

Torsemide (Demadex)

Mechanism: inhibits Na^+-K^+-Cl^- transport in loop of Henle.

3. **Thiazides**

Chlorthalidone (Thalitone)

Chlorothiazide (Diuril)

Hydrochlorothiazide (Hydrocot, HydroDiuril, Microzide, Oretic)

Methycyclothiazide (Enduron)

Polythiazide (Renese)

Mechanism: inhibits Na^+-Cl^- transport in early distal convoluted tubule.

4. **Potassium-sparing diuretics**

Amiloride (Midamor)

Spirolonalactone (Aldactone)

Triamterene (Dyrenium)

Mechanism: inhibits aldosterone in collecting tubule.

5. **Combination diuretics**

Amiloride/HCTZ (Moduretic)

Spironolactone/HCTZ (Aldactazide)

Triamterene/HCTZ (Dyazide, Maxzide)

6. **Other diuretics**

Ethacrynic Acid (Edecrine): inhibits reabsorption of a much greater proportion of filtered sodium than most other diuretics.

Indapamide (Lozol): mechanism unknown.

Metolazone (Mykrox, Zaroxolyn): inhibits sodium reabsorption at cortical diluting site and proximal convoluted tubule.

BB. Erectile stimulants

Sildenafil (Viagra): enhances the effect of nitric oxide and increased levels of cGMP in the corpus cavernosum.

Vardenafil (Levitra): blocks phosphodiesterase type 5 in human penile erectile tissue.

Yohimbine (Aphrodyne): an alkaloid.

CC. Hormones. Indications vary for each drug.

Desmopressin (DDAVP, Stimate): for diabetes insipidus, bleeding due to some hereditary coagulation defects, bed-wetting.

Estrogen (Premarin): for postmenopausal hormone replacement, contraception.

Insulin: for diabetes mellitus.

Levothyroxine (Synthroid): for hypothyroid states.

Medroxyprogesterone (Provera): for secondary amenorrhea, abnormal uterine bleeding.

Oxytocin (Pitocin): for induction of labor.

Pancrelipase (Pancrease, Cotazyme): for replacement of digestive hormones (e.g., in cystic fibrosis).

Tamoxifen (Nolvadex): for adjuvant treatment of breast cancer.

Vasopressin (Pitressin): for diabetes insipidus; local treatment of GI bleeding.

Mechanism: synthetic or natural substance that acts on hormone receptors.

DD. Inotropic agents. Indications: for patients with decreased cardiac contractility; used to increase organ perfusion.

Digoxin (Lanoxicaps, Lanoxin)

Dobutamine (Dobutrex)

Dopamine (Intopin, Dopistat)

Epinephrine (Adrenalin)

Metaraminol (Aramine)

Midodrine (ProAmatine)

Milrinone (Primacor)

Phenylephrine (Neo-Synephrine)

EE. Laxatives. Indications: for constipation, to increase passage of stool.

Ducosate sodium (Colace)

Lactulose (Chronulac)

Bisacodyl (Dulcolax)

FF. Nonopioid analgesics. Indications: for relief of pain, swelling, fever.

Some also called NSAIDs (nonsteroidal anti-inflammatory drugs). Aspirin used as antiplatelet drug as well.

Acetaminophen (Datril, Tempra, Tylenol)

Celecoxib (Celebrex), Rofecoxib (Vioxx): Cox 2 inhibitors.

Diclofenac (Cataflam, Voltaren, Voltaren XR)

Diclofenac/Misoprostol (Arthrotec)

Aspirin (Bayer, Ecotrin)

Ibuprofen (Advil, Motrin)

Nabumetone (Relafen)

Naproxen (Naprosyn)

Tramadol (Ultram)

Tramadol/Acetaminophen (Ultracet)

Mechanism: inhibits cyclooxygenase, slowing the conversion of arachidonic acid to various prostaglandins and thromboxane.

GG. Opioid analgesics. Indications: mainly used to relieve pain; other uses include sedation, cough suppression, and treatment of diarrhea.

Codeine

Methadone (Dolophine)

Fentanyl (Sublimaze)

Hydrocodone/Ibuprofen (Vicoprofen)

Hydromorphone (Dilaudid)

Meperidine (Demerol)

Methadone (Dolophine)

Morphine

Oxycodone (Endodan, Percocet, Percodan, Roxicet, Tylox)

Propoxyphene (Darvocet-N, Darvon-N, Dolene)

Mechanism: acts on specific opioid receptors in the CNS and periphery.

HH. Sedatives

Chloral hydrate (Noctec)

Midazolam (Versed)

Secobarbital (Seconal)

Triazolam (Halcion)

Zalpelon (Sonata)

Zolpidem (Ambien)

Mechanism: unclear for most drugs in this category. Benzodiazepines (Midozalam, Triazolam) act at specific receptors in the CNS to facilitate the inhibitory actions of GABA.

II. Steroids. Indications: anti-inflammatory drugs used in a wide variety of conditions, including arthritis, gout, asthma, allergic conditions, and collagen-vascular diseases.

Dexamethasone (Decadron)

Prednisone

Cortisone (Deltasone)

Hydrocortisone (Solu-Cortef)

Methylprednisolone (Depo-Medrol, Solu-Medrol)

Mechanism: acts at steroid receptors in the nucleus of cells to alter gene expression.

GG. **Thrombolytics.** Indications: acute arterial and venous thrombosis, acute MI.

Alteplase (Activase)

Reteplase (Retavase)

Streptokinase (Streptase, Kabikinase)

Tenecteplase (TNKase)

Urokinase (Abbokinase)

Mechanism: degrades fibrin by activating plasminogen to plasmin.

APPENDIX **D**

Common Drug-Drug and Drug-Herb Interactions

Adverse drug-drug interactions, including adverse reactions when prescription medications are used with certain herbal supplements, are one of the leading causes of morbidity and mortality in health care worldwide. Up to 5% of hospital admissions and several hundred deaths occur annually in the United States due to such interactions and a significant percentage of these are preventable and should be anticipated. The Centers for Education and Research on Therapeutics of the Food and Drug Administration (FDA), in an effort to promote screening by health care providers of the possibility of such reactions, has defined a high-risk patient for drug-drug interactions as any patient taking two or more medications.

Recent advances such as computer prescription entry, bar-coding, electronic medication records, and drug-drug interaction computer software have supplemented the traditional vigilance of pharmacists and others who dispense medications. The FDA's decision in 2003 to impose new rules on dietary manufacturers to make clean and accurately labeled products is welcome. Knowledge of the basic principles and common types of drug-drug interactions by physicians and allied health personnel remains essential, however, to the provision of quality health care.

An excellent listing of many, though not all, drug-drug interactions can be found in the *Washington Manual of Medical Therapeutics.* We list here examples of the most common drug-drug interactions you should be aware of, including certain precautions when patients on some herbal supplements are also prescribed medication. Before we list these interactions, we need to recall some of the basic pharmacologic principles involved in the absorption, distribution, metabolism and elimination of medications.

The major group of enzymes in the liver that metabolize drugs can be isolated in a subcellular fraction called microsomes. The most important of these is the cytochrome p450 family of enzymes. Many different isoforms of this enzyme exist but six of these have been studied best and are important to understand and recognize in terms of clinically relevant drug metabolism.

Cytochrome p450–3A, found in the gastrointestinal tract and liver, is responsible for the metabolism of most calcium channel blockers (used primarily for hypertension and angina pectoris), benzodiazepines (used as a sedative or antidepressant), protease inhibitors (used in human immunodeficiency virus disease management), hepatomethyl glutaryl CoEnzyme A reductase inhibitors (commonly known as statins, used for cholesterol lowering), and the drug cyclosporine. When cimetidine (an antiulcer agent) is given along with a calcium channel blocker, for instance, the former inhibits the cytochrome p450–3A mediated metabolism of the latter, which may lead to excess accumulation of the calcium channel blocker. Other inhibitors of cytochrome p450–3A metabolism include certain antifungal agents (fluconazole, itraconazole, ketoconazole), certain antibacterial agents (clarithromycin, erythromycin, tholeandomycin), and even grapefruit juice.

Inducers of cytochrome p450–3A metabolism, such as certain antiseizure medications (carbamazepine), certain antituberculous drugs (rifampin, rifabutin), certain antiviral agents (ritonavir), and even the herbal supplement St. John's wort, could potentially result in a lack of therapeutic efficacy of drugs commonly metablized by this route (through decreased bioavailability) if both are used concomitantly.

Some drug-drug interactions have to do with biochemical incompatibility. The antibacterial agent, gentamycin, is both physically and chemically incompatible with most beta-lactam antibacterial agents, resulting in a loss of antibiotic effect. Sucralfate (an antiulcer agent) blocks absorption of anti-bacterial agents like azithromycin, quinolones, and tetracycline. Omeprazole, lansoprazole, and other proton-pump inhibitors used as antiulcer agents reduce the absorption of ketoconazole. Cholestyramine (a cholesterol lowering agent) binds raloxifene (a hormone), thyroid hormone, and digoxin (a positive cardiac inotropic agent also used for ventricular rate control in atrial fibrillation.)

Drug/Herb	Interacting Drug/Herb	Effect
Alendronate	Calcium, Ferrous Sulfate	Decreased Alendronate absorption
Alprazolam	Clarithromycin, Diltiazem, Erythromycin, Fluconazole, Kava, Ketoconazole, Nefazadone, Verapamil	Increased Alprazolam concentrations
Antacids	Alendronate	Decreased Alendronate concentration
Antacids	Ketoconazole	Decreased Ketoconazole absorption
Antacids	Quinolones	Decreased Quinolone absorption
Antacids	Tetracycline	Decreased Tetracycline absorption
Atorvastatin	Clarithromycin, Diltiazem, Erythromycin, Fluconazole, Ketoconazole, Nefazodone, Protease Inhibitors, Verapamil	Increased Atorvastatin concentrations
Atorvastatin	CoEnzyme Q10	Decreased CoEnzyme Q10 concentrations
Beta Blockers (e.g., Carvedilol, Metoprolol, Propranolol)	Cimetidine, Fluoxetine, Paroxetine, Quinidine	Increased Beta Blocker concentrations
Beta Blockers	Carbamazepine, Phenytoin, Rifampin	Decreased Beta Blocker concentrations
Cefamandole, Cefmetazole,	Warfarin	Increased risk of bleeding

Drug/Herb	Interacting Drug/Herb	Effect
Cefoperazone, Cefotetan		
Cimetidine	Beta Blockers	Increased Beta Blocker concentrations
Cimetidine	Metformin	Increased Metformin concentrations
Cimetidine	Phenytoin	Increased Phenytoin concentrations
Cimetidine	Theophylline	Increased Theophylline concentrations
Cimetidine	Tricyclic antidepressants	Increased Tricyclic antidepressant concentrations
Cimetidine	Warfarin	Increased Warfarin concentrations
Ciprofloxacin	Antacids, Calcium, Ferrous Sulfate, Zinc	Decreased Ciprofloxacin concentrations
Clarithromycin	Alprazolam	Increased Alprazolam concentrations
Clarithromycin	Atorvastatin, Lovastatin, Simvastatin	Increased Statin concentrations
Clarithromycin	Digoxin	Increased Digoxin concentrations
Clarithromycin	Theophylline	Increased Theophylline concentrations
Clarithromycin	Triazolam	Increased Triazolam concentrations
CoEnzyme Q10	Oral hypoglycemics	Increased risk of hypoglycemia
Corticosteroids	Dehydroepiandrosterone (DHEA)	May decrease Corticosteroid concentrations
Dehydrooepiandro sterone (DHEA)	Corticosteroids	May decrease Corticosteroid concentrations
Devil's Claw	Warfarin, Gingko biloba, garlic, High-dose Vitamin E	Increased anticoagulant effect
Digoxin	Clarithromycin, Erythromycin, Quinidine, Verapamil	Increased Digoxin concentrations
Digoxin	St. John's wort, Amiodarone	May decrease Digoxin concentrations
Diltiazem	Alprazolam, Triazolam	Increased Benzodiazepine concentrations
Diltiazem	Atorvastatin, Lovastatin, Simvastatin	Increased Atorvastatin concentrations

Drug/Herb	Interacting Drug/Herb	Effect
Diltiazem	Vitamin D	May decrease Diltiazem concentrations when taken with calcium supplements
Dong Quai	Warfarin	May increase Warfarin concentrations
Ephedra	Monoamine oxidase inhibitors	May lead to severe tachycardia, hypertension, or death
Erythromycin (see Clarithromycin)		
Ferrous Sulfate	Alendronate	Decreased Alendronate concentrations
Ferrous Sulfate	Quinolones	Decreased Quinolone concentrations
Ferrous Sulfate	Tetracyclines	Decreased Tetracycline absorption
Feverfew	Ibuprofen	Increased risk of nephropathy
Fluconazole	Alprazolam, Triazolam	Increased Benzodiazepine concentrations
Fluconazole	Atorvastatin, Lovastatin, Simvastatin	Increased Statin concentrations
Fluconazole	Phenytoin	Increased Phenytoin concentrations or decreased Fluconazole concentrations
Fluconazole	Warfarin	Increased Warfarin concentrations
Fluoxetine	Beta Blockers	Increased Beta Blocker concentrations
Fluoxetine	Benzodiazepines	Increased Diazepine concentrations
Fluoxetine	Rizatriptan, Sumatriptan	Increased risk for serotonin syndrome
Fluoxetine	Tricyclic antidepressants	Increased tricyclic antidepressant concentrations
Garlic	Devil's Claw, Gingko biloba, ginger, high-dose vitamin E	Increased risk of bleeding when given with an anticoagulant
Gingko biloba	Devil's Claw, garlic, ginger, high-dose vitamin E	Increased risk of bleeding when given with an anticoagulant
Ginseng	Phenylzine	Increased risk of headache, tremulousness, and manic symptoms

Drug/Herb	Interacting Drug/Herb	Effect
Ginseng	Oral hypoglycemics	May decrease serum glucose
Green tea	Warfarin	Green tea contains vitamin K and large doses can interfere with Warfarin effectiveness
Ibuprofen	Angiotensin-converting enzyme inhibitors, diuretics, Feverfew	Increased risk of nephrotoxicity
Ibuprofen	Warfarin	Increased risk of bleeding
Itraconazole	Alprazolam	Increased Alprazolam concentrations
Itraconazole	Antacids	Decreased Itraconazole concentrations
Itraconazole	H2 Blockers, Proton pump inhibitors	Decreased Itraconazole concentrations
Itraconazole	Phenytoin	Increased Phenytoin concentrations or decreased itraconazole concentrations
Itraconazole	Statins	Decreased Itraconazole concentrations
Itraconazole	Warfarin	Increased Warfarin concentrations
Kava	Alprazolam, Diazepam, Triazolam	Increased Benzodiazepine concentrations
Ketoconazole (see Itraconazole)		
Labetolol (see Carvedilol)		
Lansoprazole	Itraconazole, Ketoconazole	Decreased Itraconazole, Ketoconazole concentrations
Lovastatin (see Atorvastatin)		
Metformin	Cimetidine	Increased Metformin concentrations
Metoprolol (see Carvedilol)		
Metronidazole	Warfarin	Increased Warfarin concentrations
Nefazodone	Alprazolam, Triazolam	Increased Benzodiazepine concentrations
Nefazodone	Atorvastatin, Lovastatin, Simvastatin	Increased Statin concentrations

Drug/Herb	Interacting Drug/Herb	Effect
Niacin	Statins	Increased risk of myopathy or rhabdomyolysis
Omeprazole	Diazepam	Increased Diazepam concentrations
Omeprazole	Itraconazole, Ketoconazole	Decreased Itraconazole, Ketoconazole concentrations
Omeprazole	Phenytoin	Increased Phenytoin concentrations
Omeprazole	Theophylline	Increased Theophylline concentrations
Paroxetine	Carvedilol, Metoprolol, Propranolol	Increased Beta Blocker concentrations
Paroxetine	Rizatriptan, Sumatriptan	Increased risk for serotonin syndrome
Phenelzine	Ginseng	Increased risk of headache, tremulousness, and manic symptoms
Phenelzine (and other monoamine oxidase inhibitors)	Ephedra	Severe Tachycardia, hypertension, or death
Phenelzine (and other monoamine oxidase inhibitors)	Meperidine	Hyperpyrexia, agitation, and seizures
Phenelzine (and other monoamine oxidase inhibitors)	Nefazodone	Serotonin syndrome
Phenelzine (and other monoamine oxidase inhibitors)	Rizatriptan, Sumatriptan, Zolmitriptan	Increased Rizatriptan, Sumatriptan, Zolmitriptan concentrations
Phenelzine (and other monoamine oxidase inhibitors)	Selective serotonin reuptake inhibitors	Serotonin syndrome
Phenytoin	Antiarrhythmics	Increased antiarrhythmic concentrations
Phenytoin	Carvedilol, Metoprolol, Propranolol	Increased Beta Blocker concentrations
Phenytoin	Cimetidine	Increased Phenytoin concentrations
Phenytoin	Corticosteroids	Decreased Corticosteroid concentrations

Drug/Herb	Interacting Drug/Herb	Effect
Phenytoin	Fluconazole, Itraconazole, Ketoconazole	Decreased anti-fungal concentrations
Phenytoin	Omeprazole	Increased Phenytoin concentrations
Phenytoin	Protease inhibitors	Decreased Protease inhibitor concentrations
Phenytoin	Quinidine, Theophylline	Decreased Quinidine, Theophylline concentrations
Phenytoin	Ticlopidine	Increased Phenytoin concentrations
Phenytoin	Warfarin	Decreased Warfarin concentrations
Pravastatin	Niacin	Increased risk of myopathy or rhabdomyolysis
Propranolol (see Carvedilol)		
Quinidine	Digoxin	Increased Digoxin concentrations
Quinidine	Nortriptyline	Increased Nortriptyline concentrations
Quinidine	Phenytoin	Decreased Quinidine concentrations
Quinidine	Tricyclic Antidepressants	Increased risk for arrhythmias
Rizatriptan	Selective Serotonin Reuptake Inhibitors	Increased risk of serotonin syndrome
Simvastatin (also see Atorvastatin)	St. John's wort	May decrease Simvastatin concentrations
St. John's wort	Digoxin	May decrease Digoxin concentrations
St. John's wort	Oral Contraceptives	May decrease Oral Contraceptive effectiveness
St. John's wort	Protease inhibitors	Decreased Protease inhibitor concentrations
St. John's wort	Simvastatin	May decrease Simvastatin concentrations
St. John's wort	Theophylline	May decrease Theophylline concentrations
St. John's wort	Warfarin	May decrease Warfarin concentrations
Sucralfate	Alendronate	Decreased Alendronate concentrations

Drug/Herb	Interacting Drug/Herb	Effect
Sucralfate	Quinolones	Decreased Quinolone concentrations
Sucralfate	Tetracyclines	Decreased Tetracycline absorption
Sumatriptan (see Rizatriptan)		
Tetracyclines	Antacids, Sucralfate	Decreased Tetracycline absorption
Tetracyclines	Ferrous Sulfate	Decreased Ferrous Sulfate absorption
Tetracyclines	Zinc	Decreased Tetracycline concentration
Theophylline	Cimetidine, Ciprofloxacin, Clarithromycin, Erythromycin, Ticlopidine, Zileuton	Increased Theophylline concentrations
Theophylline	Omeprazole, Phenytoin	Decreased Theophylline concentrations
Ticlopidine	Phenytoin	Increased Phenytoin concentrations
Ticlopidine	Theophylline	Increased Theophylline concentrations
Ticlopidine	Warfarin	Increased Warfarin concentrations
Triazolam (see Alprazolam)		
Verapamil	Atorvastatin, Lovastatin, Simvastatin	Increased Statin concentrations
Verapamil	Digoxin	Increased Digoxin concentrations
Verapamil	Triazolam	Increased Triazolam concentrations
Vitamin A (Retinol)	Warfarin	May increase Warfarin concentrations
Vitamin B$_1$ (Thiamine)	Loop Diuretics	May decrease vitamin B$_1$ concentrations
Vitamin B$_2$ (Riboflavin)	Oral Contraceptives	May decrease Riboflavin concentrations
Vitamin B$_6$ (Pyridoxine)	Levodopa (when taken alone)	May decrease Levodopa concentrations
Vitamin D	Cardizem, Diltiazem, Verapamil	May decrease Calcium Channel Blocker concentrations when taken with calcium supplements
Vitamin E, high dose	Devil's Claw, garlic, ginger, Gingko biloba,	Increased risk of bleeding when given with an anticoagulant

Drug/Herb	Interacting Drug/Herb	Effect
Warfarin	Aspirin, Cefamandole, Cefoperazone, Cefotetan, Devil's Claw, Dong Quai, Ibuprofen, garlic, ginger, high-dose vitamin E, Salicylates gingko biloba	Increased risk of bleeding
Warfarin	Cimetidine, Fluconazole, Itraconazole, Ketoconazole, Metronidazole, Sulfamethoxa-zole, Ticlopidine, vitamin A (Retinol), Zafirlukast	Increased Warfarin concentrations
Warfarin	Green tea	Green tea contains vitamin K, which can interfere with Warfarin effectiveness
Warfarin	St. John's wort	May decrease Warfarin concentrations
Zafirlukast	Warfarin	Increased Warfarin concentrations
Zileuton	Theophylline	Increased Theophylline concentrations
Zinc	Quinolones	Decreased Quinolone absorption
Zinc	Tetracyclines	Decreased Tetracycline absorption

Normal Laboratory Values

These are reference values for some of the most common laboratory tests you will encounter when managing patients. Many of these values will vary slightly by hospital. It is best to check with your hospital lab for its range of normal before deciding a test result is abnormal.

Values for each test are for adults, given in the units most commonly used in American hospitals. Many other areas of the world use SI (Système International) units; a complete list of normal values in SI units, as well as multiplication factors for converting between the two systems, can be found in the *Washington Manual of Medical Therapeutics*. Normal hematologic test values can be found in Chap. 10 of this book.

Test	Reference value
Albumin	3.6–5.0 gm/dl
Alkaline phosphatase	38–126 IU/L
Aminotransferases	
Alanine (ALT, SGPT)	7–53 IU/L
Aspartate (AST, SGOT)	11–47 IU/L
Ammonia (plasma)	9–33 μl/L
Amylase	35–118 IU/L
Bilirubin	
Total	0.3–1.1 mg/dl
Direct	0–0.3 mg/dl
Blood gases (arterial, whole blood)	
PH	7.35–7.45
PO_2	80–105 mm Hg
PCO_2	35–45 mm Hg
C-Reactive Protein	.08–3.1 mg/L
Calcium	
Total	8.6–10.3 mg/dl
Free	4.5–5.1 mg/dl
CO_2 content (plasma)	22–32 mmol/L
Chloride	97–110 mmol/L
Cholesterol, total	
Normal	< 200 mg/dl
High	> 200 mg/dl

Test	Reference value
Complement	
C3	77–156 mg/dl
C4	15–39 mg/dl
Copper	75–145 µg/dl
Creatine kinase (CK)	
Male	30–200 IU/L
Female	20–170 IU/L
MB fraction	0–7 IU/L
Creatinine	0.5–1.7 mg/dl
Ferritin	
Male	20–323 ng/ml
Female	10–283 ng/ml
Fibrinogen	150–360 mg/dl
Folate (serum)	1.7–12.6 ng/ml
Glucose (fasting, plasma)	65–109 mg/dl
Glycated hemoglobin	4.0–6.0%
Haptoglobin	30–220 mg/dl
HDL cholesterol	> 40 mg/dl
Immunoglobulins	
IgA	91–518 mg/dl
IgM	61–355 mg/dl
IgG	805–1830 mg/dl
Iron	
Total	50–175 µg/dl
Binding capacity	220–420 µg/dl
Transferrin saturation	20–50%
Lactate (plasma)	0.7–2.1 mmol/L
Lactate dehydrogenase (LDH)	100–250 IU/L
Lipase	< 100 IU/dL
Magnesium	1.3–2.2 mEq/L
Myoglobin	5–70 ug/L
Osmolality	275–300 mOsm/kg
Phosphate	2.5–4.5 mg/dl
Potassium (plasma)	3.3–4.9 mmol/L
Protein (total)	6.5–8.5 gm/dl
Sodium	135–145 mmol/L
Thyroid function tests	
TSH	0.35–6.20 µU/ml
T4 (total)	4.5–12.0 µg/dl
T3	45–132/dl
Free thyroxine	0.7–1.8 ng/dl

Triglycerides (fasting)	<250 mg/dl
Troponins	Depends on method used
Urea Nitrogen (BUN)	8–25 mg/dl
Uric acid	3.0–8.0 mg/dl
Vitamin B_{12}	187–1057 pg/ml

APPENDIX **F**

The Essential Clinical Library

As a student about to take care of patients directly for the first time, you are faced with a bewildering choice of books that can assist you. You may have a tendency either to buy no books at all or to buy every text that looks like it might be useful. Following is a list of books we have found to be particularly useful — to own or to borrow; more information about the authors and publishers can be found in the references that follow the appendices.

I. Medical dictionary. A good medical dictionary is essential for looking up new terms you come across on the wards. We recommend *Stedman's Medical Dictionary*, which has very good illustrations.

II. Major medical textbooks. Although these are expensive, every student should own at least one to use as a reference.

A. *Cecil's Essentials of Medicine* is probably the best introductory text and also available in paperback form; it is well organized, eminently readable, and easy to digest.

B. *Harrison's Principles of Internal Medicine* still sets the standard for comprehensive medical textbooks. You will learn to appreciate it more and more as you gain clinical experience. While the book is best used as a reference, the introductory chapters are worth reading in their entirety.

C. *Kochar's Concise Textbook of Medicine* is unique in that it is, in fact, concise and especially geared for medical students and residents. It contains much summative information, avoids being detailed or redundant, and students may find it useful as a quick reference resource.

III. Brief summaries and overviews. These books provide good introductions and reviews. Keep them in your locker for those times when you need a 5-minute consult before presenting a patient or starting your reading on a particular topic.

A. The *Merck Manual* is a concise treatment of common diseases. It is less complete than *Harrison's*, but more complete than *Cecil's Essentials* or *Kochar's*.

B. *Griffith's 5-Minute Clinical Consult* is an exhaustive summary of many of the topics, symptoms, and signs you will come across during your training.

IV. Books to carry on the wards and clinics

A. *Fundamentals of Clinical Medicine* (this book) is an excellent resource for medical students and students of allied health care fields as an introductory manual to patient care. It provides basic clinical information, including handy reference information found in the appendices, that you will refer to frequently as you learn the ropes and start to see, examine, and manage patients.

B. The *Washington Manual of Medical Therapeutics* is an up-to-date, relatively comprehensive summary of medical treatments pitched at the level of a medical student or intern. If you carry only one book with you once you become an intern and resident, this should be it.

C. *Problem-Oriented Medical Diagnosis* is a handy guide to the work-ups of the most common medical problems, with good diagnostic and therapeutic algorithms.

V. History and physical exam

A. *The Clinical Encounter* by Billings and Stoeckle is an excellent collection of patient interviewing techniques, especially for difficult subjects like the sexual history.

B. *Bates' Guide to Physical Examination and History Taking,* is probably the best physical diagnosis text for the novice. Its newest edition has many excellent diagrams and color pictures. Many students choose to borrow rather than purchase it, because it is useful for only a few months.

C. *DeGowin's Diagnostic Examination* is complete and authoritative, but many students may find the text too detailed for everyday use. It is, however, an excellent resource for the academically minded student.

D. *Evidence-Based Physical Diagnosis* is a scholarly, detailed compendium of physical examination techniques and clinical signs, including their historical development, background, and modern utility. It is recommended especially for those with an interest in academia or those particularly curious about the physical diagnostic techniques physicians employ today.

E. *Rapid Access Guide to Physical Examination* is a handy pocket manual that contains many black-and-white photographs, diagrams, and illustrations explaining in some detail how to perform numerous physical examination techniques. Many borrow, rather than purchase, this book since many of the techniques listed are easily learned and committed to memory.

F. *Mosby's Guide to Physical Examination* is a detailed look at how to perform a complete and thorough history and physical examination that many students own.

G. *Learning Clinical Reasoning*, while a little outdated, is an excellent book that describes many of the diagnostic reasoning processes and "tricks of the trade" used by clinicians to arrive at a diagnosis. It is ideal for the student interested in an academic career.

VI. Clinical laboratory

A. Serum chemistry and hematology. Wallach's *Interpretation of Diagnostic Tests* contains reasonably complete lists of most serum chemistry and hematology results. This book is perhaps too complete to be really useful for a student, but it can be helpful when constructing differential diagnoses of lab abnormalities.

B. ECG interpretation

1. *Dubin* is a simple and straightforward approach to ECGs. Try to borrow rather than buy this, as you will absorb it in a few evenings.

2. *Mudge* still has the best collection of abnormal ECGs of any introductory text. The unknowns are particularly helpful.

3. *The Only EKG Book You'll Ever Need* is very well written and contains many, excellent quality EKG rhythms. It is useful and very easy to read.

C. Radiology. *Squire's Fundamentals of Radiology* is the classic introductory text for diagnostic radiology, and every student should read it.

D. Differential diagnosis. While *Adler* may be more useful on the wards for interns and residents than for the novice student, this pocket "book of lists" offers dozens of causes for practically every presenting symptom or clinical finding you will encounter.

VII. Other texts

A. *Lilly* is a good treatment of pathophysiology of the heart, written by medical students for medical students.

B. *Weinberger* is an extremely well organized discussion of pulmonary diseases and a model for good writing.

C. *Cope's Early Diagnosis of the Acute Abdomen* is the classic text on clinical evaluation of the tender abdomen.

D. *Clinical Neurology* contains a great treatment of cranial nerves and neural pathways.

E. Bratman and Girman's *Handbook of Herbs and Supplements* is a useful, up-to-date listing that cites the clinical evidence for dozens of herbal remedies. It is organized into two sections: one lists the 76 common medical conditions for which herbal products are used; the other lists the 163 herbal products commonly used.

VIII. Online software resources

A. *MedsPDA* (www.medspda.com) is a website for physicians, medical students and nurses that delivers many downloadable handheld software applications, includeing *Griffith's 5-Minute Clinical Consult* and the *Washington Manual Internship Survival Guide*. Costs for the software are generally $30-$70 each.

B. *Handheld Med* (www.handheld.com) also offers downloadable handheld software applications. Its *EZReader* permits a single interface for all titles and an automatic book-linking feature that is quite useful.

C. *Collective Med* (www.collectivemed.com/freesoftware.shtml) offers a number of free medical applications for your handheld device, including *MedCalc* (which contains the most commonly used equations you are likely to require at your fingertips) and *ABGpro* (which facilitates interpretation of arterial blood gas values).

Commonly Used Herbal Medications

The sale of herbal supplements has increased by nearly 400% in the past decade and represents the fastest growing segment of retail pharmacy in the United States. More than 60 million Americans spend in excess of $4 billion on herbal supplements and more than $4 billion on nonherbal supplements each year. While the Food and Drug Administration has been reviewing prescription medications for safety since 1938, and has been reviewing drugs for both safety and efficacy since 1962, supplements are not categorized as medicines and, therefore, are not formally reviewed nor regulated.

While some supplements, and most vitamins, are relatively safe and clinical research trials are underway to prove their efficacy, caution is generally warranted for many other supplements that have not been studied or described well. Paying attention to news of such research or other cautionary statements is prudent. In 2003, for instance, the American Medical Association began an effort to have ephedra (ma huang)—which speeds up metabolism and burns fat—removed from the market following the deaths of scores of individuals taking the supplement, whether alone or in combination with caffeine.

The herbal supplements and vitamins listed below are among the most commonly used in the United States.

Herbal Supplement	Common Uses
Cartilage (Bovine, Shark)	Cancer treatment
Cat's Claw	Osteoarthritis
CoEnzyme Q10	Congestive heart failure
Creatine	Exercise enhancement
Devil's Claw	Osteoarthritis
Dehydroepiandrosterone (DHEA)	Systemic lupus erythematosus
Dong Quai	Menstrual disorders
Echinacea	Upper respiratory infections
Elderberry	Viral infections
Ephedra (Ma Huang) **Linked to deaths, especially when used with caffeine**	Weight loss, sinus congestion
Evening Primrose Oil	Diabetic neuropathy
Feverfew	Migraine headaches
Fish Oil	Rheumatoid arthritis
Garlic	Atherosclerosis, hyperlipidemia

Herbal Supplement	Common Uses
Ginger	Nausea, vomiting
Gingko biloba	Dementia, memory loss, premenstrual syndrome
Ginseng	Enhancing immunity
Glucosamine	Osteoarthritis
Green tea	Periodontal disease, cancer prevention
Kava (Kawa)	Anxiety
Melatonin	Jet lag, insomnia
Phenylalanine	Depression
Saw palmetto	Benign prostatic hypertrophy
St. John's wort	Depression
Valerian	Insomnia, anxiety
Vitamin A (Retinol)	Viral infections
Vitamin B_1 (Thiamine)	Congestive heart failure
Vitamin B_2 (Riboflavin)	Migraine headaches
Vitamin B_3 (Niacin)	Hyperlipidemia
Vitamin B_6 (Pyridoxine)	Nausea, vomiting
Vitamin B_{12} (Cobalamin)	Male infertility
Vitamin C (Ascorbic Acid)	Upper respiratory infections
Vitamin D	Osteoporosis
Vitamin E (Alpha-tocopherol)	Cancer prevention
Vitamin K	Osteoporosis
Zinc	Upper respiratory infections

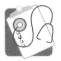

Osteopathic Musculoskeletal Examination

The principles and practices of osteopathy, now called osteopathic medicine, were first enunciated by Andrew Taylor Still, M.D., a frontier physician, in 1874. Dr. Still went on to found the American School of Osteopathy in Kirksville, Missouri in 1892. Today there are more than 50,000 osteopathic physicians and 20 colleges of osteopathic medicine in the United States.

Graduates of American osteopathic medical schools incorporate traditional medical concepts within a holistic context. Osteopathic education includes a broad range of modalities called osteopathic manipulative treatment (OMT). These techniques range from precise mobilization of a restricted joint (which may include an audible "popping" sound) to the more subtle approaches in which the physician places his or her hand around an area of dysfunction with gentle force and waits for the body's inherent biodynamic healing forces to undo tissue or strain patterns.

Osteopathic physicians are eligible for licensure to practice medicine and surgery like their allopathic (M.D.) counterparts, in all fields and specialties, in all fifty states. The **osteopathic structural examination** is performed by osteopathic physicians as part of a comprehensive, traditional history and physical examination. Its basic elements include a thorough examination of the muscles and joints, including their range of motion, and specific tests designed to diagnose asymmetries and other dysfunctions involving the spine and other associated and neurological structures. The "Thinking, Knowing, Sensing, Feeling" hands of the D.O. also may assess fluid stasis along lymphatic channels and terminations. Included here for osteopathic medical students is a brief description of some of the components that should be included in such an examination:

Somatic dysfunctions should generally be described with reference to any bony or soft tissue texture changes (bogginess, ropiness, effusions, tone), asymmetry (misalignment, luxations, or subluxations, which may be no more than fractions of an inch), range of motion abnormalities (including the quantitative and qualitative aspects of restrictions and contractures, and tenderness. Although "tenderness" may be considered subjective, a "wince" or pain upon palpation is a reliable sign. The mnemonic for these four sets of findings is **TART**. Usually two or three of these findings are used to make a diagnosis of a somatic dysfunction. The term somatic dysfunction does not fully describe the significance of one's findings because the alterations may also indicate underlying organic disorders.

Spinal somatic dysfunctions should generally include references to whether there is a continuous group curvature (scoliosis), a single vertebral abnormality, or several discontinuous vertebral units (including the associated ligaments, muscles, and fluids) that are dysfunctional. List the vertebral levels of such dysfunction (e.g., T4-T8, T5 alone) and the directions in which the vertebral segments are altered (sidebending and rotation, and whether one is more prominent in flexion or extension).

Directed testing of the musculoskeletal system, including special tests (e.g., Drawer test for assessment of anterior and posterior cruciate ligament stability of the knee joint), should be undertaken as required depending upon the pathology that is suspected as part of a comprehensive structural examination.

Specific osteopathic manipulative treatments performed, in addition to any pharmacologic intervention, should be carefully documented. These may include: 1) soft tissue treatments, such as active and passive myofascial release; 2) direct and indirect muscle energy; 3) high velocity, low-amplitude thrusting; 4) Jones' strain-counterstrain; 5) Schiowitz' facilitated positional release; 6) Chapman's neurologic reflex treatment; 7) balanced ligamentous or membranous tension; 8) Spencer's techniques; 9) Sutherland's osteopathy in the cranial field; 10) Dowling's progressive inhibition of neurologic structures; 11) Becker's biodynamic approach; or 12) Fulford's oscillatory treatment.

The sequence of examination for the osteopathic structural exam should be methodical and complete, and may either precede, occur together with, or follow examination of the traditional organ systems (depending upon the chief complaint).

A **comprehensive osteopathic structural exam** includes the following elements:

Observation for any obvious skin pathology or gross musculoskeletal asymmetries

Gait (observe the patient walk towards you, then away)

Head and craniosacral analysis

Neck/Cervical spine

Upper thoracic spine and thorax, including ribs and diaphragm

Abdomen

Upper extremities, including shoulder joints

Lumbar spine (low back pain is one of the most common reasons for occupational disability)

Pelvis/Sacrum

Lower extremities, including hip joints and assessment for leg length discrepancy

Nervous system, including central and autonomic (look for signs of hypersympathetic tone, such as vasoconstriction, piloerection, or increased sweat)

APPENDICEAL REFERENCES

Adams C: Unapproved drugs linger on the market. *Wall Street Journal*, 241(55): p. A4, March 20, 2003.

Adler SN, Gasbarra DB, Adler-Klein D: *A Pocket Manual of Differential Diagnosis*. Philadelphia, Lippincott, Williams & Wilkins, 2000.

Ahya SN, Flood K, Paranjothi S (eds): *The Washington Manual of Medical Therapeutics*, 30th ed. Philadelphia, Lippincott, Williams & Wilkins, 2001.

Andreoli TE, Carpenter CCJ, Griggs RC, et al. (eds): *Cecil's Essentials of Medicine*, 5th ed. Philadelphia, WB Saunders Co., 2001.

Bickley LS, Szilagyi PG: *Bates' Guide to Physical Examination & History Taking*, 8th ed. Philadelphia: Lippincott, Williams & Wilkins, 2002.

Billings JA, Stoeckle JD: *The Clinical Encounter: A Guide to the Medical Interview and Case Presentation*, 2nd ed. St. Louis, Mosby, 1999.

Bonadkar RA: Herb-drug interactions: what physicians need to know. *Patient Care*. pp. 58–69, January 2003.

Bratman S, Girman AM: *Mosby's Handbook of Herbs and Supplements and their Therapeutic Uses*. St. Louis, Mosby, 2003.

Braunwald E, Fauci AS, Kasper DL, et al. (eds): *Harrison's Principles of Internal Medicine*, 15th ed. New York, McGraw Hill, 2001.

Dambro MR: *Griffith's 5-Minute Clinical Consult*, 2003, 11th ed. Philadelphia, Lippincott, Williams & Wilkins, 2003.

DeGowin RL, Brown DD: *DeGowin's Diagnostic Examination*, 7th ed. New York, Mcgraw-Hill, 1999.

Dubin D: *Rapid Interpretation of EKG's*, 6th ed., Clover Publishing, 2000.

Einarson TR: Drug-related hospital admissions. *Ann Pharmacother.* 27:832–840, 1993.

Fessenden F, Drew C: Bottom line in mind, doctors sell ephedra. *NY Times*, March 31, 2003.

Friedman HH: *Problem-Oriented Medical Diagnosis*, 7th ed. Philadelphia, Lippincott, Williams & Wilkins, 2001.

Greenberg DA, Aminoff MJ, Simon RP (eds): *Clinical Neurology*, 5th ed. New York, McGraw-Hill Appleton & Lange, 2002.

Greenberg DA, Aminoff MJ, Simon RP: *Clinical Neurology*, 5th ed., McGraw-Hill/Appleton & Lange, 2002.

Juurlink DN, Mamdani M, Kopp A, et al.: Drug-drug interactions among elderly patients hospitalized for drug toxicity. *JAMA*. 289(13): 1652–1658, 2003.

Kassirer JP, Kopelman RI: *Learning Clinical Reasoning*. Philadelphia, Williams & Wilkins, 1991.

Kutty K, Schapira RM, Ruiswyk JV, et al. (eds): *Kochar's Concise Textbook of Medicine*, 4th ed. Philadelphia, Lippincott, Williams & Wilkins, 2003.

Lazarou J, Pomeranz BH, Corey PN: Incidence of adverse drug reactions in hospitalized patients: a meta-analysis of prospective studies. *JAMA*. 279:1200–1205, 1998.

Leape LL, Bates DW, Cullen DJ, et al.: Systems analysis of adverse drug events. ADE Prevention Study Group. *JAMA*. 274(1): 35–43, 1995.

Lilly LS: *Pathophysiology of Heart Disease: A Collaborative Project of Medical Students and Faculty*, 3rd ed., Philadelphia, Lippincott, Williams & Wilkins, 2002.

McGee S: *Evidence-Based Physical Diagnosis*. Philadelphia, WB Saunders Co., 2001.

McNeil DG, Day S: FDA to put new rules on dietary supplements. *NY Times*. March 8, 2003.

Mudge GH: *Manual of Electrocardiography*, 2nd ed, Philadelphia, Little Brown, 1986.

Novelline RA: *Squire's Fundamentals of Radiology*, 5th ed., Harvard University Press, 1997.

Novey DW: *Rapid Access Guide to Physical Examination,* 2nd ed. St. Louis, Mosby, 1998.

Seidel HM, Ball JW, Dains JE et al.: *Mosby's Guide to Physical Examination*, 5th ed. St. Louis, Mosby, 2002.

Silen W: *Cope's Early Diagnosis of the Acute Abdomen,* 15th ed., Oxford University Press, 2000.

Stedman TL: *Stedman's Medical Dictionary,* 27th ed. Philadelphia, Lippincott, Williams & Wilkins, 2000.

Strugatch W: Debate on ephedra, herbal stimulant, hits home. *NY Times*, November 24, 2002.

Thaler MS: *The Only EKG Book You'll Ever Need*, 4th ed. Philadelphia, Lippincott, Williams & Wilkins, 2003.

Wallach J: *Interpretation of Diagnostic Tests,* 7th ed. Philadelphia, Lippincott, Williams & Wilkins, 2000.

Weinberger SE: *Principles of Pulmonary Medicine,* 4th ed. Philadelphia, WB Saunders Co., 2004.

Weinberger SE, Fletcher J (eds): *Principles of Pulmonary Medicine,* 3rd ed. Philadelphia, WB Saunders Co., 2003.

Index

Note: Page numbers followed by f indicate figures; those followed by t indicate tables.